Integrative Geriatric Nutrition

Julie Wendt • Colleen Considine • Mikhail Kogan

Integrative Geriatric Nutrition

A Practitioner's Guide to Dietary Approaches
for Older Adults

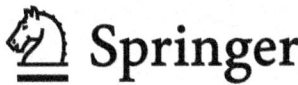 Springer

Julie Wendt
George Washington University School of
Medicine and Health Sciences
Washington, DC
USA

Colleen Considine
George Washington University
Washington, DC
USA

Mikhail Kogan
GW Center for Integrative Medicine
George Washington University
Washington, DC
USA

ISBN 978-3-030-81757-2   ISBN 978-3-030-81758-9   (eBook)
https://doi.org/10.1007/978-3-030-81758-9

This Springer imprint is published by the registered company Springer Nature Switzerland AG
The registered company address is: Gewerbestrasse 11, 6330 Cham, Switzerland

Preface

Each human being develops a relationship with food over one's lifetime; mother's milk is perfect for a baby but not sufficient for an adult. As Rumi, the Sufi mystic, precisely described back in the thirteenth century, "What is poison for one is honey to someone else." In this specific poem, Rumi goes on to describe an encounter in the desert between Moses and a shepherd. The entire poem is about the fact that "I have given each being a separate and unique way of seeing and knowing and expressing that knowledge." This core truth is applicable to food we eat just as much as to the way we pray or relate to others. In fact in modern days of industrialization, our food choices and patterns are only increasing in variety and complexity. But despite that or may be because of this, our relationship with food has changed dramatically over the last 100 years or so. We often don't give any thought to where food is coming from and how it was raised and harvested. Our consumerist society offers us immediate and easy access to food but at what cost? We have learned to select only foods we like or what we are told are healthy. We have stopped eating with the seasons which puts us out of step with the natural order of the world in which we have evolved. There are so many different dietary recommendations that one could feel completely overwhelmed. Often specific diet advocates are rather rigid in their views of what is best for us, and their opinions often divided. I was recently asked to speak at a conference where one of my very esteemed colleagues has been describing the benefits of a plant-based diet. After his excellent talk, he was confronted by a social worker who works in a very vulnerable area of a large metropolitan city. She emphasized that her patients rarely have access to quality produce. When she asked what he would recommend for them, he could only offer suggestions about how to obtain cheaper plant-based foods such as canned beans or frozen vegetables. While this is of course much better than fast food or highly processed and refined carbohydrates, the mere discussion was sadly totally off. The social worker was trying to hint at a major social divide and hoped for practical solutions, but the academician had nothing to offer except self-evident responses. Yet developing microcosms of food securities in smaller communities based on going back to one's roots is something that has been aggressively tried in so many places around the globe. When I was in residency in Montefiore, few of us had actually tried to work with the local community to grow basic vegetables just in our clinic's back-yard. We as a society have stopped thinking about food as "relationship." Food has become a commodity that we only relate to as something that comes from a super-market or from a restaurant. And even those few of us who take remarkable steps to live in a different relationship with our food suffer from being part of the culture. For over a decade, I have been keeping bees in my backyard sharing sweet honey with friends, neighbors, relatives. Yet, I am constantly aware that this is not how nature intended us to coexist with bees. We have modified our relationship with our food every step of the way, from the seed to the prepared meal. I have no doubt that the science of nutrition will keep evolving as our knowledge expands, but we must not forget our relationship with our food is much more than just calories and micronu-trients, our relationship to food anchors our place in the natural world.

Washington, DC, USA   Mikhail Kogan

Acknowledgments

"I sail with you on the ocean of my dreams to a far away distant Place of great beauty and tranquility, where suffering and pain do not exist, where we give praises for our joy and happiness, where our Love intertwines with Love for all things". Rumi

We dedicate this book to all those who want to pursue their optimal health through improvements in diet and lifestyle and to those who care for the well-being of older adults.

We also dedicate this book to all those who rose above all the difficulties of 2020 and gave their time and energy to help older adults get through the hardship of the COVID-19 pandemic.

While this book was the brainchild of Dr. Kogan and Julie Wendt, Colleen's contribution to the research and coordination of this book cannot be understated—we could not have done it without her!

We would like to extend our deep gratitude for the work done by our Springer publishing team. Thanks specifically to Cecily and Eugenia for providing the perfect amount of guidance and persistence to keep us on track through this past year that was full of unexpected delays as we all accommodated the change the pandemic brought into our work and family lives.

Dr. Kogan would personally like to thank GW University Office of Integrative Medicine and Geriatric Colleagues, including Janette Rodriguez, Drs. Leigh Frame, Marianna Ledenac, Deirdre Orceyre, Katalin Roth, Christina Prather, Robert Jayes, Tania Alchalabi, Tahira Lodhi, Elizabeth Cobbs, Karen Blackstone, and many others for never-ending support and encouragement. He specifically wants to thank his wife Angela for protecting his time.

Julie would like to thank her family for their unending support for her passion around diet and lifestyle. They are the inspiration for all that she does!

Colleen would like to sincerely thank Dr. Kogan and Julie for bringing her into this project; it has been such an invaluable experience! She would also like to thank her family and friends for supporting her throughout the writing and editing process. It truly takes a village!

Contents

Chapter 1
Introduction and Core Concepts

Contents

Since the early 2000s, the fastest-growing population in most world countries has been people over 55 years of age. The rate of growth of the aging population is staggering. According to a Brookings report, "between 2010 and 2020, the number of people over age 55 grew by 27%, which is 20 times larger than the growth rate of the collective population under 55 (1.3%). The largest driver of this divide is the baby boomer generation, who passed the age of 65 during the past decade, increasing the size of the 65- to 74-year-old age group by half [1]."

While this fact has been generally well accepted, the practice of medicine has been slow to adapt aging-specific practices across all disciplines. The field of geriatric nutrition has not fared any better. Most of the medical students and allied health professionals don't get any geriatric nutrition during their training. However, this issue has been recognized, and a number of attempts have been made to address this educational gap. In 2019, Linda Van Horn and colleagues published an extensive report covering a variety of national educational activities over the past several decades [2]. In this detailed review, the authors described multiple educational programs that have been taking place at medical schools across the country. Despite the fact that these initiatives are still too few and far between, it appears that a number of attempts have been made to assure that at least some geriatric nutrition education is required to be taught throughout all medical schools.

This book is one such attempt to offer inquisitive healthcare professionals a resource that can be used in clinical practice. While the book is written for healthcare providers, many highly intelligent patients and their families will likely find it useful as well.

While the book is centered primarily around nutrition, vitamins, herbs, and supplements, we do bring up a number of other lifestyle approaches that go hand in hand with dietary interventions. In addition, we bring case studies that showcase the approaches in action and help illuminate the real-world application of our recommendations.

Before we jump into the core aspects of the book, there are few geriatric mantras that we want to review here:

1. All interventions in older adults should follow the mantra "start low and go slow." The aging metabolism may need a lot longer to adjust to what young bodies can often adapt to rapidly. Similarly, side effects of most interventions with aging are more common and often more severe.
2. The second and surprisingly often not well-recognized geriatric mantra is "there are many more cows that look like zebras than zebras that look like zebras." Often common geriatric conditions and problems present differently from the same states in younger people and at times in puzzling ways. For example, depression often does not present as low mood but rather as isolation or even as cognitive impairment, and one must be well aware of this to recognize problems correctly.
3. Lastly, and probably firstly, most older adults are overtreated and overprescribed medical treatments to the point that what most geriatricians do in their daily practice is take their patients off medications that were prescribed by numerous specialists. This book not only recognizes this, but it attempts at giving the reader unique set of tools to try to utilize nutrition, botanicals, and supplements as tools for deprescribing and attempting and lowering the risk of iatrogenic complications that, unfortunately as of the time this book has been written, represent the third most common cause of death among older adults [3]. The mantra here is, unfortunately, before giving any new treatment to an older adult, first think about whether the given problem could be caused by a prescribed medication and, if yes, how do you deprescribe it.

A key piece of integrative nutrition is managing the behavior change process because the recommendations will be less about a magic pill that will solve the issue easily and more about fundamental changes to the patient's lifestyle that require planning, much effort, buy-in from the patient and the family, and sustained attention that allows the new state of health to be established. Appendix H includes forms that can be used to guide the change process; however, most of the provider's challenge is to spend time finding out about how ready for change their patient is and what the obstacles are that the patient is facing in implementing changes and know when additional support is indicated in order for the lifestyle plan to be effective.

We weren't always in need of nutritionists or books about nutrition in older adults. For most of our existence, we were connected to the food that we ate in a very intimate way. There weren't food scientists studying how to make food products that triggered addictive responses or marketing professionals determining the perfect shade of red that creates brand loyalty. Our food choices moved with the seasons and were inherently anti-inflammatory because we were choosing foods that were nutrient dense and picked at the peak of ripeness. Centuries of wisdom about food from cultures around the world provide the framework by which we remember that food is our first medicine. Practices from three ancient traditions appear in integrative nutrition as guiding principles: Ayurvedic, traditional Chinese medicine (TCM), and the Avicenna Islamic approach/humors.

1.1   Ayurvedic Medicine

Ayurvedic medicine originated in India over 5000 years ago. Ayurvedic medicine is holistic, treating the body and mind as a whole. The focus of ayurveda is good health through lifestyle changes including massage, meditation, yoga, herbal remedies, and dietary changes. The five elements of nature (space, air, fire, water, earth) come together in the body as doshas, or components (vata, pitta, kapha). One achieves optimal health when these three doshas are balanced [4].

Research is somewhat limited on the effectiveness of the Ayurvedic approach. A 2013 clinical trial compared two Ayurvedic formulations of plant extracts against glucosamine sulfate and celecoxib for osteoarthritis. All four products provided similar reductions in pain and improvements in function [5]. A small 2011 pilot study that compared Ayurvedic treatments (40 herbal compounds) to methotrexate showed similarly effective treatment in both arms [6].

One particular therapy prescribed often by the authors is *Triphala. Triphala* is a well-recognized and highly efficacious polyherbal Ayurvedic medicine. *Triphala* can be added to treatment regimens as a laxative, appetite stimulant, antacid, antioxidant, anti-inflammatory, immunomodulator, antibacterial, antimicrobial, adaptogenic, hypoglycemic, antineoplastic, chemoprotectant, radioprotectant, and cavity prevention [7].

Integrative nutrition at its core welcomes the influence of ancient traditions particularly when assessing the appropriate interventions in consideration of the cultural background of the patients.

1.2   Traditional Chinese Medicine

Traditional Chinese medicine (TCM) is a 2000 + −year-old comprehensive system with its own methods of diagnosis and therapy. TCM's primary goal is to ensure optimal daily functioning while also being able to address acute problems of living. Today's TCM practitioners typically evaluate and treat patients based on TCM history and physical but also combined with modern biomedical diagnostic and treatment modalities, often in integrative settings with other healthcare practitioners.

Dietary therapy is the most important part of TCM treatment armamentarium. TCM practitioners see patients even when healthy and work with a diet to prevent and treat illnesses. Diet is typically tailored to a person's constitution. Dietary prescriptions are made for acute medical problems. For example, a person with an acute, productive cough would be suggested to reduce dairy, sugar, and raw foods while adding pungent spices to food, until the condition clears [8]. For chronic conditions such as fatigue and poor appetite, recommendations will be for nutrient-dense bone broth, consumed daily over time [9].

Some of the core TCM principles of eating and a detailed overview of therapeutic approach can be found in *Integrative Geriatric Medicine* textbook [10]. The following is a short excerpt summarizing contrast between TCM general dietary recommendation and standard American diet: "TCM states that eating fresh, properly cooked light meals, without a lot of fat, salt or sugar, cooked rather than raw, is better for a weaker digestion. The standard American diet is heavy, with cloying, difficult to digest fried foods, mucus-producing dairy, and glucose and salt-enriched processed foods. It lacks in the wide variety of tastes that TCM principles state should be eaten at each meal: salty, sweet, sour, pungent or spicy, bitter, bland, astringent. In fact, the therapeutic taste of bitter is often entirely absent from the American diet."

1.3   Nutrition Challenges in the Aging Population

Unique challenges face the aging population. It is critical to appreciate these concerns in order to effectively serve the needs of this community. Barriers to proper nutrition include physical, financial, and social dynamics that are at the core of why nutrition in the aging population is, on balance, so poor. The prevalence of undernutrition in older adults ranges significantly, from 1.3% to 47.8%. It is much higher in low- and middle-income countries than high-income countries [11].

Access to quality healthcare remains a source of disparity in the United States that perpetuates the disadvantages of the underserved and vulnerable communities. The aging population is considered a vulnerable population because they rely on a fixed income and lack the financial mobility that younger patients enjoy. There are many socioeconomic forces that the provider must consider when recommending diet and lifestyle changes to the aging population. Further, the provider needs to be fully aware of the local and regional resources that are meant to serve the aging adult so that they can take advantage of the support that is in place for them.

The National Council on Aging reports that 10% of the aging population faces the threat of hunger which is worse among minorities and those who rent vs. own their house [12]. Over half of the older adults who qualify for the Supplemental Nutrition Assistance Program (SNAP) are not enrolled in the program. Providers can play a role in connecting their patients to these programs so that they can improve health outcomes by providing better access to sufficient calories. Other creative solutions include understanding ways to get healthier foods, more affordably such as through Community Supported Agriculture (CSA). Connecting patients with these resources is critical to supporting health through diet and lifestyle.

Exposure to toxins is another risk to optimal health that the aging population is more likely to experience. Toxins permeate our modern lifestyle from our drinking water to our food to the materials throughout our houses. Actively avoiding toxins wherever possible helps reduce the risks these pose such as cognitive decline, fatigue, inflammation, and gut disturbances. A resource that can help educate and guide patient's in this area is the Environmental Working Group (EWG) [13]. The EWG's mission is "to help people live healthier lives in a healthier environment" [13]. They have consumer guides on everything from water quality and filtering solutions to the best foods to get organic in order to avoid the most pesticide exposure.

Cultural competency in the field of nutrition requires an appreciation for the diversity with which the patient population presents and how culture relates to the nutritional treatment plan. Cultural norms intersect with nutritional recommendations in several ways. Religious traditions such as fasting during Ramadan, the Catholic practice of avoiding meat on Fridays during lent, and Jewish kosher guidelines represent the kind of details about a patient's life that will impact nutritional recommendations. In addition, the specific ways in which a patient engages in social gatherings and traditions can create challenges for implementing healthy habits and can actually add to a risk factor for this population – social isolation. Leaning into the cultural heritage can provide clues to establishing the ideal eating approach for an individual. In the end, the more knowledge and understanding providers bring to the individual, the more effective nutritional guidance can be.

While 95% of older adults live in the community, 2.5 million live in nursing homes or assisted living [14]. Specific challenges exist in delivering therapeutic food interventions in these institutional settings. In short, institutional settings are not set up for therapeutic dietary interventions because by design food choices follow standard guidelines and offer limited options for health such as diabetic and low-fat/low-sodium diet for cardiac health. The problem is that most of these recommendations are outdated and not actually appropriate. Internally, most of the facilities do not have processes for applying therapeutic diets. These facilities are managed by dietitians, not nutritionists, who are trained in a more traditional institutional style that focuses on preventing overt disease rather than optimizing health. The focus is primarily on macronutrients and standard doses of micronutrients according to recommended dietary allowance (RDA) which cannot address therapeutic needs. RDAs are designed to prevent medical conditions but never for treatment; thus, they are not relevant to most chronic medical care when specific micronutrients may be given at completely different magnitudes of dosing. For example, the RDA for vitamin B12 is 2.4 µg, but for depression, cognitive decline, or anemia, therapeutic doses may be 2000 µg or more.

The quality of the foods that people have access to has a direct impact on the ability of food to be used therapeutically. When most facilities spend $5/day on food per resident or when an aging adult is struggling to afford enough calories, quality foods will likely not be on the table. The policies of the government create a food economy where the foods that are most affordable are the foods which contribute the most to our chronic disease crisis.

The challenge as integrative nutrition professionals is to hold all of the challenges facing the aging adult, understand the personal history and lifestyle habits that the individual patient brings into the encounter, and allow time and space to personalize the nutrition recommendations so that the patient can achieve elevated health and improved quality of life. It's not appropriate to prioritize a specific or rigid diet paradigm over the ability of the patient to implement the diet in a way that works for them. Too often we are told this food is good and this food is bad, and this leaves the patient carrying the stress of how these choices help or hurt their health. This book seeks to create a balanced approach and highlights the need to consider all aspects of a patient's life when recommending nutrition and lifestyle changes. Above all else, integrative nutrition is about personalizing recommendations based on the unique constellation of stars that make up the individual before us.

Of course, we realize that while we are what we eat and nutrition is essential for health and quality of life at all ages, ultimately the approach to healthy aging and adding years to life is much more complex. Recently, Dr. Kogan designed the so-called AgeWise approach that combines a variety of nutrition and nonnutritional approaches. The book that describes this approach in detail is titled *Optimal Aging* and scheduled to be published by Oxford University Press in early 2022. The AgeWise approach is a combination of 13 core principles, with three of these principles centered around nutrition. First one is consuming a diet high in micronutrients and plant-based antioxidants and eating intermittently, applying principles of intermittent fasting or fast-mimicking diet. Second is knowing one's individual nutritional weak spots and supplementing with vitamins and minerals as needed. Third one is food as medicine. Know your power foods, herbs, vitamins, and minerals that can help you manage common, mostly self-resolving issues to avoid taking medications to minimize iatrogenic complications. Good examples are magnesium citrate capsules for periodic constipation, valerian root for occasional sleep disturbances, and ginger/honey tea for sore throat. Another core AgeWise principle not directly related to nutrition is to establish one's own integrative healthcare team. Obviously having a primary care doctor who can help navigate both acute and chronic problems and help with access to care to experts if more complex problems arise is critical. But we hope that one day all patients, not just those lucky to have enough income, will be able to have a health coach and nutritionist who can design the best diet approach and advise on how to improve it in one's lifestyle.

In our vision, the future of care of our elders will be fully integrated with first and primary accent made on quality of life and centered around non-pharmacological, non-interventional approaches where nutrition takes a center role, in addition to movement therapies, community engagement, and support in never stopping to redefine and re-engage in meaningful engagement in life. As Dr. Kogan summarized in first definitive *Integrative Geriatric Medicine* textbook, "Successful aging is far beyond being healthy and vibrant. It is rectifying internal conflicts, paradoxes, and redefining life's meaning, and adding years to life and life to years both" [10].

References

1. Frey M. What the 2020 census will reveal about America: Stagnating growth, an aging population, and youthful diversity [Internet]. Brookings. 2021 [cited 2021 Apr 5]. Available from: https://www.brookings.edu/research/what-the-2020-census-will-reveal-about-america-stagnating-growth-an-aging-population-and-youthful-diversity/#.
2. Van Horn L, Lenders CM, Pratt CA, Beech B, Carney PA, Dietz W, et al. Advancing nutrition education, training, and research for medical students, residents, fellows, attending physicians, and other clinicians: building competencies and interdisciplinary coordination. Adv Nutr. 2019;10(6):1181–200.
3. Xu J, Murphy SL, Kochanek KD, Bastian BA. Deaths: final data for 2013. Natl Vital Stat Rep. 2016;64(2):1–119.
4. Husney A. Ayurveda [Internet]. Michigan Medicine University of Michigan. 2020 [cited 2021 Apr 16]. Available from: https://www.uofmhealth.org/health-library/aa116840spec#:~:text=Ayurveda%2C%20or%20ayurvedic%20medicine%2C%20is,the%20use%20of%20herbal%20remedies.
5. Chopra A, Saluja M, Tillu G, Sarmukkaddam S, Venugopalan A, Narsimulu G, et al. Ayurvedic medicine offers a good alternative to glucosamine and celecoxib in the treatment of symptomatic knee osteoarthritis: a randomized, double-blind, controlled equivalence drug trial. Rheumatology (Oxford). 2013;52(8):1408–17.
6. Furst DE, Venkatraman MM, McGann M, Manohar PR, Booth-LaForce C, Sarin R, et al. Double-blind, randomized, controlled, pilot study comparing classic ayurvedic medicine, methotrexate, and their combination in rheumatoid arthritis. J Clin Rheumatol. 2011;17(4):185–92.
7. Peterson CT, Denniston K, Chopra D. Therapeutic uses of triphala in ayurvedic medicine. J Altern Complement Med. 2017;23(8):607–14.
8. Leggett D. Helping ourselves: a guide to traditional chinese food energetics. 3rd ed. Totnes, Devon: Meridian Press; 2014.
9. Flaws B. The Tao of healthy eating: dietary Wisdom according to traditional chinese medicine. 2nd ed. Boulder: Blue Poppy Press; 1999.
10. Weil A. Integrative geriatric medicine. Kogan M, editor. Oxford University Press; 2018.
11. World Health Organization. Evidence profile: malnutrition. ICOPE Guidelines; 2017.
12. The National Council on Aging [Internet]. [cited 2021 Apr 2]. Available from: https://www.ncoa.org/article/get-the-facts-on-snap-and-senior-hunger.
13. EWG. Environmental Working Group [Internet]. Environmental Working Group. 2020 [cited 2021 Apr 19]. Available from: https://www.ewg.org/.
14. Size and demographics of aging populations – providing healthy and safe foods as we age – NCBI Bookshelf [Internet]. [cited 2021 Apr 2]. Available from: https://www.ncbi.nlm.nih.gov/books/NBK51841/.

Chapter 2
Blue Zone Lessons and Longevity Diets

Contents

2.1 Introduction

Nutrition and intermittent fasting are key aspects of any and all longevity programs that are currently discussed in clinical and scientific settings. In a number of longevity circles, aging is now considered a "disease." As such, it is "treated" like any other disease, by unlocking the biochemistry, identifying the key regulator genes, and thereby highlighting possible intervention points. Using a standard multidisciplinary approach, treatment includes a variety of different strategies, including dietary.

Basic cellular activities, including regulation of metabolism, growth, and aging, interact through a complex signaling network that is highly conserved among organisms. Early studies have shown that in model organisms such as yeast and mice, downregulating (or upregulating) certain pathways modulated, for example, by insulin/insulin-like growth factor through dietary changes has the ability to demonstrably modify metabolism, stress response, and, consequently, aging [1]. These pathways, however, are susceptible to a number of factors beyond nutrition, including genetics, prenatal and childhood conditions, exercise, and other lifestyle exposures. As such, the information presented in this chapter reflects only one piece of the answer to how

© The Author(s), under exclusive license to Springer Nature
Switzerland AG 2021
J. Wendt et al., *Integrative Geriatric Nutrition*,
https://doi.org/10.1007/978-3-030-81758-9_2

and why we age [2]. As epigenetic studies continue to prove how sensitive these pathways are to external factors, there very well may be competing and contributing interventions not discussed here and not yet discovered that influence aging.

There are a variety of opinions on why we age. These include, but are not limited to, the free radical theory, the immunologic theory, the inflammation theory, and the mitochondrial theory [3]. Most theories can be classified into three major categories: program hypotheses, error theories, or combinations of the two [4]. Programmed aging theories propose there is deliberate deterioration with age because, historically, a limited life span has proven to have evolutionary benefits. Error and damage theories suggest aging is not programmed but instead the absence of selection for maintenance. With this absence, damage accumulates in an entropy-driven fashion. One prominent longevity researcher, David Sinclair, suggests that if DNA is the digital information on a CD, aging is due to scratches. Repetitive scratches result in "information mishandling." Aging, according to Sinclair, can be reversed by resetting and reprogramming genes, thereby causing cells to act younger, so as to handle information efficiently and appropriately [5]. More recently, combined theories, in which aging is considered through a more comprehensive lens, have emerged, but these theories are only in their infancy.

In this chapter, we turn to two experts in the field, Dan Buettner and Valter Longo, Ph.D., and review their research to date. Buettner is best known for his book *The Blue Zones*, where he describes unique communities around the world with a markedly high concentration of the longest-lived people in the world. By studying the very old, he brings relatively simple and universal truths to his audience as to how to live a life of both rich quantity and quality. Dr. Longo, director of the Longevity Institute at the University of Southern California and founder of create-cures.org and author of *The Longevity Diet*, turns to the other extreme. In his groundbreaking work researching juventology, the study of youth, Longo puts forth his theory on "rejuvenation from within." His longevity diet, backed by basic science, epidemiological studies, and randomized control trials, has shown promising results of dietary modifications that reduce inflammation, increase stem cell activation and regeneration to slow aging, combat disease, optimize weight, and, ultimately, improve longevity.

2.1.1 Blue Zones

Buettner begins his quest to learn the secrets of a full and long life by first locating the experts. He identifies five cities with an impressive population of these experts, or more specifically, centenarians, individuals who have either reached or surpassed the 100-year mark. These cities include Sardinia, Italy; Loma Linda, California; Nicoya, Costa Rica; Okinawa, Japan; and Ikaria, Greece. While Buettner uncovers a wealth of information supporting longevity in these populations, from family support systems to a meaningful sense of purpose, in this chapter, we will focus specifically on his nutritional findings, of which there are plenty. Table 2.1 summarizes Buettner's findings in these blue zones.

Table 2.1 Blue zones in detail [6]

	Diet	Nutritional benefits	Eating habits
Sardinia, Italy	Plant based, supplemented with fava beans, goat's milk, whole-wheat bread, pecorino cheese, mastic oil, and Sardinian wine. Meat on special occasions	*Goat's milk:* Anti-inflammatory. Contains 135 more calcium, 25 percent more vitamin B6, 47 percent more potassium, and 3x more niacin than cow's milk. May be superior at preventing iron deficiencies and mineral losses in the bone. May be protective against atherosclerosis and Alzheimer's disease *Whole wheat bread and pasta:* Complex carbohydrates which supply energy without blood sugar spikes *Pecorino cheese:* High in omega-3 fatty acids *Mastic oil:* Antibacterial and antimutagenic *Sardinian wine:* Rich in flavonoids, a group of phytonutrients well known for their antioxidative, anti-inflammatory, antimutagenic, and anticarcinogenic properties	
Okinawa, Japan	Vegetables, sweet potatoes, tofu, goya, and miso soup Meat on special occasions. If so, pork Mugwort, ginger, and turmeric	*Sweet potatoes:* High in fiber, vitamin A, potassium, vitamin C, beta-carotene, and folic acid *Goya:* Antioxidant and lowers blood sugar *Tofu and soy products, e.g., miso soup:* Phytoestrogens that improve bone health and reduce heart disease risk by lowering LDL cholesterol. When fermented, soy products enrich the diversity of our microbiome *Pork:* Rich in vitamin B1 and B2 *Mugwort:* Promotes circulation and is anti-malaria *Turmeric:* Anti-inflammatory. Can help decrease heart disease, bone loss, and Alzheimer's	Confucian adage, *Hara hachi bu:* "Eat until you are 80% full." it takes approximately 20 min for our stomachs to signal to our brain that we are full. By effectively "undereating," the Okinawans not only eat less without feeling deprived, but they slow their body's metabolism in such a way that it produces fewer damaging oxidants, which wreak damage and accelerate aging
Loma Linda, CA	Plant based, half were vegetarians Nuts, fruit, tomatoes, and legumes. Largely avoided meat	*Nuts:* Lower cholesterol and decrease risk of heart disease	Ate early and light dinners

(continued)

Table 2.1 (continued)

	Diet	Nutritional benefits	Eating habits
Nicoya, Costa Rica	Plant based, corn, beans, rice, tortillas, garden vegetables, marañon, anona, sweet lemon, banana, papaya, mango, pineapples, chicozapote, and oranges. Rarely ate pork. Hard water	*Hard water*: High levels of calcium and magnesium. The increased mineral content of their water may help promote cardiac health and improve longevity *Corn*: Infused with lime (calcium hydroxide). The high concentration of calcium makes it easier for our bodies to absorb certain amino acids and vitamins and provides complex carbohydrates, protein, and niacin *Marañon*: Red-orange fruit five times richer in vitamin C than oranges. Abundant in beta-carotenes and believed to help prevent stomach cancer	
Ikaria, Greece	Olive oil, vegetables, wild greens, fruits, legumes, goat's milk, fish, wine, coffee, sourdough bread, and honey. Low in dairy, meat, and sugar Mountain tea: Herbs, plants, and roots, including wild marjoram, sage, mint, olive tree leaf, rosemary, lemon, dandelions, chamomile, and hibiscus	*Olive oil*: Lowers LDL and raises HDL *Goat's milk*: Promotes diverse microbiome and is more easily digestible and hypoallergenic *Wild greens*: Rich in vitamins A and C, folate, calcium, fiber, phytonutrients, and antioxidants *Local wine*: When consumed with plant-based meals, it helps the body absorb more flavonoids *Coffee*: Lowers rates of diabetes, Parkinson's, and heart disease *Sourdough bread*: Helps decrease rise in blood sugar levels *Potatoes*: Heart-healthy potassium, vitamin B5, and fiber *Honey*: Controls blood sugar and LDL cholesterol *Chamomile*: Reduces clots *Peppermint*: Antiviral properties *Herbs*: Many were mild diuretics, help rid bodies of natural waste products, and reduce and control blood pressure	Ikarians say they don't have three things that cause people all the troubles in the world: They don't have work, time, and stress Ikarian's work is mostly tending to their gardens and animals. They tend to eat smaller high-protein meal early in AM before farmwork and very large meal with entire often large family, often with homemade wine and very late at night. Thus they naturally fast at least 12 h during each working day following circadian rhythm more than their watches. *of note, this is in contradiction to Bredesen's approach (see Chap. 9 for more on this. The social structure supporting large family meals likely plays a critical role in this practice.)*

2.1.2 Creating Your Own Blue Zone

Buettner wraps up his investigation of blue zones worldwide by laying out an easy-to-follow guide for building your own blue zone at home. His diet recommendations come from the tried and true practices of centenarians around the world. The summary is as follows:

- Quality is just as important, if not more than, as the quantity of our food.
- Stop eating when we are 80 percent full, thereby cutting our caloric intake by 20 percent.
- Be mindful of circumstantial eating.
- Monitor portion control by serving food and then promptly storing the remainders (out of sight, out of mind).
- Invest in smaller plates and glasses can make our food look bigger.
- Healthy foods and snacks should be easily accessible, while treats and indulgences should be out of reach.
- Eat slowly, focus on what we're eating, sit, and try to avoid eating 3–4 h before bed:

  - Note: this practice is not followed in Ikaria; see above commentary on social habits of Ikarians.

Eating a plant-based diet was common practice across all blue zones. We should aim for 4–6 servings of vegetables per day. Dr. Leslie Lytle of the UNC recommends that for those of us over 19 years of age, we need only 0.8 grams of protein for every kilogram (2.2 pounds) of our weight. This is because our body cannot store protein, so excess protein gets converted to calories, eventually becoming fat. We should, however, consume protein at every meal, as it helps us feel satiated and moderates blood sugar levels. Plant protein, found in each of the blue zone diets, can be found in legumes, garden vegetables, and tofu. Legumes have the added benefit of providing flavonoids and fiber. Tofu in addition to being high in protein is low in calories, dense in minerals, low in cholesterol, and rich in phytoestrogens, which has been shown to be cardioprotective in some women [7]. Meat was eaten rarely, if ever only a few times each month.

Nuts, found across many blue zones, are powerhouse foods rich in monounsaturated fat and soluble fiber, which aid in lowering LDL cholesterol. Incorporating nuts into our diet can help reduce the risk of heart disease. Buettner recommends incorporating almonds, peanuts, pecans, pistachios, hazelnuts, walnuts, and pine nuts into your diet for their cardioprotective benefits.

Red wine, undoubtedly, was a staple in these communities. One or two drinks daily of high-quality red wine, rich in polyphenols, have been associated with lower rates of heart disease and reduced stress levels. These benefits must be viewed in context of the obvious risk factors of alcohol. Limiting drinking to one or two glasses with meals or nuts during happy hour is most beneficial.

Buettner closes with a reminder that maintaining a healthy diet is easiest when we are surrounded by like-minded people. A *New England Journal of Medicine* study found that after following 12,067 over 32 years, subjects were more likely to become obese when their friends became obese. Creating a strong support system is not only practically beneficial but allows space for deepened relationships and intimacy.

2.1.3   The Longevity Diet

Longevity interest in the general public has led to a variety of new lifestyle directions including nutritional [8]. Over the last several decades, a number of nutritional approaches claimed to improve longevity have emerged. Instead of reviewing some that are more controversial and do not have clear science backing them up, we will concentrate in this part of the chapter on the longevity diet. Dr. Valter Longo revolutionized the study of aging by uncovering our body's innate capabilities to heal. In his book, *The Longevity Diet,* Longo discusses the how and why of both the longevity diet and fasting-mimicking diet (FMD) and the benefits of this combined routine for treating specific diseases [9].

Preclinical and clinical trials have long demonstrated the benefits of fasting for a number of diseases, including obesity, diabetes mellitus, cardiovascular disease, cancers, and neurologic disorders. Animal models have repeatedly demonstrated that fasting has the potential to increase longevity. The underlying mechanisms include both metabolic switching and increasing cellular stress resistance [10]. However, research in humans has been limited to shorter interventions, over weeks or months. Due to practical difficulties in maintaining restrictive eating habits for an extended period of time and the time required to conduct such a study, the same benefits seen in animal models have yet to be proven in humans.

The researchers began by analyzing fasting conditions among yeast. When yeast were starved by removing all the nutrients available to them and feeding them only water, the yeast lived twice as long. Dwarf yeast, in particular, with mutations in the growth gene TOR-S6K, lived up to five times longer than normal yeast [11]. Similarly, mice and rats, treated in the lab with varying longevity diets (discussed later), lived up to 40% longer and had fewer diseases compared to mice on standard diets [12]. Monkeys on a calorie-restricted diet, thereby reducing protein, fat, and carbohydrates, demonstrated a significant reduction in disease and increased longevity. Furthermore, sugar accelerates aging and death in yeast by activating two gene pathways, RAS and PKA, which inactivate protective mechanisms in our body [13]. If these findings held true in microorganisms, perhaps they would be evident in humans as well.

The next phase of the research looked into how the genetics of a small Ecuadorian population with Laron syndrome affected longevity. These individuals lacked a growth hormone receptor and, thus, had stunted growth. Despite their poor diet and otherwise unhealthy lifestyle, this population had markedly low incidence of cancer and diabetes, diseases typical of aging populations. What's more is that the Laron population had refined cognitive function into their older years. This mutation in the growth hormone receptor gene appeared to be prompting the body to "enter and stay in an alternative longevity program characterized by high protection, regeneration, and low incidence of disease" [12].

Instead of targeting diseases individually, the research focuses on targeting aging itself. Armed with the genes and pathways known to accelerate aging, such as TOR-S6K, PKA, RAS, and IGF-1, and evidence that starving microorganisms promote longevity, this would lead to further investigation into how to replicate these effects in humans [12, 14].

The longevity diet proposes that by following the recommended protocol, along with periods of fasting-mimicking diets, these "longevity genes" can be regulated and optimized to increase longevity. As with any diet, it is essential to understand its core components and the balance of macronutrients and micronutrients. Macronutrients include protein, carbohydrates, and fats. Proteins are composed of amino acids, which, when broken down, serve to build new proteins for various activities within our body. Carbohydrates are composed of sugar and are categorized as either simple or complex. Simple carbohydrates act quickly, entering our bloodstream and increasing blood sugar levels, prompting insulin spikes. Complex carbohydrates are slowly broken down into simple carbohydrates before they can be absorbed. As such, they do not have the same effect on blood sugar nor insulin, as their effect is more gradual. Fats are our body's major source of energy storage. Fat is crucial to everyday function as it is the primary component in our cell membrane and the building block of hormones. Fats are categorized as either saturated or unsaturated. Unsaturated fats can further be divided into monounsaturated fats (olive oil) and polyunsaturated fats (salmon). Polyunsaturated fats include the essential omega-3 and omega-6. They are considered essential because the human body cannot generate them on its own.

Micronutrients include vitamins and minerals. Unfortunately, between 50 and 90 percent of adults in the United States do not get enough vitamins A, D, E, and K, magnesium, calcium, or potassium. Dietary supplements, contrary to popular belief and the impressive growth of the United States supplement industry, are ineffective in preventing morbidity and mortality [15]. The best way to get these micronutrients is to eat a diet rich in vegetables, fish, nuts, and whole grains. As it can be difficult to maximize micronutrients from even the most comprehensive diets, the recommendation is to take a multivitamin every 2 to 3 days, as micronutrient excess can cause its own problems.

A Note on Supplements
A majority of supplements are full of synthetic nutrients that are inferior to what the experts are using. When prescribed by licensed practitioners, supplements can be incredibly beneficial. It is imperative to thoroughly review the quality of supplements before starting.

Calorie restriction is beneficial because high protein intake, as seen in the model organisms prior, causes activation of the growth hormone receptor, which increases the levels of insulin and insulin-like growth factor, whose altered concentrations are associated with diabetes and cancer, respectively. Proteins can also activate TOR-S6K, a set of genes that accelerates aging. PKA, shown to be activated by sugars, accelerates age-related disease. Thus, calorie restriction reduces protein and sugar intake, turning down the TOR-S6K and PKA genes. It is important to note that especially in the elderly, chronic caloric restriction can cause more harm than good. Adequate calories are required for maintaining basic metabolic functions, and increased levels are required above 65 to maximize wound healing, immune response, and temperature balance.

Putting all this together, the longevity diet was born. It is largely plant based with occasional fish (2–3 portions per week, avoiding fish with high mercury content like tuna, swordfish, mackerel, and halibut). For those over 65 losing muscle mass, one should increase protein by 10–20% by introducing more fish and other healthy protein sources such as goat's milk or eggs. Protein intake should be "low but sufficient," 0.31–0.36 g per pound of body weight per day. Animal proteins should be largely avoided, while vegetable proteins found in legumes and nuts should be maximized. Complex carbohydrates, found in whole-wheat bread, legumes, and vegetables, should always be chosen over simple sugars like those found in pasta, fruit, juice, and candy. The diet is rich in healthy unsaturated fats like olive oil, salmon, and nuts and low in saturated, hydrogenated, and trans fats. To maximize micronutrients, he recommends a multivitamin and omega-3 fish oil tablet every 2–3 days.

Building off Buettner's research, the longevity diet encourages foods that were common among our ancestors. Introducing even the healthiest foods foreign to you and your family may induce intolerances. The recommendation is to eat twice a day, plus a snack. For the elderly, they should stick to three meals a day plus one snack, acknowledging that one major meal may have to be broken down to facilitate digestion. Although not long ago there was significant excitement around the five to six small meals a day, this increases our chances of overeating, since we consistently grossly underestimate calorie counts. Breakfast should not be skipped, as this has repeatedly been associated with increased risk for numerous age-related diseases. It is important to note many of these suggestions are in contrast to intermittent fasting recommendations. Like most things, there is not a "one-size-fits-all" approach to longevity.

The longevity diet encourages observing time-restricted eating, limiting food intake to 11–12 h each day. Shorter eating windows less than 10 h can be even more effective for weight loss but harder to maintain and may increase the risk of gallstones and cardiovascular disease. At least two (and in certain cases, more) times per year, we should undergo a 5-day fasting-mimicking diet. If we follow these above points to a healthy weight and abdominal circumference, we have the opportunity to maximize longevity.

The longevity diet is built off Buettner and others' work, turning to centenarians for diet practices that have withstood the test of time. As mentioned earlier in this chapter, most centenarian diets (and therefore, the longevity diet) are plant based with lots of nuts and some fish. They are low in proteins, sugars, and both saturated and trans fats. They are high in complex carbohydrates. Most communities eat two to three times a day, with their lightest meal in the evening. Finally, by comparing the human body to complex systems (like cars and airplanes), the reader has real-life examples of how proper fuel and regular maintenance are required to support a long-lasting car, airplane, or human.

2.1.4 The Fasting-Mimicking Diet

If the longevity diet is to be followed on a regular basis, adopted as a lifestyle, how and when are we to incorporate the fasting-mimicking diet? As a reminder, in yeast, starving organisms increased longevity (the yeast lived twice as long). However, chronic starvation provides its own challenges. Perhaps brief periods of fasting might garner the same results while minimizing risk. A fasting state was defined as lower levels of IGF-1, lower levels of glucose, higher levels of ketone bodies, and higher levels of growth factor inhibitors (IGFBP1).

The 3-day, calorie-restricted diet (later known as Prolon) was first tested in 16-month-old mice, and this diet was compared to a standard mouse diet. The results were incredible: the 75 percent life span (age at which 75% of the mice were still alive) was extended by 18%. Although they ate the same quantity of food per month as the control group, the mice on the intervention diet lost weight and abdominal fat, with minimal loss of muscle mass. Age-dependent bone mineral density loss decreased. Tumors, if present, were reduced by nearly 50%, and cancer onset for most of the mice was delayed from 20 months to 26 months (the equivalent of delaying cancer in humans from 60 years to 70 years). Skin inflammatory diseases were cut in half. Stem cell populations increased. The intervention diet mice were sharper, performing better on movement and learning tasks. Fasting was destroying the damaged cells and regenerating stem cells, which by definition have the capacity to become any cell possible. What's more is that when the mice began eating again, the stem cells regenerated cells specific to the system that needed repair. These new cells exhibited characteristics of younger cells and were highly functioning.

The next step was to test these findings in humans with the Prolon diet in a 100-subject clinical trial. By fasting, cells would switch into a protective, antiaging mode. Autophagy (self-destruction) would remove damaged and unnecessary cellular components and would be replaced by newly activated stem cells. On a macrolevel, the body would shift into an abdominal/visceral fat-burning mode, which would continue beyond 5 days. The results, summarized below, were remarkable.

Obese subjects lost more than 8 pounds, primarily abdominal fat. They experienced an increase in muscle mass relative to body weight. On average, the prediabetic patients saw a 12-mg/dL decrease in glucose levels (no effect seen in patients with low fasting glucose). In subjects with moderately high blood pressure, there was a 6-mmHg decrease in blood pressure (but not in patients with low blood pressure). In subjects with high cholesterol, they experienced an average of 20-mg/dL decrease in cholesterol. In high-risk cancer patients, they saw a 55-ng/mL decrease in IGF-1 levels. Patients saw a 1.5-mg/dL decrease in C-reactive protein (CRP), a universal inflammatory marker. In patients with high triglycerides, on average, they experienced a 25-mg/dL decrease in triglycerides.

It is important to note, as the abovementioned results dictate, that the Prolon diet showed the most promising results in the highest-risk patients. It is also worth reminding that a combination of these nutritional strategies, along with conventional therapies, has proven to be most successful. In other words, there is no silver bullet.

2.1.5 Cancer

The rest of the book outlined the benefits of the longevity diet and the fasting-mimicking diet in a variety of disease states. In cancer patients, research proposed healthy cells and cancer cells exhibited a differential stress resistance; if you starve a healthy cell, it will retreat to a protective, nongrowth mode. If you starve a cancer cell, its very nature is to override nongrowth signals, and it, therefore, will grow autonomously. The benefit to this difference in response is that if chemotherapy is preceded by fasting, the chemotherapy can preferentially treat the growing cells (cancer cells) and does not touch the protected cells (healthy cells). Thus, chemotherapy can not only be more effective, but the subject would experience significantly fewer side effects.

This theory was first tested in mice, with astounding results. One group of mice with cancer was fed a water-only diet and another group a normal diet 2–3 days before chemotherapy. After chemotherapy, almost all of the fasting mice were alive and active after chemotherapy. The mice on the normal diet were ill and weak. In the following weeks, nearly all the fasting mice survived, whereas 65% of the mice on the normal diet had died.

Numerous animal trials in a variety of cancers followed showing synonymous results; fasting was not only improving the efficacy of chemotherapy but reducing side effects in breast cancer, prostate cancer, colorectal cancer, pancreatic cancer, neuroblastoma, glioma, lung cancer, mesothelioma, melanoma, and many others. Although clinical trials are smaller in number, they have now been successfully performed in humans, leading to the formulation of Chemolieve, a fasting-mimicking diet product for cancer patients.

2.1.6 Diabetes

Type 2 diabetes is defined by chronic insulin resistance. Although the pancreas produces insulin, our body's cells become desensitized to it, preventing insulin from allowing glucose to enter our cells for energy. Those who are obese or overweight with high levels of abdominal fat have a much greater chance of developing diabetes. Although there are many drugs available that lower blood sugar, these drugs treat symptoms, not the diabetes itself.

To explore the role of nutrition and diabetes incidence, the researchers returned to the Laron patients in Ecuador. Because of their mutation in the growth hormone receptor gene, they are at increased risk for obesity. Interestingly, although obesity is one of the major risk factors for diabetes, not one of the Laron subjects in Ecuador developed diabetes. As studied earlier, since protein is a key regulator of the growth hormone gene, a high protein intake may increase the risk of diabetes by increasing activity of growth hormone. Conversely, the absence of the growth hormone receptor (as in the Laron patients or a very-low-protein diet) effectively eliminates the implications of obesity on diabetes.

In the 100-patient clinical trial, results were similar. As expected, these patients who underwent three monthly cycles of the 5-day fasting-mimicking diet had lower risks of diabetes by reducing protein intake and abdominal and liver fat, promoting fat loss without muscle loss, and promoting targeted cellular autophagy and regeneration.

2.1.7 Cardiovascular Disease

Cardiac disease is responsible for approximately one in three deaths in the United States every year and becomes increasingly common in the elderly. As the Mediterranean diet showed, adhering to a diet largely plant based and packed with nuts and olive oil reduces cardiovascular events. When the fasting-mimicking diet was tested in humans, individuals demonstrated lower cardiovascular disease and inflammatory markers (CRP), after only three cycles, without any deleterious effects. They had reduced body weight and abdominal fat, reduced total and LDL cholesterol, lower triglycerides, and lower blood pressure and blood sugar. These results were most significant in patients who presented at high risk for cardiovascular disease.

2.1.8 Alzheimer's

The number one risk factor for Alzheimer's, the most prevalent subset of dementia, is age. The Spain study showed us that patients that followed the Mediterranean diet had improved cognitive performance than those on a low-fat, control diet. To maximize brain health and delay Alzheimer's onset, the longevity diet, with added olive oil and nuts, provides a more selective version of the Mediterranean diet, with additional nutrients of benefit.

Coffee and coconut oil, both controversial over the years, show promise in Alzheimer risk reduction. Coffee consumption was responsible for an approximate

30 percent risk reduction in Alzheimer's, likely due to its high polyphenol content. Coconut oil has also been shown to improve cognitive status, likely due to its high concentration of medium-chain fatty acids (MCFA). Conversely, high levels in saturated or trans fats increase the risk for dementia. Adhering to the longevity diet minimizes intake of such fats, therefore reducing dementia risk. As certain vitamins (vitamin B12, vitamin E) are known to be neuroprotective, supplementing the longevity diet with such vitamins may avoid risk and delay dementia.

In younger and middle-aged adults, increased BMI has been associated with reduced cognition and higher risk of dementia. Beyond 65 however, slightly higher BMI is associated with improved cognition and reduced mortality.

Although treating Alzheimer's with nutritional interventions has not been fully explored, the above prevention mechanisms along with alternating cycles of periodic fasting-mimicking diet may be beneficial. For more, please see Chap. 10, Neurodegenerative disease for Dale Bredesen's approach.

2.1.9 Inflammatory and Autoimmune Diseases

While we need a robust immune system to function, inappropriate activation can cause systemic inflammation, wreaking havoc on our bodies. Fat cells are known to be an important source of inflammatory markers (TNF-alpha and IL-6). Therefore, obesity, especially increased abdominal fat, could contribute to inflammatory and autoimmune diseases. High salt consumption has also been theorized to activate T cells, a prime mediator in autoimmune diseases. As a large portion of our body's immune system is located in our gut, dietary changes that influence our microbiome can help or hurt our immune system; switching to a largely plant-based diet can reduce inflammation, mitigating risk and in some cases treating both inflammatory and autoimmune disease.

In mice with multiple sclerosis, multiple cycles of the fasting-mimicking diet eliminated a portion of the damaging autoimmune cells, reduced symptoms, and promoted regeneration of the spinal cord, previously damaged by the inappropriate inflammatory response. When replicated in humans, 20 patients with multiple sclerosis completed one cycle of the fasting-mimicking diet and reported symptomatic improvement. Repetitive cycles of the FMD have the potential to reduce symptoms even more dramatically and eliminate hazardous autoimmune cells and restore healthy new progenitor cells.

Rheumatoid arthritis has responded similarly to fasting/low-calorie diets. Although it has not yet been studied, integrating the fasting-mimicking diet into the longevity diet for patients with rheumatoid arthritis should both reduce inflammation and improve symptoms.

Since *The Longevity Diet* was published, the research has continued to show promising results in human studies. In one randomized control trial in

Table 2.2 Fast-mimicking diet vs. intermittent fasting

	Fast-mimicking diet (FMD)	Intermittent fasting (IF)
Pros	Much easier to start and fewer "side effects"	Much easier overall logistics and lower cost
Cons	Cost of complexity of making it	Side effects, especially when starting. Much slower adaption and harder to implement fasts over 20 h
Efficacy	Researched mostly in animals but the number of small human trials is positive	Much longer historic use and more overall evidence
Potential	Probably greater than IF	Greater potential for implementation when money or complexity of making cannot be overcome

HER2-negative breast cancer patients, those that followed the FMD 3 days prior and during their neoadjuvant chemotherapy were more likely to have a radiologically complete or partial response and a Miller-Payne 4 out of 5 pathological response (indicating 90–100% tumor cell loss) compared to their regular diet. The FMD showed no difference in toxicity and significantly reduced chemotherapy-induced DNA damage in T lymphocytes [16]. In a more recent 100-person randomized study of healthy US participants, subjects who followed the FMD for 5 consecutive days each month over 3 months had lower body and trunk weight and total body fat, lowered blood pressure, and decreased IGF-1 than those randomized to an unrestricted diet. After 3 months, the control diet participants crossed over to the FMD program. Subjects in both FMD arms proved that body mass index, blood pressure, fasting glucose, IGF-1, triglycerides, total and low-density lipoprotein cholesterol, and C-reactive protein were more beneficial in participants at higher risk for disease than healthy subjects [17].

Many leaders in longevity research promote low-animal-protein, methionine-restricted plant-based protein diet [18]. We do not advocate for these approaches for older adults given the fact that protein deficiency can lead to sarcopenia and functional decline [19]. Table 2.2 describes key differences between the fast-mimicking diet and intermittent fasting.

2.2 Nutritional Supplements to Promote Longevity

There is preclinical and possibly some clinical evidence that intake of the below supplements may support longevity. As we do not all live in blue zones, it is our opinion that adding these supplements, as captured in Table 2.3, supports a similar lifestyle.

Table 2.3 Nutritional supplements to promote longevity

Anti-inflammatory herbs and supplements	Curcumin, quercetin, *Boswellia*, omega-3 s, green tea (EGCG), Saffron, glucosamine, chondroitin, MSM, and vitamin D
Mitochondrial function and energy production and metabolic support	L-carnitine, nicotinamide riboside, nicotinamide mononucleotide, and vitamin D
Antioxidants and scavengers	Resveratrol, alpha lipoic acid, NAC, glutathione, vitamin C, multivitamins, and CoQ10
Adaptogenic herbs and mushrooms	Holy basil, schizandra, rhodiola, cordyceps, reishi, and lion's mane
Minerals and trace minerals	Magnesium, calcium, potassium, lithium, silica, boron, vanadium, and molybdenum

References

1. Santos J, Leitão-Correia F, Sousa MJ, Leão C. Dietary restriction and nutrient balance in aging. Oxidative Med Cell Longev. 2016;2016:4010357.
2. Passarino G, De Rango F, Montesanto A. Human longevity: genetics or lifestyle? It takes two to tango. Immun Ageing. 2016;13:12.
3. Tosato M, Zamboni V, Ferrini A, Cesari M. The aging process and potential interventions to extend life expectancy. Clin Interv Aging. 2007;2(3):401–12.
4. da Costa JP, Vitorino R, Silva GM, Vogel C, Duarte AC, Rocha-Santos T. A synopsis on aging-theories, mechanisms and future prospects. Ageing Res Rev. 2016;29:90–112.
5. Sinclair D. The Sinclair lab [internet]. The Sinclair Lab, Harvard Medical School: Blavatnik Institute Genetics. 2019 [cited 2021 Apr 2]. Available from: https://genetics.med.harvard.edu/sinclair/research.php.
6. Buettner D. The blue zones, Second Edition: 9 lessons for living longer from the people who've lived the longest. second ed. National Geographic; 2012.
7. Park D, Huang T, Frishman WH. Phytoestrogens as cardioprotective agents. Cardiol Rev. 2005;13(1):13–7.
8. Lang FR, Rupprecht FS. Motivation for longevity across the life span: an emerging issue. Innov Aging. 2019;3(2):igz014.
9. Longo V. The longevity diet: discover the new science behind stem cell activation and regeneration to slow aging, fight disease, and optimize weight. Illustrated. New York: Avery; 2018.
10. de Cabo R, Mattson MP. Effects of intermittent fasting on health, aging, and disease. N Engl J Med. 2019;381(26):2541–51.
11. Longo VD. Mutations in signal transduction proteins increase stress resistance and longevity in yeast, nematodes, fruit flies, and mammalian neuronal cells. Neurobiol Aging. 1999;20(5):479–86.
12. Guevara-Aguirre J, Balasubramanian P, Guevara-Aguirre M, Wei M, Madia F, Cheng C-W, et al. Growth hormone receptor deficiency is associated with a major reduction in pro-aging signaling, cancer, and diabetes in humans. Sci Transl Med. 2011;3(70):70ra13.
13. Longo VD, Mitteldorf J, Skulachev VP. Programmed and altruistic ageing. Nat Rev Genet. 2005;6(11):866–72.
14. Fabrizio P, Pozza F, Pletcher SD, Gendron CM, Longo VD. Regulation of longevity and stress resistance by Sch9 in yeast. Science. 2001;292(5515):288–90.
15. Enough Is Enough | Annals of Internal Medicine [Internet]. [cited 2021 Apr 2]. Available from: https://www.acpjournals.org/doi/10.7326/L14-5011.
16. de Groot S, Lugtenberg RT, Cohen D, Welters MJP, Ehsan I, Vreeswijk MPG, et al. Fasting mimicking diet as an adjunct to neoadjuvant chemotherapy for breast cancer in the multicentre randomized phase 2 DIRECT trial. Nat Commun. 2020;11(1):3083.

17. Wei M, Brandhorst S, Shelehchi M, Mirzaei H, Cheng CW, Budniak J, et al. Fasting-mimicking diet and markers/risk factors for aging, diabetes, cancer, and cardiovascular disease. Sci Transl Med. 2017;9(377):eaai8700.

18. Brandhorst S, Longo VD. Protein quantity and source, fasting-mimicking diets, and longevity. Adv Nutr. 2019;10(Suppl_4):S340–50.

19. Volkert D, Sieber CC. Protein requirements in the elderly. Int J Vitam Nutr Res. 2011;81(2–3):109–19.

Chapter 3
Gastrointestinal Health

Contents

Aging affects the digestive tract in every capacity, as demonstrated in Fig. 3.1. Effective management of all health conditions requires a well-functioning gastrointestinal tract as the gut is the foundation of health. In Table 3.1, we discuss the more common changes associated with aging along with the nutritional considerations [2].

Many medications have direct effects on the gut. Table 3.2 highlights these side effects along with any known associated nutrient deficiencies.

The Institute for Functional Medicine (IFM) established a framework called the five Rs for repairing the gut that recognizes the prevalent dysfunctions and addresses the underlying causes that allow for complete gut repair:

Used with permission from the Institute for Functional Medicine (IFM), a global leader in functional medicine and a collaborator in the transformation of healthcare. IFM is a 501(c)(3) nonprofit organization that believes functional medicine can help every individual reach their full potential for health and wellbeing. Under

© The Author(s), under exclusive license to Springer Nature
Switzerland AG 2021
J. Wendt et al., *Integrative Geriatric Nutrition*,
https://doi.org/10.1007/978-3-030-81758-9_3

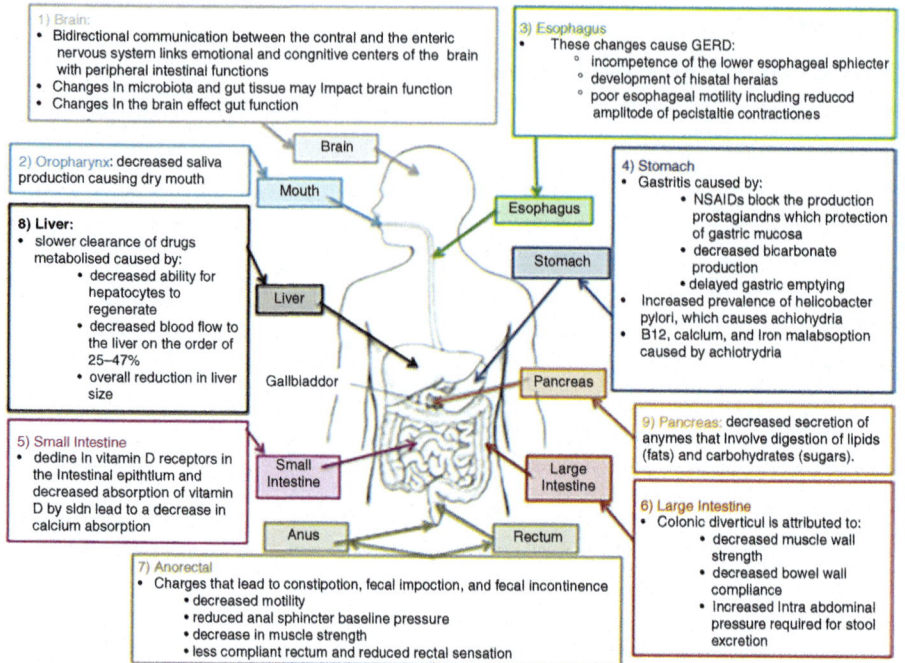

Fig. 3.1 Physiologic and pathological changes of the aging gut [1]

Remove eliminate sources of inflammation in the gut which can be related to pathogenic infections, inflammatory foods, food allergies or sensitivities, dysbiosis, and medications. The use of testing and elimination diets is key aspect of this step.

Replace evaluate for insufficient digestive capacity related to hydrochloric acid, digestive enzymes, and bile acids and replace any that are deficient using supplements.

Reinoculate establish a balanced microbiome by encouraging the growth of beneficial bacteria, yeast, and spores. Research on the use of probiotic supplements has been extensive with mixed outcomes causing confusion over their efficacy for general health vs. specific conditions that have been studied; however, it's advisable to approach the use of probiotic supplements in a clinical setting using a moderate dose (20 billion CFU), multi-strain probiotic for any patient presenting with a disrupted gut microbiome [50]. Additionally, fermented foods are natural sources of probiotics and should be encouraged as part of a regular diet. Fermented foods include yogurt, sauerkraut (raw and cultured), kombucha, kimchi, and other fermented vegetables.

Table 3.1 Common changes in the GI tract with age [2]

Area	Concern	Clinical nutrition implications
Mouth	Dentition	Inability to chew certain foods and pain
	Gingivitis	Balancing oral microbiome through food and supplements
	Decreased saliva	Dry mouth, choking, change in types of food that are safe to eat, and difficulty swallowing pills
	Change in taste	Decreased appetite for healthy foods, cravings for unhealthy foods, and difficulty following therapeutic diets
Esophagus	Ineffective LES (lower esophageal sphincter)	Decreased tone in lower esophageal sphincter (LES) coupled with a reduction in stomach acid production creates heartburn which leads to pain associated with certain foods and eating and an avoidance of eating resulting in lower nutritional status
	Poor motility	Slowed and more labored swallowing requires dietary modifications, and eating time increases. Tendency toward liquids and away from solid foods and predisposition to constipation
Pancreas	Decreased secretion of enzymes	Maldigestion of fats and carbohydrates and subsequent nutrient depletion
Stomach	Hypochlorhydria	Root cause of GERD in many cases, pain, inability to tolerate certain acidic foods, increased susceptibility to pathogens passing via food and water intake, and reduced ability to digest proteins, vitamin B12, calcium, and iron
Small intestine	Slowing of migrating motor complex (MMC)	Delayed gastric emptying reduces appetite and volume of food intake. Decreased clearance of pathogen increasing carbohydrate maldigestion and SIBO (small intestinal bacterial overgrowth) risk, constipation/diarrhea, and resulting inflammation and toxicity
	Decreased vitamin D receptors	Impaired calcium metabolism and decreased immune response
Large intestine	Decreased muscle wall strength and compliance	Increased risk of constipation and resulting inflammation and toxicity
Brain	Increased BBB permeability	Bidirectional communication between the gut and the brain creates a reliant pathway that links emotions, cognition, and intestinal function having direct impact on gut health

Repair and regenerate create a healing regimen that will allow the intestinal mucosal barrier to recover. The single cell wall of the gastrointestinal tract is interconnected via protein gates called tight junctions, which act as a selective entry for larger molecules that cannot diffuse through the cell wall. In an environment of inflammation, the intercellular tight junctions fail and become rogue entry points for molecules that enter the bloodstream, interact with our immune cells, and create systemic inflammation. During the repair and regenerate phase, the use of key gut-healing nutrients promotes proper barrier function to be re-established, restores the function of the brush border enzymes, and creates an environment conducive to optimal health. Key supplements are L-glutamine, marshmallow root, deglycerized licorice, aloe, vitamin A, prebiotic fibers, and zinc carnosine.

Table 3.2 Common medications that have direct impact on digestive tract [2–5]

Medication	Side effect	Associated nutrient deficiencies
Antacids	*GI*: constipation (aluminum inhibits motor activity of GI tract) and diarrhea (magnesium stimulates muscle contractions) *Metabolic*: milk-alkali syndrome [6], [7]	B12 [8]
Azithromycin, clarithromycin, and erythromycin	*GI*: nausea, vomiting, diarrhea, and abdominal pain (dose-related effect on motilin receptors) *Hepatobiliary*: hepatotoxicity [9] *Cardiac*: QT prolongation [9]	None reported
Anticholinergics	*General*: hyperthermia and anhidrosis *CV*: tachycardia, flushing, and arrhythmias *GI*: constipation, dysphagia, xerostomia (inhibits parasympathetic response), reduced gut motility, and vomiting *GU*: urinary retention *HEENT*: blurred vision, mydriasis, narrow-angle glaucoma, and potentially vision loss *MSK*: diminished muscle contraction [10]	None reported
Anticonvulsants	*GI*: anorexia, nausea, and vomiting *Metabolic*: hyponatremia *MSK*: bone loss *Derm*: SJS, TEN, DRESS *Psych*: suicidality [11]	None reported
Antidiabetics	*Neuro*: headache *HEENT*: sore throat *Respiratory*: upper respiratory tract infections *Cardiovascular*: heart failure and myocardial infarction *Endocrine*: hypoglycemia and bone fractures *GI*: anorexia, diarrhea, nausea, constipation, indigestion, vomiting, weight changes, and flatulence *GU*: UTIs, genital infections, and yeast infections *Skin*: rash [12–15]	Folic acid, vitamin B12, and dibencozide [16]

Table 3.2 (continued)

Medication	Side effect	Associated nutrient deficiencies
Bisphosphonates	*HEENT*: ocular side effects *Endo*: hypocalcemia *Cardiovascular*: atrial fibrillation *MSK*: osteonecrosis of the jaw, atypical femur fractures, and musculoskeletal pain *GI*: pill esophagitis, gastric ulcers, nausea, and dysphagia (direct gastric/esophageal irritation) [17] *Renal*: renal impairment and acute renal failure [18]	Transient hypocalcemia [19]
Calcium channel blockers	*GI*: constipation and dysphagia [20] *Cardiovascular*: edema [20]	None reported
Cardiovascular drugs (antiarrhythmics, diuretics)	*Skin*: rash *MSK*: myalgias *GI*: anorexia, esophagitis, nausea, diarrhea, abdominal bloating, and discomfort [21–23]	None reported
Colchicine	*GI*: anorexia, diarrhea, vomiting, and nausea [24]	None reported
Furosemide	*Cardiovascular*: orthostatic hypotension *CNS*: dizziness, headache, paresthesia, restlessness, and vertigo *Skin*: rash *GI*: abdominal cramps, xerostomia, anorexia, constipation, diarrhea, gastric irritation, pancreatitis, nausea, and vomiting *Otic*: deafness *Renal*: interstitial nephritis and renal disease [25]	Hypokalemia, hyponatremia, hypomagnesemia, and hypocalcemia [26, 27]
H2 blockers	*GI*: achlorhydria, dysphagia, *C. difficile* infection, microscopic colitis, atrophic gastritis, and malabsorption (inhibit gastric acid secretion and alter pH of the stomach) [28]	Hypomagnesemia [29] and B12 depletion [30]
Iron supplements	*GI*: constipation, esophagitis, abdominal pain, darkening of stools, heartburn, nausea, flatulence, and diarrhea [31]	Do not take with calcium. Inhibits absorption when taken with food [32]
Lithium	*Endo and metabolic*: hypothyroidism, diabetes insipidus, hypercalcemia, and weight changes *GI*: dysgeusia, ageusia, anorexia, abdominal pain, and nausea *Neuro*: hyperactive DTRs and hypertonia [33]	None reported

(continued)

Table 3.2 (continued)

Medication	Side effect	Associated nutrient deficiencies
Metronidazole	*Neuro*: seizures, neuropathy, dizziness, vertigo, weakness, insomnia, headache, ataxia, confusion, encephalopathy, irritability, and tremors *GI*: dysgeusia, ageusia, nausea, diarrhea, vomiting, constipation, and cramping *GU*: deep red-brown urine *Disulfiram-like reaction*: flushing, tachycardia, palpitations, nausea, and vomiting [34]	Iodine and vitamin K [35]
NSAIDs	*GI*: diverticular disease, pill esophagitis, anorexia, dyspepsia, peptic ulcer disease, bleeding (mucosal damage via COX-1 inhibition), gastric damage, and mucosal damage *Renal*: acute renal failure *Hepatic*: livery injury [36, 37]	Folic acid, glutathione, and vitamin B12 [38]
Opioids	*Neuro*: myoclonus *Respiratory*: respiratory depression *GI*: constipation, diverticular disease, nausea, and vomiting [39]	None reported
Oral steroids	*Skin*: thinning and ecchymoses *General*: weight gain and Cushingoid features *HEENT*: cataracts, increased intraocular pressure, and exophthalmos *CV*: fluid retention and HTN and arrhythmias *GI*: peptic ulcer disease, gastritis, and diverticular disease *Bone and muscle*: steoporosis, osteonecrosis, and myopathy *Neuropsychiatric*: mood disorders, psychosis, and memory impairment *Metabolic*: hyperglycemia and HPA suppression *Immune*: impaired immunity *Hematologic*: leukocytosis [40]	Potassium [41], calcium, chromium, magnesium, and vitamin D [42]
Potassium chloride	*CV*: arrhythmias, conduction disturbance, and edema *Endocrine and metabolic*: fluid and electrolyte disturbance, and hypervolemia *GI*: esophagitis (direct irritant effect), cramps, distress, pain, diarrhea, flatulence, irritation, ulcer, nausea, and vomiting [43]	Parenteral administration may cause hyponatremia; risk may be increased in elderly patients [44]

Table 3.2 (continued)

Medication	Side effect	Associated nutrient deficiencies
Proton pump inhibitors	*GI*: *C. difficile* diarrhea and malabsorption *Renal*: acute and chronic kidney disease and acute interstitial nephritis *Electrolytes*: hypomagnesemia *Respiratory*: *Endocrine*: pneumonia and bone fracture *Neurod*: dementia [28, 45, 46]	B12 deficiency
SSRIs	*Cardiovascular*: orthostatic hypotension and QTc prolongation *Neuro*: agitation and drowsiness *GI*: peptic ulcer disease, upper GI bleeding, and appetite changes [47]	Sodium [48]
Tricyclic antidepressants	*Cardiac*: QTc prolongation *Neuro*: anticholinergic effects (xerostomia, appetite changes, constipation) and seizures *Endocrine*: antihistaminic effects (weight gain) *MSK*: bone fractures [49]	None reported

Rebalance and retain assess lifestyle factors that impact gut health: diet,exercise, sleep, stress management, and social connections. The connection between our sense of well-being and our gut function is wired via our vagus nerve which transmits messages relayed by the two branches of our autonomic nervous system: parasympathetic and sympathetic. The bidirectional pathway of the brain-gut axis predicts the impact that our sense of well-being has on the health of our gut and, if out of balance, will lead to the very concerns the five-R protocol attempts to address: intestinal permeability, visceral sensitivity, and alteration in GI motility that subsequently causes imbalance in the gastrointestinal tract. Promoting regular exercise, sleep, mindfulness, and social connections in the context of a nutrient-dense diet is key to a healthy gut.

3.1   Condition-Specific Care

Functional and integrative medicine offers a range of diagnostic approaches to gastrointestinal disorders that help the clinician identify the root cause of the dysfunction that when addressed allows the natural healing capacity of the body to restore balance. In the following section, we address common gastrointestinal conditions that are prevalent in older patients and provide a spectrum of choices to address them.

3.1.1   Irritable Bowel Syndrome (IBS)

As a diagnosis of exclusion, IBS affects 10% of the general population, with hallmark symptoms of gas, pain, bloating, and alteration in bowel habits (constipation, diarrhea, or both) [51]. Adults over 50 report milder pain but overall worse quality of life [52]. Adults over 65 are more likely to wait for over 1 year before consulting a physician [53]. As a functional disorder, IBS often goes underdiagnosed in the elder population due to the frequent occurrence of polypharmacy in this age-group with its known negative impact on the GI tract [2]. Additionally, IBS is commonly attributed to small intestinal bacterial overgrowth (SIBO) which can be diagnosed via lactulose breath testing for hydrogen and methane [54]. If SIBO is the underlying driver of the bowel irregularity, then symptoms will only resolve following appropriate treatment using a combination of a low-FODMAP or elemental diet, antimicrobial herbs or antibiotics, and motility support. Predisposing factors in SIBO development include anatomic abnormalities, diabetes, hypochlorhydria, food poisoning, PPI or narcotic use, recurrent antibiotics, achlorhydria, and slowed motility [55, 56]. While it is prevalent in the elder population, not all IBS is caused by SIBO, but rather it is related to poor eating habits (insufficient fiber or water intake), low microbial diversity, food intolerances, or genetic predispositions [57]. Patients suffering from SIBO require support in a variety of areas, including digestion, liver and gallbladder function, colon health, intestinal motility, small intestine bacteria reduction, and dietary intervention. For guiding principles on SIBO treatment, please see Table 3.3.

3.1.2   Inflammatory Bowel Disease (IBD)

Certain elder patients will have been living with IBD much of their life, but 15% of them will have a new diagnosis for IBD when they are over 65 years old [62]. As an autoimmune disease, integrative medicine's approach to addressing IBD focuses on three aspects: resolving increased intestinal permeability, identifying triggers and removing them, and optimizing epigenetic expression. Often these triggers are related to foods; the standard approach to identifying food triggers is an elimination

Table 3.3 Mainstays of SIBO treatment [56, 58, 59]

Intestinal motility	Prokinetics: octreotide (50 ug SC) × 3 weeks and cisapride (10 mg TID) [60]
Small intestine bacteria reduction	Antibiotics: rifaximin (550 mg BID) × 14 days *or* rifaximin + neomycin (500 mg BID) × 14 days *or* rifaximin + Flagyl (250 mg TID) × 14 days *Botanicals:* berberine, dill, oregano, and thyme [61]
Dietary intervention	Elemental diet, low-FODMAP diet, and supplementation of B12 and fat-soluble vitamins (A, D, E, K)

diet coined by Dr. Sarah Ballantyne. The autoimmune protocol (AIP) diet removes the most common triggers for all autoimmune diseases and then slowly reintroduces the foods to see what is causing symptoms [63]. A promising prospective study on the effects of AIP on active IBD patients showed an improvement in index scores for both UC and CD, a decrease in fecal calprotectin, and an improvement in endoscopic scores after the 11-week trial [64]. See Chap. 11 for more details on the AIP diet [65].

3.1.3 Gastroesophageal Reflux Disease (GERD)

Due to the loss of esophageal sensitivity in older adults, GERD can be difficult to diagnose as the hallmark complaint of heartburn is often lacking [66]. The use of proton pump inhibitors (PPIs), the conventional approach to treatment, is not without its drawbacks and often serves to mask the underlying issue creating the reflux of acid into the esophagus. PPIs have a long list of side effects likely due to the fact that drop in gastric acidity not only shifts how pancreatic enzymes work [67] but also negatively impacts gut microbiome and as result increases risk of different infections and nutritional deficiencies and even causes chronic inflammation [68].

Treating GI concerns requires a comprehensive approach. See Table 3.4 for proposed start.

3.1.4 Traveler's Diarrhea

S. boulardii and other probiotics during traveling can reduce the risk of traveler's diarrhea. It is recommended to take nonrefrigerated probiotics if traveling to areas with food safety concerns. Although many probiotics require refrigeration, not all do [72].

3.2 Healing Foods for the GI Tract

All foods interact with the human body in significant ways to alter biochemistry, physiology, microbiome composition, mood, energy levels, and more. Many foods provide added benefit for the body which goes above and beyond the macronutrient and micronutrient lists, and we refer to these as functional foods. While they are not defined by the FDA, functional foods play an important role in supporting healing and balance in the body [73]. For optimal gut health, consider these functional foods and supplements as described in Tables 3.5 and 3.6, respectively.

Table 3.4 Integrative approach to common GI complaints

Condition	Lifestyle functional medicine prevention	Medications and supplements	Nutrition therapy
Gastroesophageal reflux	Smaller meals Avoid eating 2–3 h before going to bed Elevation of head of bed or using wedge pillow Weight management Quitting smoking Drinking 8–10 glasses of water daily Assess for hypochlorhydria	*Medications*: Antacids H2 blockers Proton pump inhibitors *Supplements*: A. vera juice DGL, 2–4 tablets 380 mg before meals Rice bran oil, 150 mg TID Slippery elm, 2 tbsp in water after meals and bedtime Betaine HCl if hypochlorhydria, taken 20 min before meal Digestive enzymes with meals	Avoid offending foods and beverages (alcohol, caffeine, fatty foods, spicy foods) and high intake of simple carbs and in some cases gluten Elimination diet to identify food triggers (see Chap. 11) If hypochlorhydria is suspected, add 1–2 tbsp of raw apple cider vinegar in 3 ounces of water 20 min before meal to help trigger LES closure
Gastric ulcers	Eating breakfast and regular meals Avoiding caffeine and alcohol Avoid NSAIDs and steroids Regular exercise Adequate sleep	*Medications*: Antacids H2 blockers Proton pump inhibitors *Supplements*: DGL: 2–4 tabs (380 mg) before meals Mastic gum: 500 mg TID Slippery elm: 2 tbsp mixed in water after meals and at bedtime A. vera juice: 1/2 a cup TID Cabbage juice: one glass BID Chamomile tea: three cups daily Turmeric: 600 mg 5× daily Vitamin C: 1200–5000 mg daily to suppress *H. pylori* (no more than 500 mg a dose, up to 4 weeks total) Zinc: 30–50 mg daily as arginate or hydrate form for 3–6 weeks, supplement with at least 1–2 mg copper daily Glutamine: 1600–3000 mg in 3–4 divided doses for 4 weeks Fish oil and black currant oil: 1 g of each daily for 8 weeks for suppression of *H. pylori*	Fresh cabbage juice, 2–4 ounces taken before each meal [69] Demulcents: almonds, barley, chia, coconut oil, figs, flaxseed, oats, okra, parsley, pomegranate seeds, prunes, and pumpkin [70]

Table 3.4 (continued)

Condition	Lifestyle functional medicine prevention	Medications and supplements	Nutrition therapy

Colon cancer	High-fiber, Mediterranean-type diet
	Avoid smoking
	Regular exercise
	Maintain BMI under 30
	Maintain adequate vitamin D levels
		Medications:
		  Anti-inflammatories including NSAIDs and aspirin
		Supplements:
		  Calcium and vitamin D
		  B6
		  Caffeine: three cups daily
		  Garlic, 2.4 mL daily for 12 months
		  Magnesium
		  Fish oil
		  Selenium
		  Curcumin
		  Folate
			Diet high in fruits and vegetables offers protection from colorectal cancer
			Avoid processed meats
			High-polyphenol (>700) olive oil
			Daily intake of cruciferous vegetables (broccoli, cauliflower, kale, brussels sprouts, cabbage, collard greens)
			At least 5–11 servings of fruits and vegetables daily

Constipation	Adequate hydration
	30-g fiber daily
	Regular exercise
	Tea or coffee in moderation
	Bowel-habit diary
	Review medications that may be constipating
	Rule out SIBO
		Laxatives:
		  Docusate and milk of magnesia, 1–2 tbsp daily
		  Magnesium citrate: 350–500 mg a day in chelated form
		  Polyethylene glycol, sorbitol, lactulose, and bisacodyl
		  Senna, tea with ½ tsp of senna in cup of water 1–2× daily
		  Saline or mineral oil enema
		Supplements:
		  A. vera, short-term use only, less than 1 week; juice, ½ cup TID; and capsule, 40- to 170-mg dehydrated juice in capsule
		  Cascara: short-term use only, less than 1 week, 250 mg BID or TID
		  Vitamin C: 500–2000 mg a day
		  Wheat or corn bran: 1 tbsp daily
		  Probiotic bifidobacteria: at least 4 billion units BID or TID
			Fruits and vegetables 5–11 servings daily
			Fiber and other bulk-forming agents – such as psyllium, methylcellulose, or calcium polycarbophil. However, they may not be useful in slow-transit constipation

(continued)

Table 3.4 (continued)

Condition	Lifestyle functional medicine prevention	Medications and supplements	Nutrition therapy
Diarrhea	Handwashing Care with food and water when traveling Cautious in the use of antibiotics (*C. difficile* risk) Screen for gut infections and food sensitivities	*World Health Organization's rehydration formula*: 3.5-g sodium chloride, 2.9-g trisodium citrate, or 2.5-g sodium bicarbonate, 1.5-g potassium chloride, 20-g glucose, or 40-g sucrose. Solution prepared at home using ½ tsp of salt, ½ tsp of baking soda, 4 tbsp of sugar, and 1 L of water *Antimotility agents*: Loperamide (Imodium): 4 mg to start and 2 mg after each unformed stool to a maximum of 16 mg daily no more than 2 days Diphenoxylate (Lomotil): 4 mg up to QID daily for no more than 2 days Caution: use either sparingly and avoid if fever or bloody diarrhea *Antibiotics*: Ciprofloxacin, levofloxacin, trimethoprim/sulfamethoxazole, doxycycline, azithromycin, erythromycin, and vancomycin *Antiparasitics*: Metronidazole *Supplements*: Bilberry: capsules, 240–600 mg per day, or tincture, 1–2 ml BID, and juice, ½ cup BID or TID Ginger: 500 mg BID or 1–2 cups of ginger tea Glutamine: 1000–3000 mg TID Red raspberry, blackberry, or blueberry leaf: tea, one to two teaspoons of dried leaves in cup of boiling water, and capsule, 5–10 mg daily Slippery elm: tea, three cups daily, and capsule, 500 mg daily for 3 days Avoid magnesium citrate/oxalate and vitamin C during diarrhea Probiotics: to re-establish bacterial balance, two to six capsules of *Lactobacillus* and bifidobacteria at least 4 billion units daily Bulk-forming agents: Kaopectate, Metamucil, and psyllium Lactase (Lactaid) if dairy/lactose intolerance is suspected (chronic diary)	Regular intake of fermented foods, yogurt, prebiotics, and probiotics Avoid sugar alcohols (ending in -ol) Olive oil

Table 3.4   (continued)

Condition	Lifestyle functional medicine prevention	Medications and supplements	Nutrition therapy
Diverticulosis	Maintain healthy weight Regular exercise Prevent constipation May not be necessary to avoid seeds and nuts	*Antibiotics*: Ciprofloxacin (Cipro): 500 mg BID Metronidazole (Flagyl): 500 mg TID Other options: amoxicillin-clavulanate, clindamycin, or moxifloxacin *Supplements*: Gamma oryzanol: 100 mg TID for 3–6 weeks L-glutamine: up to 8 g daily in 3–4 divided doses Slippery elm bark: 1–2 cap. TID or make a tea with 1 tsp in two cups of water A. vera: (short-term use only, less than 1 week; juice, ½ cup TID; and capsule, 40–170 mg of dehydrated juice in capsule Probiotics to prevent infection: *Acidophilus*/bifidobacteria: 1 cap. BID for prevention or 2 cap. TID for flare-ups	Maintain high-fiber intake 25–30 g daily when acute condition subsides Soluble fiber such as psyllium and ground flaxseed (2–3 tbsp daily) Trial of low-fat diet

(continued)

Table 3.4 (continued)

Condition	Lifestyle functional medicine prevention	Medications and supplements	Nutrition therapy
Irritable bowel syndrome	Avoid NSAIDs and COX-2 inhibitors Reduce alcohol intake Reduce caffeine intake Regular exercise Stress management Screen for SIBO, celiac disease, and food sensitivities	*Antispasmodics*: Dicyclomine (Bentyl): 20 mg up to QID Hyoscyamine (Levsin): 0.125–0.25 mg TID or QID Sustained-release hyoscyamine (Levbid): 0.375–0.75 mg q 12 h *Antidepressants*: Amitriptyline, desipramine, imipramine, and nortriptyline: dosing is variable based on response and side effects Paroxetine: 20 mg daily Fluoxetine: 20 mg daily Sertraline: 100 mg daily *Anti-diarrheals*: loperamide (Imodium), 2–4 mg as needed not to exceed 16 mg a day *Anxiolytics for short-term use* only: Lorazepam (Ativan): 0.5–1 mg up to TID Diazepam (Valium): 1–10 mg up to TID Oxazepam (Serax): 10–30 mg TID *Serotonin antagonists* for relief of abdominal pain and discomfort: Ondansetron (Zofran): 4–8 mg 1–2 times daily Granisetron (Granisol): 2 mg daily Lubiprostone (Amitiza): 8 mcg BID for women >18 with constipation variety IBS *Supplements*: Peppermint oil: 1–2 enteric-coated cap. TID Caraway oil: enteric-coated volatile oil 0.05–0.2 ml TID and can be taken with peppermint oil Fennel: 1 tsp with food Ginger: 250–500 mg TID or QID Chamomile: one cup of tea TID Iberogast: 20 drops TID for 4 weeks Probiotics: 25 billion units of bifidobacteria and 25 billion units of *Lactobacillus* for 4–6 weeks then 10 BU daily	High-fiber diet and balancing soluble and insoluble fiber based on symptoms Anti-inflammatory diet Regular intake of fermented foods, yogurt, prebiotics, and probiotics, if SIBO is ruled out Dietary modifications: lactose, gluten, carbohydrates, food allergy, and gas-producing foods Fiber (insoluble vs. soluble): psyllium, wheat bran or polycarbophil, and methylcellulose (trial of ½–1 tbsp daily to start). Soluble fiber as flaxseed 2–3 tbsp daily If SIBO breath test is positive, then low-FODMAP diet should be done (see Chap. 12)

Table 3.4 (continued)

Condition	Lifestyle functional medicine prevention	Medications and supplements	Nutrition therapy

Inflammatory bowel disease	Anti-inflammatory diet
	Avoid NSAIDs and COX-2 inhibitors
	Consider food allergy and sensitivity, e.g., gluten and dairy, as contributing or exacerbating factors
	Reduce alcohol intake
	Regular exercise
	Stress management
		Supplements:
		  Aloe: ½ cup TID
		  Rice bran oil: 100 mg TID for 3–6 weeks
		  Boswellia: 550 mg TID
		  Curcumin: 1 mg BID
		  Fish oil: 6 g daily at least 3.2 g of EPA and 2.2 g of DHA
		  Glutamine: 1600–3000 mg daily divided in 3–4 doses
		  Wheatgrass juice: 3.5 ounces daily for a month
		Supplements to replace malabsorbed nutrients: calcium, 1200 mg daily; magnesium, 350 mg daily; iron, 300 mg daily; selenium, 200 mcg daily; zinc, 30 mg daily; vitamin A, 5000 IU daily; vitamin B1, 50 mg daily; vitamin B6, 50 mg daily; folic acid, 400 mcg daily; vitamin B12, 50 mcg daily; and vitamin D, 2000 IU daily
		Antioxidants:
		  Beta carotenoids: 10000 IU daily
		  Vitamin C: 250–500 mg daily
		  CoQ10: 50–100 mg daily
		Probiotics (mixed species): start with 1 BU TID and gradually increase over a month to 20–30 BU daily
		  Saccharomyces boulardii, 250 mg TID
		  Fecal transplant therapy
			Elemental diet for 3–14 days to give bowel rest and reduce inflammation
			Regular intake of fermented foods, yogurt, prebiotics, and probiotics
			High-fiber diet when non-acute phase [71]

Hemorrhoids	Adequate hydration
	Use stool softeners if needed for constipation
	Maintain a healthy weight
	Using topical moisturized towelettes for anal hygiene to decrease irritation
		Conservative treatment with fiber and increased fluids
		Application of topical hydrocortisone for up to a week with pain and itching
		Supplements:
		  Horse chestnut: 300 mg BID or TID
		  Bioflavonoid complex: 1000 mg TID during flares
		  Butcher's broom: 100 mg TID
		  Application of topical gels or creams containing 2% aescin
		  Topical witch hazel
		  Soluble fiber such as psyllium or ground flaxseed 2–3 tbsp daily
			Maintain high-fiber intake 25–30 g daily

Table 3.5 Nutritional recommendations for GI health

Food	Function	Prescription
High-fiber foods: aspberries, pear, apple, banana, orange, strawberries, peas, broccoli, turnip greens, barley, bran, quinoa, oats, beans, and lentils	Food for beneficial bacteria and bulking agents	For men, 35 grams of fiber/day, and for women, 30 grams of fiber/day
Fermented foods: kombucha, kimchi, sauerkraut, lacto-fermented vegetables, yogurt, and kefir	Improve microbiome health by inoculating the gut with beneficial yeast and bacteria [74]	Daily intake of one serving of fermented food/day
Cruciferous vegetables: broccoli, cabbage, arugula, cauliflower, brussels sprouts, and mustard greens [75]	Improves composition of gut microbiome via phytochemicals such as glucosinolates	One serving/day
Demulcents: aloe, almonds, barley, chia, coconut oil, figs, flaxseed, oats, okra, parsley, pomegranate seeds, prunes, pumpkin, and honey	Help restore mucosal barrier along GI tract and soothe inflammation	As needed or after meals/before bed [76]
Spices: turmeric, black pepper, and ginger [77]	Antioxidant and anti-inflammatory actions	Condiment with spices. Turmeric and black pepper should be used at the same time

Table 3.6 Herbs and supplements to support malnourishment

	MOA	Daily dose	Food sources
Bitters	Cephalic vagal reflex increases saliva and vagal stimulation to the digestive organs. Local reflex increases digestive secretions. This improves blood circulation to the abdominal organs [78]	1000 mg [78]	Roasted coffee (*Coffea arabica semen*), gentian (*Gentiana lutea radix*), and wormwood (*A. absinthium herba*) [78]
Apple cider vinegar	Probiotic. Assists in protein utilization and stimulates digestion [79]	1–2 tsp 3× daily [79]	Source
Fermented vegetables	Probiotic. Aid in digestion [80]	2–3 servings per day [81]	Kimchi and sauerkraut [81]
Probiotics	Assists in bowel movement	At least 4 billion units per day	Yogurt, cultured buttermilk, cheese, miso, tempeh, sauerkraut, beer, sour dough, bread, chocolate, kimchi, olives, pickles, and kefir [82]
Bone broth	Contains collagen, which breaks down into amino acids and minerals	One cup	Source

3.3   Special Diets for Gut Health

3.3.1   Low-FODMAP Diet

The role of diet in the treatment of IBS drastically changed as Dr. Pimentel's research brought to light the relationship between certain types of fermentable carbohydrates and the hallmark symptoms of IBS – gas, pain, bloating, and altered bowel habits. Research out of Monash University provides specific food lists to guide the elimination diet that can be helpful in confirming the underlying cause of 80% of all IBS cases – SIBO [83]. Used in conjunction with antimicrobial treatment, the low-FODMAP diet provides welcome relief from symptoms, usually within a week of starting the elimination diet. It's critical to note that this is an elimination diet which has a specified removal and then reintroduction timeline. Because these are the very same fibers that feed the healthy microbiome in the colon, long-term restriction of these fermentable carbohydrates will ultimately reduce the abundance and diversity of the microbiome and lead to poor health [84]. Thus, limiting the elimination diet to on average 3 months and no longer than 6 months is critical. Once the underlying overgrowth is resolved in the small intestine, the patient should be able to tolerate these important foods. For details on the diet, refer to Chap. 12.

3.3.2   Elemental Diet

A long-standing remedy for rapid gut healing is complete bowel rest. Epithelial cells lining the GI tract live just about 3 days which allows for rapid healing when sources of inflammation such as pathogens or triggering foods are removed. There are only a few products on the market today that allow for bowel rest outside the inpatient setting by supplying an elemental diet which is defined as containing all macronutrients in a readily absorbed form. The critical elements include complete amino acid profile, medium-chain fats, and simple carbohydrates in a hypoallergenic formula. The elemental diet is the ideal choice for treating complex gut issues such as SIBO as well as the hypersensitive patient that reacts to most of the common foods [85]. A 2–3-week course of 100% liquid elemental diet is the standard of care with a slow reintroduction of soups/stews while gradually adding in more solid food over the course of a week [86]. In addition, patients suffering from advanced malabsorption may benefit from ongoing intake of elemental diet as a portion of their normal intake.

3.3.3 Autoimmune Paleo (AIP)

A growing body of evidence suggests that autoimmune disease requires two conditions: a genetic predisposition and a trigger that activates the immune system to attack self-tissue. A common stressor that can both perpetuate and trigger the autoimmune process is food. After years of research, Dr. Sarah Ballantyne created the AIP diet to address the most common food triggers that patients with autoimmune disease find help to interrupt the immune attack [63]. AIP is also an elimination diet that should be applied with a timeline in mind rather than a long-term dietary approach. While full nutrition can be accessed from the AIP, the restrictive nature of the diet can have negative social and physiological impacts on the patient. For details on the diet, refer to Chap. 12.

3.3.4 Gluten-Free

The pioneering work of Dr. Alessio Fasano has shed light on the spectrum of gluten sensitivity, explaining the connection between the protein that is found in wheat, barley, and rye and systemic gut inflammation. Dr. Fasano identified the protein, zonulin, that regulates the tight junctions between colonocytes with a high sensitivity toward the gluten protein which stimulates the opening of the tight junctions, allowing large particles into the bloodstream that in turn stimulate the immune system and create systemic inflammation and symptoms [87]. A reliable first-line recommendation for highly inflamed patients, with or without GI symptoms (see Table 3.7), is to remove gluten from the diet for 2–4 months to see if symptoms improve. See Chap. 12 for details on the gluten-free diet.

Tables 3.8 and 3.9 summarize key micronutrients and supplements (respectively) that in our opinion are most beneficial to overall GI health.

3.4 Cases

3.4.1 Case 1: IBS

Sandy, a 68-year-old retired clerk, presents with decades of intermittent abdominal pain, gas, and alternating diarrhea and constipation. She often describes being bloated soon after eating, especially high-carbohydrate meals. Over the years, she

Table 3.7 Common symptoms associated with gluten sensitivity [88, 89]

GI: nausea, constipation, abdominal bloating, gastrointestinal discomfort, abdominal pain, diarrhea and flatulence, and aphthous stomatitis
Extraintestinal: inability to concentrate, fatigue, headache, anxiety, numbness, joint/muscle pain, and skin rash

Table 3.8 Micronutrients and their impact on GI health [90–92]

Micronutrient	Function	Source	Deficiency	RDA[a] male (>70 years)	RDA female (>70 years)
Vitamin A (includes retinol, retinal, retinoic acid, and retinyl esters) (ug/d)	Contributes to maintenance of epithelial tissue and immune function and supports microbiome [93]	Liver, meat, eggs, dairy products, cod liver oil, carrots, pumpkins, mangoes, and papayas	Impaired immunity and diarrhea	900	700
Vitamin C (mg/d)	Reducing agent and scavenger of free radicals. Supports microbiome. Possible protective effect against esophageal cancer [94]	Fresh fruit (citrus, cantaloupe, mango, berries)	Scurvy	90	75
Vitamin D (ug/d)	Immune health. Assists with calcium absorption, important role in regulating cellular proliferation, differentiation, and apoptosis. Possible protective role in CRC [95]	Liver, egg yolk, saltwater fish, and sun	Rickets	20	20
Vitamin E (mg/d)	Antioxidant and scavenger of free radicals. Supports microbiome [96]	Vegetable oils, various oil seeds, and wheat germ	Rare	15	15
Thiamine (mg/d)	Aldehyde transfer reactions, oxidative decarboxylation reactions, and transketolase reactions. Improved IBD fatigue syndrome [97]	Yeast, meat, and legumes	Mild GI discomfort	1.2	1.1

(continued)

Table 3.8 (continued)

Micronutrient	Function	Source	Deficiency	RDA[a] male (>70 years)	RDA female (>70 years)
Niacin (mg/d)	Constituent of NAD and NADP [98]	Yeast, meat, liver, peanuts, and legumes	Diarrhea	16	14
Vitamin B6 (mg/d)	Supports amino acid metabolism and microbiome. May be protective against CRC and benefit celiac disease patients [99]	Liver, fish, whole grains, nuts, legumes, egg yolk, and yeast	Stomatitis and glossitis	1.7	1.5
Folate (ug/d)	Supports microbiome and may be protective against CRC by preventing DNA synthesis errors [100]	Liver, spinach, and black-eyed peas	Megaloblastic anemia, weakness, and fatigue. Common in IBD	400	400
Vitamin B12 (ug/d)	Cofactor for methionine synthase and methylmalonyl CoA mutase [101]	Fish, meat, poultry, eggs, and milk	Pernicious anemia, megaloblastic anemia, neurologic dysfunction. Increased risk of deficiency in vegans or patients with ileal resection (UC or CD). Increased risk of deficiency in celiac patients	2.4	2.4
Zinc (mg/d)	Enzyme constituent. Facilitates carbohydrate metabolism and supports microbiome [102]	Meat, nuts, beans, wheat germ, oyster, crab, and lobster	Anemia, immune dysfunction, and leaky gut	11	8

Table 3.8   (continued)

Micronutrient	Function	Source	Deficiency	RDA[a] male (>70 years)	RDA female (>70 years)
Magnesium (mg/d)	Anti-inflammatory. Supports microbiome [103]	Almonds, spinach, cashews, and peanuts	Anorexia, nausea, vomiting, fatigue, weakness, neurologic changes, arrhythmias, hypocalcemia, and hypokalemia	420	320
Magnesium citrate (mL)	Treats constipation [92]	PO solution	Diarrhea	195–300	195–300
Selenium (ug/d)	Antioxidant. Supports microbiome [104]	Brazil nuts, tuna, halibut, sardines, ham, and shrimp	Inflammation, leaky gut, and IBD	55	55
Iron (mg/d)	Supports microbiome [105]	Oysters, white beans, chocolate, liver, lentils, and spinach	GI disturbances, weakness, fatigue, and immune dysregulation	8	8

[a]*RDA* recommended dietary allowance

had complete comprehensive workup with several colonoscopies, abdominal CT, and trial of a gluten-free diet which helped somewhat for a few months, but eventually symptoms got worse. Patient's gastroenterologist described her condition as irritable bowel syndrome and recommended the patient to stay on regular fiber. While fiber helped with decreasing frequency of constipation, most of the symptoms remained. What is the patient's condition and how would you handle it?

Dx: SIBO breath test and comprehensive functional GI test

Treatment: depending on severity of SIBO, starting with a low-FODMAP diet in combination with an antimicrobial herbal regimen is likely the safest and most evidence-based approach for this patient. Detailed history taking may even reveal an inciting incident, such as food poisoning or an offending medication, such as long-term use of a PPI. See Table 3.10 for further diagnostic reasoning.

Please see Neurodegenerative chapter, Case 2, for correlative case.

3.4.2 Case 2: IBD

Nancy was a vibrant 81-year-old woman who had ulcerative colitis since her 20s. Disease was intermittent and mostly mild. After the birth of her second daughter, her disease went into prolonged remission until 2 years ago when it flared up again after her younger daughter was diagnosed with metastatic breast cancer. Patient was started on oral Lialda and rectal steroids. While bloody diarrhea improved, Lily continued to lose weight and develop mild memory loss. Her physical examination showed MOCA of 24, consistent with mild memory loss, loss of 15 lbs from exam 12 months earlier, and mild diffuse tenderness on abdominal palpation. Basic blood work revealed B12 and iron deficiency anemia with no other significant findings. Gastroenterologist suggested initiating Humira, targeted biologic medication. Additionally, the patient and her family requested nutritional consultation to try changing diet and natural approaches such as probiotics. What evidenced adjunctive nutritional therapies could help this patient?

Table 3.9 Top ten supplements to support GI health [106]

Supplement	MOA	Daily dose	Food source	Provider notes/ comments
Fish oil	Revert the microbiota composition and increase the production of anti-inflammatory compounds, like short-chain fatty acids [107]	4 g [107]	Fatty fish, flax-/hemp-/ chia seeds, and nuts	Animal model studies show that the interplay between gut microbiota, omega-3 fatty acids, and immunity helps to maintain the intestinal wall integrity and interacts with host immune cells [107]
Probiotics and/or prebiotics	To re-establish bacterial balance	*Mixed species best at* least 10 billion CFUs BID or TID and over up to 60 billion CFU daily needed for severe cases	Fermented foods (kimchi, sauerkraut, kombucha), yogurt, kefir, and natto	Can cause sepsis, fungemia, and GI ischemia (generally critically ill patients in intensive care units) [108]
Zinc	Protective effect on the epithelial barrier (tight junctions). Protects against chronic alcohol exposure, heat stress, diarrhea, CFS, colitis, other GI ailments, and even some neurological conditions [109]	30–50 mg daily as carnosine forms for 3–6 weeks	Oysters, crab, and lobster [102]	Can enhance the effects of other beneficial molecules, such as whey-derived growth factor and quercetin [109]

Table 3.9 (continued)

Supplement	MOA	Daily dose	Food source	Provider notes/comments
Gut-healing herbs (marshmallow, aloe, slippery elm, turmeric, DGL)	Varies and supports immune regulation; anti-inflammatory, antioxidant activity; inhibition of leukotriene and NF-kappa B; and antiplatelet activity [110, 111]	300 mg of marshmallow root 300 mg of DGL 100 mg of slippery elm 50 mg of aloe vera [111] 500 mg 5× daily	Source	Turmeric: constipation, dyspepsia, diarrhea, distension, gastroesophageal reflux, nausea, and vomiting. Higher bioavailability in GI tract than elsewhere in the body [112] Marshmallow: may have antiplatelet effects Aloe: rare Slippery elm: rare DGL: headache, nausea, and vomiting, contact dermatitis (topical), diarrhea, itching, nausea, and rash (IV) [113]
Ginger	Anti-inflammatory, antioxidant, antitumor, and antiulcer. Decreases pressure on lower esophageal sphincter, reduces intestinal cramping, and prevents dyspepsia, flatulence, and bloating [114]	Ginger: 250 to 500 mg TID or QID or 1–2 cups of ginger tea	Source	Rare. Minor GI upset [114]
CoQ10	Antioxidant. Generates cellular bioenergy	30–90 mg, taken in divided doses, but up to 200 mg per day [115]	Oily fish (salmon and tuna), organ meats (liver), and whole grains [115]	May experience diarrhea or rash [115]

(continued)

Table 3.9 (continued)

Supplement	MOA	Daily dose	Food source	Provider notes/ comments
Glutamine	Promotes enterocyte proliferation, regulates tight junctions, suppresses pro-inflammatory pathways, and protects cells against apoptosis and cellular stresses [116]	7 g TID [117] of L-glutamine form	Beef, skim milk, white rice, corn, tofu, and egg [116]	Short-term supplementation appears to have the most benefit. No long-term supplementation benefit is seen yet in humans [116]
Vitamin C	Suppresses *H. pylori*, supports gut barrier function, and is an antioxidant [118]	500–2000 mg daily (no more than 500 mg a dose, up to 4 weeks in total)	Red and green pepper, orange juice, orange, grapefruit juice, kiwifruit, and broccoli [119]	Best with vitamin E [118]
Butyric acid	Increases 5-HT concentration, increases brain-derived neurotrophic factor, and upregulated occludin and zonula protein levels (helps restore BBB) [120]	900 mg TID with meals	Produced in the gut with resistant starch (cooked and cooled grain, starchy veggies, beans)	Controversial impact on obesity [121]. The total amount of short-chain fatty acids (SCFAs) is higher in obese individuals. Butyric acid is able to increase lipid synthesis from acetyl-CoA or ketone bodies, which can contribute to obesity. Butyric acid not only provides the substrate for energy expenditure but contributes to signaling pathways involved in glycolipid metabolism

1. *Course of elemental diet.*
2. *Probiotics, specifically brands that have been studied in more detail: VSL#3 and others.*
3. *How should B12 and iron deficiency be addressed: oral* vs. *other forms of B12. Iron supplements are often very hard on the system; review alternative iron supplements such as Floradix and others. Review activated forms of B12 injections over cyanocobalamin.*

Table 3.10 Diagnostic tests for IBS Case 1

SIBO breath test [58]	Comprehensive digestive stool analysis [122]
Lactulose breath testing captures a 3-h picture of small intestine function. When bacteria digest food, they naturally produce gas (such as hydrogen and methane), which travels through the intestinal walls, into the bloodstream, and to the lungs and is eventually released by exhaling. The breath test checks for levels of hydrogen and methane, which indicates where bacteria are fermenting and how much gas they are creating. Humans cannot digest lactulose, but bacteria specific to the small intestine can. Thus, high levels of hydrogen and methane released in the breath indicate bacterial overgrowth in the small intestine. *The test*: after a 24-h preparatory diet, the lactulose sample is swallowed. Breath samples are collected every 20 min for 3 h. Samples are shipped to the testing facility	The Comprehensive Digestive Stool Analysis (CDSA) can be used to evaluate maldigestion, malabsorption, IBS, altered GI immune function, bacterial overgrowth, and chronic dysbiosis. The CDSA samples stool for markers specific to digestion and absorption (chymotrypsin, SCFA, fiber, fats), metabolism (SCFA, n-butyrate, beta-glucuronidase, pH, lactoferrin, blood, mucus), and microbiology (bacteria, mycology) *The test*: stool sample is collected by the patient and shipped to the testing facility

3.4.3 Case 3: GERD/Gluten Sensitivity

Steve, a 66-year-old executive, was brought to see Dr. Kogan after his wife got increasingly upset about his medical care. Just a few years ago, Steve was in his best health, running half marathon in under 2 h and 30 min, still managing his real estate business, and never complaining of being tired. Over the last decade, Steve has been periodically complaining about acid reflux that usually would go away with tums or avoidance of spicy foods that seem to trigger it. However, gradually acid reflux symptoms increased in frequency, and eventually Steve had EGD that diagnosed GERD and gastritis. A course of omeprazole mildly improved GERD symptoms, and since he felt better, he was kept on low daily dose. About 6 months later, symptoms got progressively worse, and omeprazole was switched to pantoprazole with very minimal improvement. Around the same time, diagnosis of hypertension was made, and Steve was started on hydrochlorothiazide (HCTZ). Three months later, Steve cancelled his planned half marathon race due to inability to run even 6 miles and increasing fatigue. At this point, his wife brought him to see Dr. Kogan. Dietary history revealed increased carb cravings and increase in grain intake in the last 12 months as opposed to his previous low-grain, paleo-style of eating. His physical exam revealed a well-developed, younger than stated age, man who appeared to be healthy. Comprehensive blood work revealed normal serum but low RBC magnesium, low normal vitamin B12 level, and low ferritin despite normal blood counts and iron level. Celiac blood work test was negative. What is going on here and how should we help Steve?

Given the history and blood work suspicious of malabsorption, we have restarted Steve on a gluten-free diet in combination with home subcutaneous twice weekly

Fig. 3.2 Weaning protocol
for proton pump inhibitors
[123]

Weaning Protocol for Proton Pump Inhibitors
(pantoprazole, omeprazole, etc.)

*Skip dose every 3rd day substituting ranitidine 150 mg or
famotidine 20 mg or other H2 blocker for two weeks.*

*If you tolerate this, skip every other day with substitution
every other day for two weeks.*

*If this is tolerated, at the end of a month, switch entirely to
ranitidine, famotidine of other H2 blocker and keep
pantoprazole or other PPI in reserve for flare-ups of
heartburn.*

*May also consider DGL or Aloe as an alternative to H2
blockers or to assist in the taper*

injections of 2.5 mg of methylcobalamin and topical magnesium in addition to B100 complex and omega-3 fatty acids. Within 3 months, Steve stated that his acid reflux all but resolved and his blood pressure decreased by steady 10–15 points. In addition to stopping HCTZ, we started to taper off his pantoprazole. On the next follow-up in 3 months, Steve was off both medications, felt a lot less fatigue, started running again, and signed up for a half marathon. This case demonstrates how mild cases of gluten sensitivity can present as acid reflux and lead to overprescribing of proton pump inhibitors (PPIs). PPIs can cause or worsen B12 and magnesium deficiency. In the case of magnesium, adding diuretics can worsen the issue even more. Addressing underlying cause while replenishing missing nutrients returned this patient to his baseline, eliminating need for any medications. See Fig. 3.2 for proposed weaning protocol for PPIs.

References

1. Levenstein S, Ackerman S, Kiecolt-Glaser JK, Dubois A. Stress and peptic ulcer disease. JAMA. 1999;281(1):10–1.
2. Dumic I, Nordin T, Jecmenica M, Stojkovic Lalosevic M, Milosavljevic T, Milovanovic T. Gastrointestinal tract disorders in older age. Can J Gastroenterol Hepatol. 2019;2019:6757524.
3. Firth M, Prather CM. Gastrointestinal motility problems in the elderly patient. Gastroenterology. 2002;122(6):1688–700.
4. Fligiel SE, Relan NK, Dutta S, Tureaud J, Hatfield J, Majumdar AP. Aging diminishes gastric mucosal regeneration: relationship to tyrosine kinases. Lab Investig. 1994;70(5):764–74.
5. Saraf AA, Petersen AW, Simmons SF, Schnelle JF, Bell SP, Kripalani S, et al. Medications associated with geriatric syndromes and their prevalence in older hospitalized adults discharged to skilled nursing facilities. J Hosp Med. 2016;11(10):694–700.
6. Vakil N. Antiulcer medications: mechanism of action, pharmacology, and side effects [Internet]. UpToDate. 2020 [cited 2021 Mar 4]. Available from: https://www.uptodate.com/contents/antiulcer-medications-mechanism-of-action-pharmacology-and-

side-effects?search=Antacids&source=search_result&selectedTitle=1~150&usa
ge_type=default&display_rank=1#H3816583453.

7. Erckenbrecht J, Kienle U, Zöllner L, Wienbeck M. Effects of high dose antacids on bowel motility. Digestion. 1982;25(4):244–7.

8. Jung SB, Nagaraja V, Kapur A, Eslick GD. Association between vitamin B12 deficiency and long-term use of acid-lowering agents: a systematic review and meta-analysis. Intern Med J. 2015;45(4):409–16.

9. Graziani AL. Azithromycin and clarithromycin [Internet]. UpToDate. 2020 [cited 2021 Mar 4]. Available from: https://www.uptodate.com/contents/azithromycin-and-clari thromycin?search=azithromycin&source=search_result&selectedTitle=2~145&usa ge_type=default&display_rank=5#H2.

10. Ghossein N, Kang M, Lakhar AD. Anticholinergic medications. StatPearls; 2020.

11. Schachler S. Antiseizure drugs: mechanism of action, pharmacology, and adverse effects. [Internet]. UpToDate. 2020 [cited 2021 Mar 4]. Available from: https://www.uptodate.com/contents/antiseizure-drugs-mechanism-of-action-pharmacology-and-adverse-effects?search=topiramate&source=search_result&selectedTitle=2~148&usa ge_type=default&display_rank=1#H1780224909.

12. McCulloch D. Alpha-glucosidase inhibitors and lipase inhibitors for treatment of diabetes mellitus [Internet]. UpToDate. 2019 [cited 2021 Mar 4]. Available from: https://www.uptodate.com/contents/alpha-glucosidase-inhibitors-and-lipase-inhibitors-for-treatment-of-diabetes-mellitus?search=acarbose&source=sea rch_result&selectedTitle=3~26&usage_type=default&display_rank=2#H6.

13. Exenatide [Internet]. UpToDate. 2020 [cited 2021 Mar 4]. Available from: https://www.upto-date.com/contents/exenatide-drug-information?search=exenatide&topicRef=1772&source= see_link.

14. Dungan K. Glucagon-like peptide 1 receptor agonists for the treatment of type 2 diabetes mellitus. [Internet]. UpToDate. 2020 [cited 2021 Mar 4]. Available from: https://www.upto-date.com/contents/glucagon-like-peptide-1-receptor-agonists-for-the-treatment-of-type-2-diabetes-mellitus.

15. Mayo Clinic. Diabetes treatment: medications for type 2 diabetes [Internet]. Mayo Clinic. 2018 [cited 2021 Mar 3]. Available from: https://www.mayoclinic.org/diseases-conditions/type-2-diabetes/in-depth/diabetes-treatment/art-20051004.

16. TRC. Metformin [Internet]. TRC Natural Medicines. 2021 [cited 2021 Mar 12]. Available from: https://naturalmedicines-therapeuticresearch-com.proxygw.wrlc.org/tools/nutrient-depletion.aspx#P.

17. Miller RG, Bolognese M, Worley K, Solis A, Sheer R. Incidence of gastrointestinal events among bisphosphonate patients in an observational setting. Am J Manag Care. 2004;10(7):207–15.

18. Rosen HN. Pharmacology of bisphosphonates [Internet]. UpToDate. 2019 [cited 2021 Mar 4]. Available from: https://www.uptodate.com/contents/pharmacology-of-bisphosphonates.

19. Kennel KA, Drake MT. Adverse effects of bisphosphonates: implications for osteoporosis management. Mayo Clin Proc. 2009;84(7):632–7; quiz 638.

20. Bloch MJ. Major side effects and safety of calcium channel blockers [Internet]. UpToDate. 2020 [cited 2021 Mar 4]. Available from: https://www.uptodate.com/con-tents/major-side-effects-and-safety-of-calcium-channel-blockers?search=calcium%20 channel%20blockers&source=search_result&selectedTitle=2~135&usa ge_type=default&display_rank=2#H4248664106.

21. Giardina. Amiodarone [Internet]. UpToDate. 2020 [cited 2021 Mar 4]. Available from: https://www.uptodate.com/contents/amiodarone-adverse-effects-potential-toxicities-and-approach-to-monitoring?search=amiodarone&source=search_result&selectedTitle=2~148& usage_type=default&display_rank=1#H17.

22. Giardina. Major side effects of class 1 antiarrhythmic drugs [Internet]. UpToDate. 2019 [cited 2021 Mar 5]. Available from: https://www.uptodate.com/contents/major-side-effects-of-class-i-antiarrhythmic-drugs.

23. Spironolactone: Drug Information [Internet]. UpToDate. 2020 [cited 2021 Mar 5]. Available from: https://www.uptodate.com/contents/spironolactone-drug-information?search=spironolactone&source=panel_search_result&selectedTitle=1~148&usage_type=panel&kp_tab=drug_general&display_rank=1#F222826.

24. Colchicine: Drug Information [Internet]. UpToDate. 2020 [cited 2021 Mar 5]. Available from: https://www.uptodate.com/contents/colchicine-drug-information?search=colchicine&source=panel_search_result&selectedTitle=1~148&usage_type=panel&kp_tab=drug_general&display_rank=1#F154270.

25. Furosemide: Drug Information [Internet]. UpToDate. 2020 [cited 2021 Mar 5]. Available from: https://www.uptodate.com/contents/furosemide-drug-information?search=furosemide&source=panel_search_result&selectedTitle=1~148&usage_type=panel&kp_tab=drug_general&display_rank=1#F174805.

26. Greenberg A. Diuretic complications. Am J Med Sci. 2000;319(1):10–24.

27. Oh SW, Han SY. Loop diuretics in clinical practice. Electrolyte Blood Press. 2015;13(1):17–21.

28. Wolfe MM. Proton pump inhibitors: overview of use and adverse effects in the treatment of acid related disorders [Internet]. UpToDate. 2020 [cited 2021 Mar 5]. Available from: https://www.uptodate.com/contents/proton-pump-inhibitors-overview-of-use-and-adverse-effects-in-the-treatment-of-acid-related-disorders?sectionName=ADVERSE%20EFFECTS&search=H2%20blockers&topicRef=32&anchor=H59974871&source=see_link#H59974871.

29. Kieboom BCT, Kiefte-de Jong JC, Eijgelsheim M, Franco OH, Kuipers EJ, Hofman A, et al. Proton pump inhibitors and hypomagnesemia in the general population: a population-based cohort study. Am J Kidney Dis. 2015;66(5):775–82.

30. Force RW, Nahata MC. Effect of histamine H2-receptor antagonists on vitamin B12 absorption. Ann Pharmacother. 1992;26(10):1283–6.

31. Ferrous sulfate: Drug Information [Internet]. UpToDate. 2020 [cited 2021 Mar 5]. Available from: https://www.uptodate.com/contents/ferrous-sulfate-drug-information?search=iron%20supplements&selectedTitle=1~140&usage_type=panel&display_rank=1&kp_tab=drug_general&source=panel_search_result#F170881.

32. Cook JD, Dassenko SA, Whittaker P. Calcium supplementation: effect on iron absorption. Am J Clin Nutr. 1991;53(1):106–11.

33. Lithium: Drug Information [Internet]. UpToDate. 2020 [cited 2021 Mar 5]. Available from: https://www.uptodate.com/contents/lithium-drug-information?search=lithium&source=panel_search_result&selectedTitle=1~148&usage_type=panel&kp_tab=drug_general&display_rank=1#F189309.

34. Johnson M. Metronidazole: an overview [Internet]. UpToDate. 2019 [cited 2021 Mar 5]. Available from: https://www.uptodate.com/contents/metronidazole-an-overview?search=metronidazole&source=search_result&selectedTitle=2~145&usage_type=default&display_rank=1#H13.

35. TRC. Metronidazole [Internet]. Natural medicines TRC. 2021 [cited 2021 Mar 12]. Available from: https://naturalmedicines-therapeuticresearch-com.proxygw.wrlc.org/tools/nutrient-depletion.aspx.

36. Feldman M. NSAIDs (including aspirin): Pathogenesis of gastroduodenal toxicity [Internet]. UpToDate. 2019 [cited 2021 Mar 5]. Available from: https://www.uptodate.com/contents/nsaids-including-aspirin-pathogenesis-of-gastroduodenal-toxicity?search=NSAIDs&topicRef=7989&source=see_link.

37. Solomon D. Nonselective NSAIDs: overview of adverse effects [Internet]. UpToDate. 2020 [cited 2021 Mar 5]. Available from: https://www.uptodate.com/contents/nonselective-nsaids-overview-of-adverse-effects?search=nsaid%20side%20effects&source=search_result&selectedTitle=2~149&usage_type=default&display_rank=1#H4.

38. TRC. Ibuprofen [Internet]. TRC natural medicines. 2021 [cited 2021 Mar 12]. Available from: https://naturalmedicines-therapeuticresearch-com.proxygw.wrlc.org/tools/nutrient-depletion.aspx#N.

39. Oxycodone: Drug Information [Internet]. UpToDate. 2020 [cited 2021 Mar 5]. Available from: https://www.uptodate.com/contents/oxycodone-drug-information?search=opioids%20side%20effects&selectedTitle=1~143&usage_type=panel&display_rank=1&kp_tab=drug_general&source=panel_search_result#F204871.

40. Saag KG. Major side effects of systemic glucocorticoids [Internet]. UpToDate. 2020 [cited 2021 Mar 5]. Available from: https://www.uptodate.com/contents/major-side-effects-of-systemic-glucocorticoids?search=glucocorticoid%20side%20effects&source=search_result&selectedTitle=1~150&usage_type=default&display_rank=1#H11.

41. Veltri KT, Mason C. Medication-induced hypokalemia. P T. 2015;40(3):185–90.

42. TRC. Prednisone [Internet]. TRC Natural Medicines. 2021 [cited 2021 Mar 12]. Available from: https://naturalmedicines-therapeuticresearch-com.proxygw.wrlc.org/tools/nutrient-depletion.aspx#A.

43. Castell DO. Medication-induced esophagitis [Internet]. UpToDate. 2018 [cited 2021 Mar 5]. Available from: https://www.uptodate.com/contents/medication-induced-esophagitis?search=potassium%20chloride%20esophagitis&source=search_result&selectedTitle=1~150&usage_type=default&display_rank=1#H2.

44. UpToDate. Potassium chloride [Internet]. UpToDate. 2021 [cited 2021 Mar 4]. Available from: https://www.uptodate.com/contents/potassium-chloride-drug-information?search=potassium%20chloride&source=panel_search_result&selectedTitle=1~148&usage_type=panel&kp_tab=drug_general&display_rank=1#F211796.

45. Schoenfeld AJ, Grady D. Adverse effects associated with proton pump inhibitors. JAMA Intern Med. 2016;176(2):172–4.

46. Gomm W, von Holt K, Thomé F, Broich K, Maier W, Fink A, et al. Association of proton pump inhibitors with risk of dementia: a pharmacoepidemiological claims data analysis. JAMA Neurol. 2016;73(4):410–6.

47. Hirsch M. Selective serotonin reuptake inhibitors: pharmacology, administration, and side effects [Internet]. UpToDate. 2020 [cited 2021 Mar 5]. Available from: https://www.uptodate.com/contents/selective-serotonin-reuptake-inhibitors-pharmacology-administration-and-side-effects?search=SSRI%20side%20effects&source=search_result&selectedTitle=2~138&usage_type=default&display_rank=2#H176537802.

48. TRC. Fluoxetine [Internet]. TRC Natural Medicines. 2021 [cited 2021 Mar 12]. Available from: https://naturalmedicines-therapeuticresearch-com.proxygw.wrlc.org/tools/nutrient-depletion.aspx#S.

49. Hirsch M. Tricyclic and tetracyclic drugs: pharmacology, administration, and side effects [Internet]. UpToDate. 2020 [cited 2021 Mar 5]. Available from: https://www.uptodate.com/contents/tricyclic-and-tetracyclic-drugs-pharmacology-administration-and-side-effects?search=TCA%20side%20effects&source=search_result&selectedTitle=3~144&usage_type=default&display_rank=3#H24.

50. Kothari D, Patel S, Kim S-K. Probiotic supplements might not be universally-effective and safe: a review. Biomed Pharmacother. 2019;111:537–47.

51. Lewis ED, Antony JM, Crowley DC, Piano A, Bhardwaj R, Tompkins TA, et al. Efficacy of Lactobacillus paracasei HA-196 and Bifidobacterium longum R0175 in alleviating symptoms of irritable bowel syndrome (IBS): a randomized, placebo-controlled study. Nutrients. 2020;12(4)

52. Tang Y-R, Yang W-W, Liang M-L, Xu X-Y, Wang M-F, Lin L. Age-related symptom and life quality changes in women with irritable bowel syndrome. World J Gastroenterol. 2012;18(48):7175–83.

53. Talley NJ, Boyce PM, Jones M. Predictors of health care seeking for irritable bowel syndrome: a population based study. Gut. 1997;41(3):394–8.

54. Pimentel M. A new IBS solution: bacteria-the missing link in treating irritable bowel syndrome. First printing. Sherman Oaks: Health Point Press; 2006.
55. Ghoshal UC, Shukla R, Ghoshal U. Small intestinal bacterial overgrowth and irritable bowel syndrome: a bridge between functional organic dichotomy. Gut Liver. 2017;11(2):196–208.
56. Dukowicz AC, Lacy BE, Levine GM. Small intestinal bacterial overgrowth: a comprehensive review. Gastroenterol Hepatol (N Y). 2007;3(2):112–22.
57. Chang L. Symptoms and causes of irritable bowel syndrome [Internet]. NIH National Institute of Diabetes and Digestive and Kidney Diseases. 2017 [cited 2021 Mar 5]. Available from: https://www.niddk.nih.gov/health-information/digestive-diseases/irritable-bowel-syndrome/symptoms-causes.
58. Rezaie A, Pimentel M, Rao SS. How to test and treat small intestinal bacterial overgrowth: an evidence-based approach. Curr Gastroenterol Rep. 2016;18(2):8.
59. Ginnebaugh B, Chey WD, Saad R. Small intestinal bacterial overgrowth: how to diagnose and treat (and then treat again). Gastroenterol Clin N Am. 2020;49(3):571–87.
60. Madrid AM, Hurtado C, Venegas M, Cumsille F, Defilippi C. Long-term treatment with cisapride and antibiotics in liver cirrhosis: effect on small intestinal motility, bacterial overgrowth, and liver function. Am J Gastroenterol. 2001;96(4):1251–5.
61. Chedid V, Dhalla S, Clarke JO, Roland BC, Dunbar KB, Koh J, et al. Herbal therapy is equivalent to rifaximin for the treatment of small intestinal bacterial overgrowth. Glob Adv Health Med. 2014;3(3):16–24.
62. Benchimol EI, Mack DR, Nguyen GC, Snapper SB, Li W, Mojaverian N, et al. Incidence, outcomes, and health services burden of very early onset inflammatory bowel disease. Gastroenterology. 2014;147(4):803–813.e7; quiz e14.
63. Ballantyne S. The paleo approach: reverse autoimmune disease and heal your body. 1st ed. Las Vegas: Victory Belt Publishing; 2014.
64. Konijeti GG, Kim N, Lewis JD, Groven S, Chandrasekaran A, Grandhe S, et al. Efficacy of the autoimmune protocol diet for inflammatory bowel disease. Inflamm Bowel Dis. 2017;23(11):2054–60.
65. Stepaniuk P, Bernstein CN, Targownik LE, Singh H. Characterization of inflammatory bowel disease in elderly patients: a review of epidemiology, current practices and outcomes of current management strategies. Can J Gastroenterol Hepatol. 2015;29(6):327–33.
66. Devault KR. Management of reflux disease in elderly patients. Gastroenterol Hepatol (N Y). 2007;3(7):527–9.
67. Ketwaroo GA, Graham DY. Rational use of pancreatic enzymes for pancreatic insufficiency and pancreatic pain. Adv Exp Med Biol. 2019;1148:323–43.
68. Fossmark R, Martinsen TC, Waldum HL. Adverse effects of proton pump inhibitors-evidence and plausibility. Int J Mol Sci. 2019;20:5203. https://doi.org/10.3390/ijms20205203.
69. Cheney G. Rapid healing of peptic ulcers in patients receiving fresh cabbage juice. Calif Med. 1949;70(1):10–5.
70. Lipski E. Digestive wellness: strengthen the immune system and prevent disease through healthy digestion, fourth edition. 4th ed. New York: McGraw-Hill; 2011.
71. Brotherton CS, Taylor AG, Bourguignon C, Anderson JG. A high-fiber diet may improve bowel function and health-related quality of life in patients with Crohn disease. Gastroenterol Nurs. 2014;37(3):206–16.
72. Weil A. Integrative geriatric medicine. Kogan M, editor. Oxford University Press; 2018.
73. Food Labeling & Nutrition [Internet]. US Food and Drug Administration. 2020 [cited 2021 Mar 5]. Available from: https://www.fda.gov/food/food-labeling-nutrition.
74. Dimidi E, Cox SR, Rossi M, Whelan K. Fermented foods: definitions and characteristics, impact on the gut microbiota and effects on gastrointestinal health and disease. Nutrients. 2019;11(8):1806. https://doi.org/10.3390/nu11081806.
75. Li F, Hullar MAJ, Schwarz Y, Lampe JW. Human gut bacterial communities are altered by addition of cruciferous vegetables to a controlled fruit- and vegetable-free diet. J Nutr. 2009;139(9):1685–91.

76. Sarris J, Wardle J. Clinical naturopathy: an evidence-based guide to practice. 1st ed. Churchill Livingstone Australia; 2010.

77. Bustamante MF, Agustín-Perez M, Cedola F, Coras R, Narasimhan R, Golshan S, et al. Design of an anti-inflammatory diet (ITIS diet) for patients with rheumatoid arthritis. Contemp Clin Trials Commun. 2020;17:100524.

78. McMullen MK, Whitehouse JM, Towell A. Bitters: time for a new paradigm. Evid Based Complement Alternat Med. 2015;2015:670504.

79. Gunnars K. 6 health benefits of Apple Cider Vinegar, backed by Science [Internet]. Healthline. 2020 [cited 2021 Mar 4]. Available from: https://www.healthline.com/nutrition/6-proven-health-benefits-of-apple-cider-vinegar.

80. Fermented foods can add depth to your diet [Internet]. Harvard Health Publishing. 2018 [cited 2021 Mar 4]. Available from: https://www.health.harvard.edu/staying-healthy/fermented-foods-can-add-depth-to-your-diet.

81. BBC. Will a daily dose of fermented foods boost your health? [Internet]. BBC Food. 2021 [cited 2021 Mar 4]. Available from: https://www.bbc.co.uk/food/articles/fermented_foods.

82. Syngai GG, Gopi R, Bharali R, Dey S, Lakshmanan GMA, Ahmed G. Probiotics - the versatile functional food ingredients. J Food Sci Technol. 2016;53(2):921–33.

83. Halmos EP, Power VA, Shepherd SJ, Gibson PR, Muir JG. A diet low in FODMAPs reduces symptoms of irritable bowel syndrome. Gastroenterology. 2014;146(1):67–75.e5.

84. Whelan K, Martin LD, Staudacher HM, Lomer MCE. The low FODMAP diet in the management of irritable bowel syndrome: an evidence-based review of FODMAP restriction, reintroduction and personalisation in clinical practice. J Hum Nutr Diet. 2018;31(2):239–55.

85. Pimentel M, Constantino T, Kong Y, Bajwa M, Rezaei A, Park S. A 14-day elemental diet is highly effective in normalizing the lactulose breath test. Dig Dis Sci. 2004;49(1):73–7.

86. Hunter J. Elemental diet and the nutritional treatment of Crohn's disease. Gastroenterol Hepatol Bed Bench. 2015;8(1):4–5.

87. Fasano A. Zonulin, regulation of tight junctions, and autoimmune diseases. Ann N Y Acad Sci. 2012;1258:25–33.

88. Roszkowska A, Pawlicka M, Mroczek A, Bałabuszek K, Nieradko-Iwanicka B. Non-celiac gluten sensitivity: a review. Medicina (Kaunas). 2019;55(6):222. https://doi.org/10.3390/medicina55060222.

89. Barbaro MR, Cremon C, Stanghellini V, Barbara G. Recent advances in understanding non-celiac gluten sensitivity. [version 1; peer review: 2 approved]. F1000Res. 2018;7

90. Mach N, Clark A. Micronutrient deficiencies and the human gut microbiota. Trends Microbiol. 2017;25(8):607–10.

91. Masri OA, Chalhoub JM, Sharara AI. Role of vitamins in gastrointestinal diseases. World J Gastroenterol. 2015;21(17):5191–209.

92. Magnesium Citrate [Internet]. Lexicomp. 2020 [cited 2021 Mar 5]. Available from: https://www.uptodate.com/contents/magnesium-citrate-drug-information?search=magnesium+citrate.

93. NIH. Vitamin A [Internet]. Vitamin A. 2020 [cited 2021 Jan 30]. Available from: https://ods.od.nih.gov/factsheets/VitaminA-HealthProfessional/.

94. NIH. Vitamin C [Internet]. 2020 [cited 2021 Jan 30]. Available from: https://ods.od.nih.gov/factsheets/VitaminC-HealthProfessional/.

95. NIH. Vitamin D [Internet]. NIH National Institutes of Health Office of Dietary Suppolements. 2020 [cited 2020 Dec 31]. Available from: https://ods.od.nih.gov/factsheets/VitaminD-HealthProfessional/.

96. NIH. Vitamin E [Internet]. NIH Office of Dietary Supplements. 2020 [cited 2021 Jan 30]. Available from: https://ods.od.nih.gov/factsheets/VitaminE-HealthProfessional/.

97. NIH. Thiamin [Internet]. National Institues of Health Office of Dietary Supplements. 2020 [cited 2021 Jan 16]. Available from: https://ods.od.nih.gov/factsheets/Thiamin-HealthProfessional/#:~:text=Food%20sources%20of%20thiamin%20include,major%20source%20of%20the%20vitamin.

98. NIH. Niacin [Internet]. NIH Office of Dietary Supplements. 2021 [cited 2021 Mar 5]. Available from: https://ods.od.nih.gov/factsheets/Niacin-HealthProfessional/.
99. NIH. Vitamin B6 [Internet]. National Institutes of Health Office of Dietary Supplements. 2020 [cited 2020 Dec 30]. Available from: https://ods.od.nih.gov/factsheets/VitaminB6-HealthProfessional/#:~:text=The%20richest%20sources%20of%20vitamin,1%2C3%2C5%5D..
100. NIH. Folate [Internet]. National Institutes of Health Office of Dietary Supplements. 2020 [cited 2020 Dec 30]. Available from: https://ods.od.nih.gov/factsheets/Folate-HealthProfessional/.
101. Vitamin B12 [Internet]. NIH National Institutes of Health Office of Dietary Supplements. 2020 [cited 2021 Jan 2]. Available from: https://ods.od.nih.gov/factsheets/VitaminB12-HealthProfessional/.
102. NIH. Zinc [Internet]. NIH Office of Dietary Supplements. 2020 [cited 2021 Feb 5]. Available from: https://ods.od.nih.gov/factsheets/Zinc-HealthProfessional/.
103. NIH. Magnesium [Internet]. National Institutes of Health Office of Dietary Supplements. 2020 [cited 2020 Dec 30]. Available from: https://ods.od.nih.gov/factsheets/Magnesium-HealthProfessional/#:~:text=Magnesium%20is%20widely%20distributed%20in,cereals%20and%20other%20fortified%20foods.
104. NIH. Selenium [Internet]. NIH Office of Dietary Supplements. 2020 [cited 2021 Jan 30]. Available from: https://ods.od.nih.gov/factsheets/Selenium-HealthProfessional/.
105. NIH. Iron [Internet]. NIH Office of Dietary Supplements. 2020 [cited 2021 Mar 5]. Available from: https://ods.od.nih.gov/factsheets/Iron-HealthProfessional/.
106. Dossett ML, Davis RB, Lembo AJ, Yeh GY. Complementary and alternative medicine use by US adults with gastrointestinal conditions: results from the 2012 National Health Interview Survey. Am J Gastroenterol. 2014;109(11):1705–11.
107. Costantini L, Molinari R, Farinon B, Merendino N. Impact of omega-3 fatty acids on the gut microbiota. Int J Mol Sci. 2017;18(12)
108. Didari T, Solki S, Mozaffari S, Nikfar S, Abdollahi M. A systematic review of the safety of probiotics. Expert Opin Drug Saf. 2014;13(2):227–39.
109. Skrovanek S, DiGuilio K, Bailey R, Huntington W, Urbas R, Mayilvaganan B, et al. Zinc and gastrointestinal disease. World J Gastrointest Pathophysiol. 2014;5(4):496–513.
110. Triantafyllidi A, Xanthos T, Papalois A, Triantafillidis JK. Herbal and plant therapy in patients with inflammatory bowel disease. Ann Gastroenterol. 2015;28(2):210–20.
111. Myers A. Restore gut health with 6 herbs and nutrients [Internet]. Amy Myers MD. 2021 [cited 2021 Mar 12]. Available from: https://www.amymyersmd.com/article/restore-gut-health-herbs-nutrients/.
112. Hewlings SJ, Kalman DS. Curcumin: a review of its effects on human health. Foods. 2017;6(10):92. https://doi.org/10.3390/foods6100092.
113. TRC. Foods, herbs & supplements [Internet]. TRC Natural Medicines. 2021 [cited 2021 Mar 12]. Available from: https://naturalmedicines-therapeuticresearch-com.proxygw.wrlc.org/databases/food,-herbs-supplements.aspx.
114. Nikkhah Bodagh M, Maleki I, Hekmatdoost A. Ginger in gastrointestinal disorders: a systematic review of clinical trials. Food Sci Nutr. 2019;7(1):96–108.
115. Saini R. Coenzyme Q10: the essential nutrient. J Pharm Bioallied Sci. 2011;3(3):466–7.
116. Kim M-H, Kim H. The roles of glutamine in the intestine and its implication in intestinal diseases. Int J Mol Sci. 2017;18(5):1051. https://doi.org/10.3390/ijms18051051.
117. Den Hond E, Hiele M, Peeters M, Ghoos Y, Rutgeerts P. Effect of long-term oral glutamine supplements on small intestinal permeability in patients with Crohn's disease. JPEN J Parenter Enteral Nutr. 1999;23(1):7–11.
118. Traber MG, Buettner GR, Bruno RS. The relationship between vitamin C status, the gut-liver axis, and metabolic syndrome. Redox Biol. 2019;21:101091.
119. NIH. Vitamin C [Internet]. National Institutes of Health Office of Dietary Supplements. 2020 [cited 2020 Dec 30]. Available from: https://ods.od.nih.gov/factsheets/VitaminC-HealthProfessional/.

120. Sun J, Wang F, Hong G, Pang M, Xu H, Li H, et al. Antidepressant-like effects of sodium butyrate and its possible mechanisms of action in mice exposed to chronic unpredictable mild stress. Neurosci Lett. 2016;618:159–66.

121. Liu H, Wang J, He T, Becker S, Zhang G, Li D, et al. Butyrate: a double-edged sword for health? Adv Nutr. 2018;9(1):21–9.

122. GDX. Gastrointestinal Test: Comprehensive Digestive Stool Analysis (CDSA) [Internet]. Genova Diagnostics. 2020 [cited 2021 Mar 3]. Available from: https://www.gdx.net/product/comprehensive-digestive-stool-analysis-cdsa#:%7E:text=The%20Comprehensive%20 Digestive%20Stool%20Analysis,Digestion%2FAbsorption%20Markers.

123. Kogan M, Weil A. Integrative gastroenterology. Integrative geriatric medicine. Oxford University Press; New York, 2017.

Chapter 4
Immune

Contents

The manifestations of immune system imbalance and disease cross every body system which can make the diagnosis and treatment of immune dysfunction arduous. Looking at the varied implications of immune dysfunction – seasonal and environmental allergies, autoimmune disease, and resistance to and resolution of bacterial and viral infections – gets to the core of functional medicine as we see the impact of all aspects of health at play.

© The Author(s), under exclusive license to Springer Nature
Switzerland AG 2021
J. Wendt et al., *Integrative Geriatric Nutrition*,
https://doi.org/10.1007/978-3-030-81758-9_4

4.1 Allergies

4.1.1 Allergies and Delayed Hypersensitivity Reaction (HSR)

Environmental and food-based allergies are present in 10% of adults over the age of 65 [1]. While IgE-mediated allergies will often improve with an integrative approach to wellness, the more likely target of care is with IgG-mediated responses that trigger an inflammatory response. While delayed-type HSR is not a known allergic response triggering IgE antibodies, it is recognized to cause inflammatory states and can be assessed using IgG markers. We will focus this section on the IgG-mediated responses called food sensitivities. The integrative medical view of allergies will look to address root causes such as toxic burden, inflammation, and gut imbalance while treating acute symptoms with herbal and nutraceutical support. This approach is highly effective. Symptoms and conditions that may be caused or exacerbated by a food sensitivity are captured in Table 4.1 (reproduced with permission from Alan Gaby to use Table 7-1 on page 24 of *Nutritional Medicine*) [2].

4.1.2 Allergies and Asthma

Asthma and allergies share a number of commonalities, especially through childhood. Atopic dermatitis (eczema) and seasonal rhinitis (hay fever) often precede full-blown asthma, a sequence defined as the "atopic march" [3]. The

Table 4.1 Symptoms and conditions that may be caused or exacerbated by food allergy [2]

Cardiovascular	Angina, arrhythmias, hypertension, and thrombophlebitis
Dermatological	Acne vulgaris, eczema, psoriasis, purpura, stasis ulcers, and urticaria
Ear, nose, and throat	Hearing loss, hoarseness, Meniere's disease, nasal polyps, nosebleeds (epistaxis), olfactory dysfunction, otitis externa, otitis media, sinusitis, sore throats, taste disorders, vasomotor rhinitis, and vertigo
Gastrointestinal	Abdominal pain, constipation, Crohn's disease, diarrhea, eosinophilic esophagitis, gallbladder disease, gastritis, GERD, irritable bowel syndrome, non-ulcer dyspepsia, pancreatitis, peptic ulcer, proctitis, rectal bleeding, ulcerative colitis, and vomiting
Neurological	Ataxia, epilepsy, migraine, multiple sclerosis, restless leg syndrome, and tension-type headache
Ophthalmologic	Conjunctivitis and uveitis
Pediatric	Colic, enuresis, and growing pains
Psychiatric	Anxiety, ADHD, autism, bipolar disorder, depression, dysthymia, panic attacks, and schizophrenia
Pulmonary	Asthma, COPD, and cough
Renal	Glomerulonephritis and nephrotic syndrome
Rheumatological	Juvenile rheumatoid arthritis, psoriatic arthritis, rheumatoid arthritis, systemic lupus erythematosus, and vasculitis
Urological	Dysuria, urethritis, urinary frequency, and urinary tract infection

Reprinted with permission: Gaby AR. *Nutritional Medicine*, Second Edition. Concord, NH, 2017, doctorgaby.com, Chap. 7

pathogenesis of both allergies and asthma starts at the mucosal level, where environmental allergens interact with epithelia. In asthma, this interaction occurs in the airways, triggering airway inflammation through interaction between epithelia and sentinel antigen-processing cells [3]. It is not uncommon to have asthma as a child, to resolve symptoms, and only to see it return later in life. As asthma shares obstructive lung pathology with other common pulmonary diseases of the elderly, including COPD, it can be difficult to differentiate on clinical symptoms alone.

Whereas a conventional approach to allergies focuses on antihistamine drugs that suppress H1 receptors found throughout the body in the airways, blood vessels, GI tract, brain, and spinal cord, the integrative approach will use food and nutraceuticals to balance the histamine response and avoid the negative side effects such as drowsiness and cognitive decline associated with long-term use in older adults [4]. Patients that display hyper-reactivity to foods and the environment may also be assessed for histamine intolerance (HIT) which results from an imbalance between histamine production and degradation [5]. While there is currently no diagnostic gold standard for HIT, one can consider an elimination diet, measuring blood DAO (diamine oxidase) activity, and measuring blood and urine histamine [6]. For more information, consult *What HIT me? Living with Histamine Intolerance* by Genny Masterman.

There are several sources of increased histamine to consider:

- Dysbiosis in the gut that creates an additional histamine burden due to an overgrowth of histamine-producing bacteria, most especially *Proteobacteria* and *Bifidobacteriaceae* [7]. Being mindful of these strains in any probiotic supplement is critical.
- Genetic SNPs that create a decreased efficiency of diamine oxidase (DAO) and histamine N-methyltransferase (HNMT) enzymes, creating higher levels of histamine [8].
- High-histamine foods: products of microbial fermentation, such as aged cheese, sauerkraut, wine, and processed meat as well as fish and animal products high in histidine [8].

Altered histaminergic responses can result in gut dysbiosis and inappropriate responses to toxins (mold) and trigger prior infections that the body is unable to process. Careful selection of probiotics should ensure selected strains do not produce but rather disable histamine [9]. Please see Table 4.2 for our recommendations on choosing probiotics with histamine in mind.

Table 4.2 Histamine and probiotics

Histamine-producing probiotic strains	Histamine-disabling probiotic strains
Lactobacillus reuteri, L. bulgaricus, L. lactis, L. casei, and *L. helveticus Streptococcus thermophilus* [10]	*Lactobacillus plantarum, L. rhamnosus*, and *L. salivarius* *Bifidobacterium infantis, B. bifidum, B. longum, B. lactis*, and *B. breve*

Histamine can be modified by not only the immune system but the nervous system as well.

The nervous system and immune system are closely connected, in large part due to the mast cell-nerve interaction [11]. Regulating the nervous system by activating the parasympathetic response can help lower inflammatory reactivity [12]. Behavioral interventions to engage the parasympathetic response and reduce psychological stress, such as meditation training, can help manage histamine levels downstream [13].

Nervines can also be used for nervous system support. Nervines are herbs that act therapeutically on the nervous system. In addition to providing key nutrients to the nervous system, they can provide sedative properties to calm the mind. Table 4.3 summarizes key nervines and their actions in the body.

Other dietary intolerances that can manifest with a similar symptom picture as histamine intolerance include oxalate, sulfate, salicylate, and lectin intolerances. While removing foods high in these compounds may provide short-term symptomatic relief, they are not appropriate interventions in the long term as they do not address the underlying issue of gut dysbiosis and inflammation. Table 4.4 lists sources of these dietary histamine triggers.

4.1.2.1   Treating Histamine Intolerances

Foods naturally high in quercetin and DAO can help lower histamine as follows:

- Quercetin rich: onions, apples, grapes, berries, pomegranate, broccoli, and tea [24]
- DAO rich: pea shoots, apples, pomegranate, and perilla seed oil

Table 4.3 Nervines

Nervine	Action
Lemon balm	Cholinergic effect and possible GABA mimetic effect [14]
Magnesium glycinate	Interacts with NMDA receptor and blocks excitatory signaling [15]
Ashwagandha	GABA mimetic effect. Promotes formation of dendrites [16]
L-theanine	Modulates alpha activity and provides beneficial effects on mental state and sleep quality [17]
GABA	Major neurotransmitter that exerts inhibitory activity in the CNS [18]
Lavender	Inhibits LPS-induced inflammatory reaction and antioxidant, modulates GABA and DA transmission, and may inhibit the sympathetic nervous system [19]
Chamomile	Sedative effects may be due to the flavonoid and apigenin that binds to benzodiazepine receptors in the brain [20]
Passionflower	Elicits GABA currents [21]
Valerian	GABA mimetic effect [22]

Table 4.4 Dietary triggers for histamine intolerance

Trigger	Source	Further reading
Oxalate	Spinach, beets, sweet potatoes, Swiss chard, almonds, rhubarb, and plantains	https://www.allergylink.co.uk/allergy-blog/2016/10/26/oxalate-sensitivity/
Sulfate	Shrimp, lobster, cod, crab, beef, sausages, dried fruits, potatoes, horseradish, alcohol, and fruit juices [23]	https://my.clevelandclinic.org/health/articles/11323-sulfite-sensitivity
Salicylate	Alcohol, granny smith apples, cherries, strawberries, asparagus, raw tomatoes, tomato puree, coffee, and numerous spices [23]	https://www.allergylink.co.uk/allergy-blog/2017/02/16/salicylate-intolerance-aspirin-sensitivity/
Lectins	Grains, potatoes, tomatoes, squashes, and legumes	https://www.allergylink.co.uk/allergy-blog/2018/07/03/lectins/

Table 4.5 Food sensitivity testing

Benefits	Limitations
Personalization of elimination diet	Research is mixed
Increased efficiency in resolving symptoms	Reliability is questionable due to different methods and complexity of pathways
Data-driven approach may inspire reluctant patient to overcome hesitation for elimination diet	Reduces the opportunity for patient to tune into their body and looks to outside authority

4.2   Diagnosing Food Sensitivities

The gold standard in both diagnosis and treatment of food sensitivities is an elimination diet with systematic reintroduction [25]. Through this diet, common foods that cause reactivity are removed, gut inflammation and immune reactivity is reduced, and systemic symptoms lessen and resolve. Typically, after 3 weeks (or longer based on symptom resolution), various food groups are slowly reintroduced. The duration of this elimination phase will vary by individual. Once triggers are identified, those foods are avoided for an additional 3–6 months to allow the immune system to reset, the gut to heal, and inflammation to resolve. Only then, are trigger foods introduced, individually, to ensure tolerability [26]. In one clinical case report, a variation of the elimination diet gave some patients suffering from allergies experienced a reduction in asthma symptoms, decreased dependence on pharmacological therapies, and increased quality of life [27]. See Appendix for more details on the elimination diet. For those patients that present as "reacting to everything," consider a 1–2-week trial of an elemental diet to reset the gut and hasten immune system balancing. See Appendix for more details on the elemental diet.

Food sensitivity testing is one tool commonly used in the integrative community to widen the clinicians' understanding of particular foods that may be at the root of symptoms for a specific patient. While it is tempting to want to believe that a test could reveal food sensitivities, the reality is these tests are compromised by the inherent complexity of the interaction between the food, the gut, and the immune system. In Table 4.5, we consider the pros and cons of food sensitivity testing to support an informed decision on how and when to utilize this tool.

4.2.1 Sample Food Sensitivity Panel [28]

Standard food allergy testing has low sensitivity and can miss actionable diagnoses. Figure 4.1, the IgG Food Antibody Assessment (Genova Diagnostics), shows a sample result panel, including severity of intolerance. The higher the IgG present in serum, the greater the food sensitivity.

4.2.1.1 Case 1

A 69-year-old female patient presented with a 50-year history of chronic rhinosinusitis (CRS) that was worse in the winter, postnasal drip, frequent sore throats, gastrointestinal complaints, headaches, and yeast infections. Two sinus surgeries (in years 2000 and 2002) and multiple courses of antibiotics had not resolved her sinus symptoms. In addition to CRS and inflammatory bowel syndrome, this patient was noted to have intestinal overgrowth of *Candida albicans*, multiple food sensitivities, and leaky gut syndrome.

Antifungal medication and dietary changes over the course of 8 months resulted in the resolution of her CRS and IBS. Her IgG Food Antibody Assessment panel is displayed in Fig. 4.2, highlighting the near-complete resolution of documented

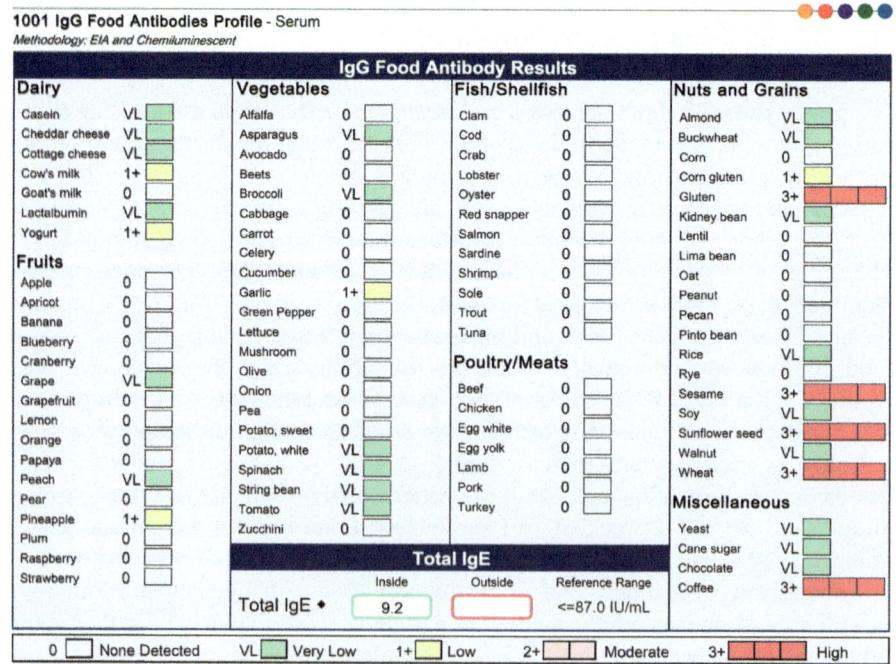

Fig. 4.1 Food sensitivity panel [28] (Weil 2018)

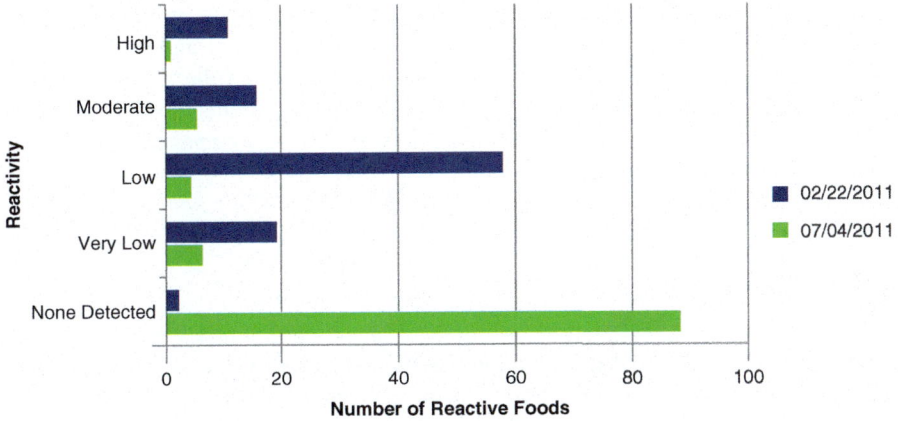

Fig. 4.2 IgG food antibody assessment panel [29] (Weil 2018)

Table 4.6 Recommendations and interventions

Removed	Continued	Added
Antibiotics	Vitamin D3	Raw garlic, nasal lavage, nystatin, probiotic, yeast-free, and anti-inflammatory diet

reactive foods. For full details of the case, please review the published article [29]. Specifics of diet and medication alterations are summarized in Table 4.6.

4.3 Autoimmune Disease

The aging immune system contributes to increased development of autoimmune responses [30]. This is in large part due to immunosenescence or immune dysregulation. This includes a reduction in immune response, an increase in the inflammatory and oxidative processes, and an increase in production of autoantibodies [31]. From recent British data, patients subjectively improve when foods that cause these reactions are removed, and we see their biomarkers of inflammation improve [32]. Rather than focusing on symptom control and immune suppression, integrative approaches to autoimmune disease focus on gut microbial balance, food sensitivities, stealth infections, and molecular mimicry [33].

As many autoimmune conditions share pathologies consistent with aging, they are frequently seen in the elderly population. These common origins include inflammation, oxidative stress, mitochondrial dysfunction, decreased proteasome activity, cellular senescence, and gut microbiota alterations [34]. As such, autoimmune diseases such as rheumatoid arthritis, osteoarthritis, osteopenia, psoriasis, and macular degeneration become dietary food choices, and nutritional balance demonstrates positive and negative effects, both short and long term on the immune system [35].

Anti-inflammatory diets that are high in phytonutrients and low in glycemic load have repeatedly shown to impact autoimmune disease trajectory and improve overall health. Conversely, specific food antigens often represent the most significant trigger of autoimmune phenomena [35]. By addressing associated nutrient deficiencies and imbalances, autoimmune disease can be more easily managed and, in some cases, eliminated [35].

4.3.1 Case 2

Alexis, a 66-year-old woman with a long-standing history of RA, hypertension, and obesity, was referred to Dr. Kogan for consultation about "alternative treatments" for her RA. Patient has been taking methotrexate but was noticed to have progression of the disease over past 12 months, and rheumatologist suggested to add tofacitinib. After reviewing side effects of this medication, the patient adamantly refused it and requested to try "natural" approaches first. Upon additional questions, patient was noted to consume diet high in dairy, gluten, and sweets. On presentation, patient was found to be moderately obese with BMI of 31; she had typical RA joint findings. In addition to methotrexate, the patient was taking HCTZ and lisinopril for blood pressure. She was taking 2000 units of vitamin D and multivitamin. Upon additional workup, she was noted to have vitamin D-OH level of 23 ng/ml, B12 level of 335 ng/ml, and magnesium RBC level of 4.4 ng/ml, and her high-sensitivity C-reactive protein (hs-CRP) was 8.5 mg/L and ESR 62 mm/h. On additional nutritional analysis, patient's omega-3 index was 3.5 (normal >4 with optimal range of 8–10), and she had positive tissue transglutaminase IgA (tIgA) and endomysial IgA. After review of prior history, exam, and laboratory results, the following interventions were made, as captured in Table 4.7.

At 3-month follow-up, the patient reported losing 25 lbs of weight, her joint pains and swelling much improved, and she also noted dramatic energy improvement. On repeat blood work in 3 months, her vitamin D-OH level was 41 ng/ml,

Table 4.7 Case study 2 interventions

Intervention	Details
Diet	Autoimmune paleo (AIP), 16-h nighttime fast
B100 complex	800-mcg methylfolate, 1000-mcg methylcobalamin, and 25,000-mcg methylcobalamin subcutaneous injections twice weekly
Oral liquid fish oil	3000-mg EPA + DHA
Vitamin D	5000 IU daily in combination with 100-mcg vitamin K2 (MK7)
Multivitamin	Multimineral formula containing Mg, Ca, Zn, and a number of other microminerals
Turmeric	One teaspoon mixed with oil-containing food
Added spices	Pinch of ground black pepper daily, ginger, saffron, matcha green tea, and tart cherry juice concentrate
Exercise	Core-strengthening program and Pilates every other day

Table 4.8 Most common autoimmune diseases in the elderly

Disease	Signs and symptoms
Psoriasis	Red patchy skin with thick, silvery scales; dry, cracked skin; itching; burning; soreness; thickened/pitted/ridges nails; and swollen/stiff joints [36]
IBD (see GI chapter)	Diarrhea, fatigue, abdominal pain, cramping, blood in stool, reduced appetite, and unintended weight loss [37]
Celiac	Diarrhea, fatigue, weight loss, bloating and gas, abdominal pain, nausea and vomiting, and constipation [38]
Rheumatoid arthritis	Tender, warm, swollen joints, joint stiffness, fatigue, fever, and loss of appetite [39]
Polymyalgia rheumatica	Body aches or pain, stiffness (particularly in AM), and limited range of motion [40]
Temporal arteritis	Persistent, severe head pain in the temple area, scalp tenderness, jaw pain, fever, fatigue, unintended weight loss, and vision loss or double vision [41]

B12 level was over 2000 ng/ml, magnesium RBC was 5.1 ng/ml, and hs-CRP was 1.4 mg/L and ESR 36 mm/h. At that point, patient was asked to stop B12 injections and take 5000 IU of vitamin D with K2 every other day; the rest of her treatment stayed the same. After 6 months, patient reported losing an additional 15 lbs with a resulting BMI of 26. Her RA was well controlled on methotrexate in combination with the above integrative regimen. After 12 months, the patient's methotrexate was discontinued with RA staying in remission.

Some autoimmune diseases are more common in the elderly than others. Table 4.8 highlights the most common pathologies and their associated findings.

Autoimmune issues and allergies often go hand in hand. Table 4.9 summarizes common supplements often used for both indications.

4.4 Infections

4.4.1 SARS-CoV-2

An impaired immune system invites opportunity for foreign pathogens such as viruses, bacteria, and yeast to invade and wreak havoc throughout the body. Most recently, research surrounding nutraceutical and botanical approaches to combating the novel SARS-CoV-2 virus, responsible for COVID-19, has exploded. Although this field is rapidly evolving, a brief summary of findings to date will be described.

Optimization of the immune system is critical in mitigating risk in the elderly with an otherwise waning immune system. Supplementing with vitamin C, vitamin D, vitamin A, zinc, selenium, and honey, garlic, and probiotics can boost symptom relief and help shorten duration of illness [85]. Beta-glucans are known to modulate immune activity. They are responsible for priming the innate immune system through pattern recognition receptors (PRRs) and inducing viral eradication or inactivation. 250–500 mg daily of beta-glucans has been shown to reduce cold and

Table 4.9 Supplements for autoimmune health and allergies

Supplement	Daily dose of supplement	Autoimmune indication (MOA)	Allergy indication
Bone broth	One cup	Gut healing and anti-inflammatory	Provides amino acids and antioxidants that can help reduce inflammation, specifically in the respiratory system Contraindicated for histamine intolerance
Quercetin	500–1000 mg [42]	Antihistamine	Antihistamine
Bromelain	200–400 mg [43]	Anti-inflammatory	None reported
Boswellia	150–250 mg BID [44]	Anti-inflammatory	None reported
Curcumin	Curcuminoid (active ingredient) [45] 500–2000 mg [46]	Anti-inflammatory	Antihistamine
	Raw turmeric root (contains 2–6% of active curcuminoid) 26,300 mg		
Vitamin C	75–90 mg [47]	Antioxidant	Antihistamine [48]
Beta-glucan	100–500 mg	Anti-inflammatory	Restoring equilibrium among T-lymphocyte subpopulation
Probiotics	1–10 billion CFU [49]	Gut microbiome balance	Modulate immune system back from Th2 response to Th1 response [50]. Pay careful attention to histamine content, as some probiotic strains are high in histamine
Optimized vitamin D-OH[a]	(40–80 ng/mL)	Modulates cytokine levels and inhibits NF-kB, prostaglandins, and other immune cells (Liu, 2018)	Inhibits both Th1- and Th2-type responses [51]
Tart cherry extract	480 mL	Polyphenols reduce inflammation and oxidative stress [52]	None reported
Green tea/EGCG (epigallocatechin gallate)	400 mg *or* four cups *or* 1 tsp of matcha powder	Polyphenols reduce inflammation and oxidative stress [53]	EGCG is an abundant antioxidant which helps prevent immune response to wide range of allergens
Pomegranate	100–500 mL of juice [54]	Antioxidant [55]	Reduces IgE binding to cashew nut allergens [56]
Omega-3 and omega-6 (GLA 500–100 mg/d)	Omega-3: 1.1–1.6 g Omega-6: 500–1000 mg [57]	Reduce cytokine and chemokine production and modulate neutrophil function and T- and B-cell activation [58]	Anti-allergic metabolites generated in the gut and impairment of mast cell degranulation [59]
Zinc	8–11 mg [60]	Decreases oxidative stress biomarkers and inflammatory cytokines [61]	May decrease airway inflammation [62]

Table 4.9 (continued)

Supplement	Daily dose of supplement	Autoimmune indication (MOA)	Allergy indication
Stinging nettle	500–1000 mg every 2–4 h, as needed	Antioxidant activity toward iron-promoted oxidation of phospholipids, fatty acids, and sugar	May decrease IFN-gamma levels and histamine release in allergic rhinitis [63]
DAO	20,000 HDU	None reported	Aids in GI degradation of histamine [64]
Black cumin seed	10 mg/kg [65]	Antioxidant. Significantly reduces levels of pro-inflammatory mediators [66]	Subjectively improved symptoms in patients with allergic rhinitis, bronchial asthma, and atopic eczema
Lemon balm	300–500 mg dried, 3× daily or as needed [67]	Antioxidant, anti-inflammatory, immunomodulatory effects through high amounts of flavonoids, rosmarinic acid, gallic acid, and phenolic contents [68, 69]	Antihistamine, especially topically in atopic dermatitis
Angelica	6–15 g [70]	Anti-inflammatory. Decreases IL-6, TNF-alpha, G-CSF, VEGF, and various LPS pathways [71]	Inhibits mast cell activation [72], inhibits production of prostaglandin E2 and NO, and reduces release of histamine [73]
Garlic	4 g (one to two cloves) raw garlic One 300-mg dried garlic powder 2–3× 7.2 g aged garlic extract [74]	Conflicting data on both pro- and anti-inflammatory responses. Antioxidative effects likely due to prevention of glutathione depletion and removal of peroxides and inhibition of NF-kB [75]	Antihistamine
Rosemary	200 mg [76]	Limits production of pro-inflammatory mediators while promoting anti-inflammatory mediators [76]	Symptomatic relief and decrease in neutrophils and eosinophils
Horseradish	20 g	Reduces nitric oxide, TNF alpha, IL-6, COX-2, and NF-kB [77]	None reported
Local raw honey[b] [78, 79]	1 tbsp/day	High phenol and flavonoid levels contribute to antioxidative effects [80]	Can improve symptoms of allergic rhinitis [81]. Quercetin reduces inflammation and pollen allergy symptoms and stabilizes cell membranes to prevent histamine release. Bee pollen and bee propolis boost the immune system and build immunity to allergens [82]

[a]Vitamin D deficiency: vitamin D deficiencies predispose patients to both autoimmune and allergic conditions [83, 84].
[b]Local raw honey: bees will travel a maximum of 2 miles. For maximum immune benefit, find a bee-keeper within 2 miles of where the patient lives. The pollen in trees and flowers that trigger allergic symptoms are also in the local raw honey. Consuming local raw honey boosts immunity to nearby pollen.

flu symptoms and upper respiratory tract infections compared to placebo [86]. The leaves of *A. paniculata* have been used in traditional Eastern medicine to treat and prevent upper respiratory tract infections, coughs, and sinusitis. *Andrographis*, in particular, is one of many agents shown to decrease the activity of furin protease, a required step in SARS-CoV-2 spike protein activation and insertion into mucosal epithelial cells [86]. Standardized extract, 100–600 mg daily of *Andrographis*, has been shown to reduce COVID-19 symptoms by inhibiting furin protease, priming innate immune function, and promoting viral eradication or inactivation. Echinacea has been shown to stimulate macrophage activation, natural killer cell activity, and increased cytokine expression [86]. The strongest evidence suggests echinacea's positive role in preventing infection, with conflicting evidence on treatment success [86].

T-cell exhaustion, high viral load, and high levels of TNF alpha, IL-1 beta, IL-6, and IL-10 have been associated with severe COVID-19. Cytokine and antigen overstimulation are possibly responsible for poor humoral response to the virus. Lower cellular redox states, which lead to pro-inflammatory states mediated by TNF alpha, are also impacted. Both in vivo and in vitro studies have demonstrated N-acetylcysteine (inhaled and systemic) to be an effective method of improving redox status, replenishing glutathione stores, and increasing the proliferative response of T cells [87]. NAC (N-acetylcysteine) may serve a therapeutic role in optimizing redox and anti-inflammatory states in patients affected with COVID-19.

Another proposed explanation for severity in COVID-19 cases is glutathione deficiency. Glutathione is the most abundant antioxidant that plays a critical role in antioxidant defense. Many factors affect glutathione stores, including age, comorbidities, gender, smoking, and diet. In one study, patients with moderate and severe COVID-19 illness had lower levels of glutathione and higher ROS and ROS/GSH ratio in plasma than patients with mild disease [88], pointing to glutathione's potentially therapeutic role.

Vitamin D in particular may have a variety of actions on cells and tissues in COVID-19 progression, specifically by decreasing the incidence of acute respiratory distress syndrome. Calcifediol rapidly increases serum 25OHD concentration. In a study of 76 consecutive patients hospitalized with COVID-19, of the 50 treated with calcifediol, one required admission to the ICU (2%). Of the 26 untreated patients, 13 required admission to the ICU (50%). Calcifediol appears to reduce the severity of the disease, thereby reducing the need for ICU treatment [89].

4.4.1.1 Supplements with Possible Therapeutic Benefits Against SARS-CoV-2

Disclaimer: we acknowledge the supplements in Table 4.10 may be not adequate to combat infections alone. They should be added to our arsenal of tools in healing our body and restoring our immune system. Supplements can help manage both short- and long-term consequences of infection. Inclusion of food sources reminds the

Table 4.10 Micronutrients, supplements, and impact on general immune health [86]

Supplement	Food source	Daily dose	Impact of supplementation [91]	Impact of deficiency [91]
Vitamin C	Red and green pepper, orange juice, orange, grapefruit juice, kiwifruit, and broccoli [47]	Varies greatly, ≥10 g [92]	Antioxidant properties protect leukocytes and lymphocytes from oxidative stress Possible reduction in incidence and duration of pneumonia	Increased oxidative damage Increased incidence of severity of pneumonia and other infections Decreased resistance to infection and cancer, decreased delayed-type hypersensitivity response, and impaired wound healing
		COVID dose: 1–3 g PO QD or in divided doses	Favorably modulate cellular defense and repair mechanisms and favorably modulate viral-induced pathological cellular processes	
Vitamin D	Cod liver oil, trout, sockeye salmon, mushrooms, and milk [93]	0.266–0.532 mg [89]	Reduced acute respiratory tract infections	Increased susceptibility to infections, especially respiratory tract infections (RTI) Increased morbidity and mortality, increased severity of infections, reduced number of lymphocytes, and reduced lymphoid organ weight Increased risk of autoimmune disease
		COVID dose: 5000 IU PO QD in the absence of serum levels	Activation of macrophages, stimulation of antimicrobial peptides, modulation of defensins, modulation of TH17 cells, reduction in viral-induced cytokine expression, and modulation of TGF beta	
NAC	Broccoli, brussels sprouts, egg yolks, garlic, oats, onions, poultry, red bell peppers, wheat germ, and yeast [94]	600–1200 mg [95]	Replenishes intracellular glutathione and cysteine levels and treats wide range of infections by restoring antioxidants [96]	Liver damage and oxidative stress
Glutathione (Inhaled)	Inhaled (COVID-19 only) Meat, fish, broccoli, cabbage, garlic, onions, cereals, and dairy products [97]	500–1000 mg [98]	Protects host immune cells through antioxidant mechanism and provides optimal functioning of lymphocytes and other immune cells [97]	Chronic inflammation [97]
Zinc	Oysters, crab, and lobster [60]	15–30 mg [99]	Maintains integrity of skin and mucosal membranes and suppresses common cold [60]	Increased bacterial, viral, and fungal infections (particularly diarrhea and pneumonia) and diarrheal and respiratory morbidity Increased thymic atrophy and consequent risk of infection
		COVID dose: 30–60 mg daily, in divided doses	Favorably modulate cellular defense and repair mechanisms and favorably modulate viral-induced pathological cellular processes	
Specialized pro-resolving mediators (SPM) (resolvins)	Omega-3-rich foods (fatty fish, flax-/hemp-/chia seeds)	2–6 g [100]	Resolve inflammation, protect organs, and stimulate tissue regeneration [101]	Chronic inflammation [101]

(continued)

Table 4.10 (continued)

Supplement	Food source	Daily dose	Impact of supplementation [91]	Impact of deficiency [91]
Curcuminoids [102]	Turmeric (2.5–6% curcumin) and curry [103]	6–7 g [104]	Antioxidant and anti-inflammatory	None reported
		COVID dose: 500–1000 mg PO BID	Modulation of inflammasome activation	None reported
Melatonin	Egg, salmon, chicken, pork, beef, and lamb [105] *Generally difficult to get high-enough melatonin through food alone, so we tend to supplement at higher doses	0.1–5 mg [106]	Immune buffer. Acts as a stimulant under basal or immunosuppressive conditions or as an anti-inflammatory compound in the presence of acute inflammation [107]	Reduced granulocytes, macrophages, natural killer cells, and CD4+ cells [108]
		COVID dose: 5–20 mg QD	Modulation of inflammasome activation	
Vitamin A	Beef liver, sweet potato, spinach, and carrots [109]	900 mcg [109]	Affects many immune functions, including number and killing activity of NK cells and neutrophil cells, neutrophil function, macrophage ability to phagocytose pathogens, growth and differentiation of B cells, and decreasing number and distribution of T cells	Increased susceptibility to infections
		COVID dose: up to 10,000–25,000 IU/d	Modulation of helper T cells, modulation of sIgA, and modulation of viral-induced cytokine production	
Vitamin E	Vegetable oils, almonds, peanuts, sunflower seeds, spinach, and broccoli [110]	15 mg [110]	Reduced RTI	Deficiency rare in humans Impaired both humoral and cell-mediated aspects of adaptive immunity, including B- and T-cell function
Vitamin B6	Chickpeas, beef liver, tuna, salmon, and chicken breast [111]	1.5–1.7 mg [111]	Promotes lymphocyte and IL-2 production [111]	Lymphocytopenia, reduced lymphoid tissue weight, reduced responses to mitogens, general deficiencies in cell-mediated immunity, and lowered antibody responses
Vitamin B12	Clams, beef liver, trout, salmon, tuna fish, and nutritional yeast [112]	2.4 mg [112]	Immunomodulation and augmentation of CD8 T lymphocytes and NK cell activity [113]	Depressed immune responses (delayed-type hypersensitivity response, T-cell proliferation)

Table 4.10 (continued)

Supplement	Food source	Daily dose	Impact of supplementation [91]	Impact of deficiency [91]
Folate	Beef liver, spinach, black-eyed peas, and breakfast cereal [114]	400 mcg [114]	Restoration of thymulin activity, increased numbers of cytotoxic T cells, reduced numbers of activated helper T cells, increased natural killer cell cytotoxicity, and reduced incidence of infections	Depressed immune responses (delayed-type hypersensitivity response, T-cell proliferation) Decreased lymphocyte number and function, particularly T cells, increased thymic atrophy, and altered cytokine production that contributes to oxidative stress inflammation
Iron	Breakfast cereals (fortified), oysters, white beans, chocolate (dark), beef liver, and lentils [115]	8 mg [115]	May enhance or protect from infection with bacteria, viruses, fungi, and protozoa depending on the level of iron	Reduced capacity for adequate immune response (decreased delayed-type hypersensitivity response, mitogen responsiveness, NK cell activity), decreased lymphocyte bactericidal activity, and lower IL-6 levels
Copper	Beef liver, oysters, baking chocolate, potatoes, and mushrooms [116]	900 mcg [116]	Supports T-cell and neutrophil proliferation [117]	Abnormally low neutrophil levels. Potentially increased susceptibility to infection
Selenium	Brazil nuts, tuna, halibut, sardines, ham, and shrimp [118]	55 mcg [118]	Improves cell-mediated immunity and enhances immune response to viruses in deficient individuals but may worsen allergic asthma and impair the immune response to parasites	Impaired humoral and cell-mediated immunity Increased viral virulence Suppression of immune function
Quercetin	Apples, berries, brassica vegetables, capers, grapes, onions, and shallots [42]	500–1000 mg [42]	Inhibition of proteasome activity	None reported
		COVID dose: 1 gm PO BID. Phytosome, 500 mg BID	Promotes viral eradication or inactivation, inhibits viral replication, modulates inflammasome activation, and modulates mast cell stabilization	
Epigallo-catechin Gallate (EGCG)	Green tea	800 mg [119]	Antioxidant and anti-inflammatory	None reported
		COVID dose: 4 c daily or 225 mg PO QD	Modulation of inflammasome activation	

(continued)

Table 4.10 (continued)

Supplement	Food source	Daily dose	Impact of supplementation [91]	Impact of deficiency [91]
Resveratrol	Grapes, wine, peanuts, and soy [120]	Diet: 6–8 mg daily Nutraceutical dose: 20–500 mg [120]	Reduces inflammation and oxidative stress and reduces ROS generation, NF-kB binding capability, and pro-inflammation signaling [120]	None reported
		COVID dose: 100–150 mg PO QD	Modulation of inflammasome activation	
Elderberry	Elderberry	650–1500 mg [121]	Modulate complement system and NO production [122]	None reported
		COVID dose: 500 mg PO QD	Favorably modulate cellular defense and repair mechanisms and favorably modulate viral-induced pathological cellular processes	
Palmitoyle-thanolamide (PEA)	Milk, beans, peas, tomatoes, corn, soy, and peanuts [123]	600 mg BID [124]	Modulates mast cell activation and degranulation [123]	None reported
		COVID dose: 300 mg PO BID to prevent infection and 600 mg PO TID × 2 weeks to treat infection	Favorably modulate cellular defense and repair mechanisms and favorably modulate viral-induced pathological cellular processes	

clinician that food is part of the therapeutic equation and it is often just as important to consider what the patient is not eating as much as what they are. For example, sinus infections will be well served by the exclusion of dairy products, and someone with chronic sinus infections should consider eliminating dairy completely. Also, the role of added sugar and colorants/preservatives to suppress immune function cannot be understated [90].

4.4.1.2   Specific Antiviral Nutritional Supplements for COVID-19 Support [86]

COVID-19 "Long Haulers"

A large percentage of patients with COVID-19 that required hospitalizations or had at least moderately severe disease continue to have persistent long-term symptoms. These symptoms include shortness of breath, cough, severe fatigue, joint pains, headaches, brain fog, confusion, and changes in or loss of smell and taste (World

Table 4.11 Integrative approach to chronic infections

Blood thinners	Aspirin 81 mg and/or nattokinase or boluoke
Anti-inflammatory	High dose of quercetin, bromelain, *Boswellia*, turmeric, fatty acids, balanced omega-6/omega-3 intake, SPM oil, inhaled glutathione, green tea (EGCG), NAC, glutathione, ginger, cinnamon, and montelukast. Nasal VIP and melatonin 3–10 mg
Constitutional support (general recovery support)	Bone broth, shitake, maitake, lion's mane, chaga, reishi, cordyceps, eleuthero, ginseng, *Andrographis*, and astragalus
Mitochondrial support	L-carnitine (or acetyl-L-carnitine if delivery to the CNS), CoQ10, Alpha-linolenic acid (ALA), methylated high-potency B complex (B100++) [should include minimum of 1000 mcg methyl B12], magnesium, zinc, selenium, nicotinamide riboside, and resveratrol
Dietary support	Anti-inflammatory diet is most balanced and widely accepted, but autoimmune protocol and paleo are also reasonable options. Cruciferous vegetables and extracts, caffeine, mushrooms, and bone broth. If GI system was involved during acute COVID-19, patient can consider the following remedies: warm water with lemon juice/apple cider vinegar, etc.
Others	IV vitamin C and IV ozone

Health Organization, 2020). There are a number of proposed pathophysiologic mechanisms that could possibly contribute to this, including but not limited to a chronic unresolving inflammatory response, prolonged immune dysregulation, alterations in mitochondrial energy production, possible changes in blood viscosity and increased clot formation, and hormonal shifts.

While the best approaches to treating these patients have yet to be understood, integrative approaches used to combat other chronic infections are included in Table 4.11.

4.4.1.3 COVID-19 Prophylactic Interventions [99]

As of the writing of this book, no integrative measures have been validated in human trials as effective specifically against preventing COVID-19. However, in understanding the role of inflammation in COVID-19 pathophysiology, the interventions in Table 4.12 may mitigate risk given their anti-inflammatory actions.

4.4.2 Cold and Flu

As cold and flu symptoms most often result from bacterial and viral infections, adding antibacterial and antiviral foods and supplements (highlighted in Table 4.13) can help support the body's ability to manage the infection without the use of antibiotics, which have a negative impact on the microbiome, creating additional need for support [126].

Table 4.12 Integrative interventions for COVID-19

Intervention		Mode	Impact
Lifestyle		Adequate sleep, meditation, and breathing exercises	Sleep deprivation increases CXCL9 levels, a monokine which increases lymphocytic infiltration and inflammasome activation. Adequate sleep ensures secretion of melatonin Stress management reduces activated NF-kB and may reduce C-Reactive protein (CRP)
Zinc		Supplement (15–30 mg daily)	May prevent COVID-19 entry into cells, appears to reduce virulence, and provides direct protective effects in the upper respiratory tract
Vitamin C		Supplement (500–3000 mg daily)	Inhibits inflammasome activation and shortens frequency, duration, and severity of common cold and incidence of pneumonia
Vitamin D3 [125]		Supplement (10,000 IU daily) for up to 2–3 months, if longer, must monitor vitamin D level	Decrease inflammasome activation
Melatonin		Supplement (0.3–20 mg daily)	Inhibits NF-kB activation and inflammasome activation and reduces oxidative lung injury and inflammatory cell recruitment during viral infections
Vegetables and fruits +/− flavonoids	*Sambucus nigra*	Elderberry	Reduce inflammasome signaling and inflammatory cascades
	Dihydroquercetin and quercetin	Onions and apples	
	Myricetin	Tomatoes, oranges, nuts, and berries	
	Apigenin	Chamomile, parsley, and celery	
	Curcumin	Turmeric root	
	EGCG	Green tea	
	Baicalin and wogonoside	Chinese skullcap	
	Liquiritigenin	Licorice	

Table 4.13 Supplements for common cold, influenza, UTI, bronchitis, sinusitis, and *Candida*

Supplement	Daily dose
A. paniculata	15.75–1200 mg [127]
Gan Mao Ling (TCM)	900–1800 mg, 3× daily
Echinacea	10.2 g for the first 24 h and 5.1 g for the following days [128]
Sambucus canadensis (elderberry)	600–900 mg [121]
Garlic (allicin powder)	180 mg
Ginseng	400 mg (2 × 200 mg) [129]
Pelargonium sidoides	60 mg [130]

Garlic Lemonade
Best for respiratory infections

- 1 quarts water
- Four garlic cloves, chopped
- Juice of one lemon
- Local raw honey to taste

Boil 1 qt of water. Place chopped garlic in 1 quart canning jar or other heat-resistant, nonreactive container. Pour boiling water over, cover, and let steep for 10 min. Add lemon and honey. Enjoy.

Fire Cider
Take preventatively throughout the fall and winter, 1 oz daily

- 1/2 cup freshly peeled and grated ginger root
- 1/2 cup freshly grated horseradish root
- One medium onion, chopped
- Ten cloves of garlic, crushed or chopped
- Two organic jalapeño peppers, chopped
- One lemon, zest and juice
- 2 tablespoons of dried rosemary leaves
- 1 tablespoon of turmeric powder or 2 tablespoons of freshly grated turmeric root
- 1/4 teaspoon cayenne powder
- Organic unfiltered apple cider vinegar
- 1/4 cup raw honey or to taste
  1. Add ginger, horseradish, onion, garlic, jalapeño peppers, lemon zest and juice, rosemary, turmeric, and cayenne powder into a quart-sized jar.
  2. Pour apple cider vinegar in the jar until all the ingredients are fully covered and the vinegar reaches the top of the jar. You want to be sure all the ingredients are covered to prevent spoilage.
  3. Use a piece of natural parchment paper under the lid to keep the vinegar from touching the metal, or use a plastic lid if you have one.
  4. Shake jar to combine all the ingredients and store in a dark, cool place for 4–6 weeks, remembering to shake the jar a few seconds every day.
  5. After 1 month, use a mesh strainer or cheesecloth to strain out the solids, pouring the vinegar into a clean jar. Be sure to squeeze out as much of the liquid as you can. This stuff is liquid gold! The solids can be used in a stir-fry or you can compost/discard them.

6. Add honey to the liquid and stir until incorporated.
7. Taste your fire cider and add more honey if needed until you reach your desired sweetness.
8. Store in a sealed container in the refrigerator or in a cold, dark place.
9. Drink 1–2 tablespoons when needed.

4.4.3   UTI

Laura, a 71-year-old homebound woman living in the community, was referred to our home-based primary care program for geriatric consultation. Past medical history included hypertension, diabetes, and stroke that left her with hemiparesis making her wheelchair bound. Laura lives with her daughter who assists her with bathing, dressing, transportation, and all IADLs. The patient had been having 2–3 UTIs/year with recently increasing frequency requiring multiple rounds of antibiotics which led to *C. difficile* colitis on two different occasions. Upon detailed discussion with the patient and daughter, the following preventive treatment was initiated: one scoop of specialized powder containing 2 gm of D-mannose/day and 750 mg capsule of cranberry concentrate twice daily in a large glass of water. For the following 3 years, she did not have any confirmed urinary tract infection despite several episodes of UTI-like symptoms that were managed by increasing the frequency of above treatment to 4 times/day for 2 weeks. See Table 4.14 above for common supplements for UTIs like Laura's.

Beyond standard treatments for mild skin infections (such as antibiotics and steroids), Table 4.15 summarizes effective supplements to replace (or add to) your regimen.

Table 4.14 Supplements for UTI

Supplement	Dose
D-mannose	2 g [131]. Conflicting evidence in some studies show D-mannose inhibits macrophage activity, slowinhg infection clearance [132]
Dried cranberry juice extract	240–300 ml [133]
Probiotic	*L. rhamnosus* and *L. fermentes* 10^9 CFU once or twice daily [134]

Table 4.15 Supplements for skin infections

Supplement	Dose
Manuka honey	1–2 tbsp
Topical cannabis	Gram-positive bacteria only and dosing data is limited
Tea tree oil	3.30% topical solution [135]
Shea butter and cocoa butter	Topical, as needed [136]

4.4.4 Traveler's Diarrhea

S. boulardii and other probiotics during traveling can reduce the risk of traveler's diarrhea. It is recommended to take nonrefrigerated probiotics if traveling to areas with food safety concerns. Although many probiotics require refrigeration, not all do [137].

4.4.5 Lyme

Lyme disease is the most commonly transmitted tick-borne infection in the United States and among the most commonly diagnosed worldwide [138]. Treating chronic Lyme disease is complex, as Lyme disease tends to affect a number of systems in a variety of ways. Conventional medicine treatment includes doxycycline to fight the infection and eliminate the bacteria. Other treatment options include inflammation control, decreasing immune dysregulation, reducing toxic load, and reducing auto-immune activity [139].

There are many chronic Lyme patients that need better treatment. Best first steps include starting with diet and supportive supplements and engaging a network of providers who are willing to work with such patients.

4.4.6 Candida Infections

Candida is an opportunistic yeast that can become pathogenic when immunity wanes. High levels of *candida* colonization are not only associated with a number of gastrointestinal issues but delay healing of inflammatory lesions, promoting further colonization. While rooted in immune dysregulation, *candida* pathologies often manifest themselves in the gut. Please see *Immune Health, Case 1* for a practical example and the GI chapter for further information [140]. Table 4.16 summarizes supplements shown to have an effect in candida infections.

See Appendix for further details.

	Supplement	Dose
Table 4.16 Supplements for candida infections	*S. boulardii* [141]	10^5–10^10 CFU
	Systemic enzymes	64,000 CU
	Olive leaf	500–1000 mg [142]
	Berberine	500 mg

4.5   Therapeutic Diets

4.5.1   Autoimmune Protocol Diet

The autoimmune protocol (AIP) diet is a modification of the Paleolithic diet which focuses on an initial elimination phase of food groups including grains, legumes, nightshades, dairy, eggs, coffee, alcohol, nuts and seeds, refined/processed sugars, oils, and food additives [143].

See Appendix for details.

4.5.2   Elimination Diet (Anti-inflammatory)

An anti-inflammatory diet sets out to re-establish hormonal and genetic balance to naturally generate satiety instead of constant hunger. The diet is rich in omega-3s and polyphenols and aims to minimize omega-6s and stabilize insulin [144].

See Appendix for details.

4.5.3   Anti-candida Diet

One of the triggers of immune dysregulation is disruption in the gut microbiota. Commensal yet opportunistic pathogens such as *Candida albicans* may start to overgrow, leading to bloating, indigestion, nausea, diarrhea, and gas. To treat gut dysbiosis, the anti-candida diet recommends avoiding added sugars; eating non-starchy vegetables, low-sugar fruits, and lots of fermented food; minimizing caffeine and gluten; and reducing alcohol [145].

References

1. De Martinis M, Sirufo MM, Viscido A, Ginaldi L. Food allergies and ageing. Int J Mol Sci. 2019;20(22):5580. https://doi.org/10.3390/ijms20225580.
2. Gaby A. Nutritional medicine. 2nd ed; Concord, NH: Fritz Perlberg Publishing. 2017.
3. Locksley RM. Asthma and allergic inflammation. Cell. 2010;140(6):777–83.
4. Gray SL, Anderson ML, Dublin S, Hanlon JT, Hubbard R, Walker R, et al. Cumulative use of strong anticholinergics and incident dementia: a prospective cohort study. JAMA Intern Med. 2015;175(3):401–7.
5. Maintz L, Novak N. Histamine and histamine intolerance. Am J Clin Nutr. 2007;85(5):1185–96.
6. Burkhart A. Histamine intolerance: symptoms, diet & treatment [Internet]. The Celiac MD. 2020 [cited 2021 Mar 9]. Available from: https://theceliacmd.com/histamine-intolerance-causing-symptoms/#:%7E:text=At%20this%20time%20there%20are,to%20correlate%20significantly%20with%20symptoms.

7. Schink M, Konturek PC, Tietz E, Dieterich W, Pinzer TC, Wirtz S, et al. Microbial patterns in patients with histamine intolerance. J Physiol Pharmacol. 2018;69(4). https://doi.org/10.26402/jpp.2018.4.09.

8. Kovacova-Hanuskova E, Buday T, Gavliakova S, Plevkova J. Histamine, histamine intoxication and intolerance. Allergol Immunopathol (Madr). 2015;43(5):498–506.

9. O'Hara B. Histamine lowering probiotics for people with mast cell activation syndrome and histamine intolerance [Internet]. Mast Cell 360. 2020 [cited 2021 Mar 9]. Available from: https://mastcell360.com/histamine-lowering-probiotics-for-people-with-mast-cell-activation-syndrome-and-histamine-intolerance/#:~:text=Lactobacillus%20rhamnosus%20has%20been%20shown,Activation%20Syndrome%20or%20Histamine%20Intolerance.

10. Thomas CM, Hong T, van Pijkeren JP, Hemarajata P, Trinh DV, Hu W, et al. Histamine derived from probiotic Lactobacillus reuteri suppresses TNF via modulation of PKA and ERK signaling. PLoS One. 2012;7(2):e31951.

11. Forsythe P. The parasympathetic nervous system as a regulator of mast cell function. Methods Mol Biol. 2015;1220:141–54.

12. Pavlov VA, Wang H, Czura CJ, Friedman SG, Tracey KJ. The cholinergic anti-inflammatory pathway: a missing link in neuroimmunomodulation. Mol Med. 2003;9(5–8):125–34.

13. Ito C. The role of brain histamine in acute and chronic stresses. Biomed Pharmacother. 2000;54(5):263–7.

14. Scholey A, Gibbs A, Neale C, Perry N, Ossoukhova A, Bilog V, et al. Anti-stress effects of lemon balm-containing foods. Nutrients. 2014;6(11):4805–21.

15. Kirkland AE, Sarlo GL, Holton KF. The role of magnesium in neurological disorders. Nutrients. 2018;10(6):730. https://doi.org/10.3390/nu10060730.

16. Singh N, Bhalla M, de Jager P, Gilca M. An overview on ashwagandha: a Rasayana (rejuvenator) of Ayurveda. Afr J Tradit Complement Altern Med. 2011;8(5 Suppl):208–13.

17. Hidese S, Ogawa S, Ota M, Ishida I, Yasukawa Z, Ozeki M, et al. Effects of L-theanine administration on stress-related symptoms and cognitive functions in healthy adults: a randomized controlled trial. Nutrients. 2019;11(10):2362. https://doi.org/10.3390/nu11102362.

18. Shi Y, Dong J-W, Zhao J-H, Tang L-N, Zhang J-J. Herbal insomnia medications that target GABAergic systems: a review of the psychopharmacological evidence. Curr Neuropharmacol. 2014;12(3):289–302.

19. Koulivand PH, Khaleghi Ghadiri M, Gorji A. Lavender and the nervous system. Evid Based Complement Alternat Med. 2013;2013:681304.

20. Srivastava JK, Shankar E, Gupta S. Chamomile: a herbal medicine of the past with bright future. Mol Med Rep. 2010;3(6):895–901.

21. Elsas SM, Rossi DJ, Raber J, White G, Seeley CA, Gregory WL, et al. Passiflora incarnata L. (Passionflower) extracts elicit GABA currents in hippocampal neurons in vitro, and show anxiogenic and anticonvulsant effects in vivo, varying with extraction method. Phytomedicine. 2010;17(12):940–9.

22. Murphy K, Kubin ZJ, Shepherd JN, Ettinger RH. Valeriana officinalis root extracts have potent anxiolytic effects in laboratory rats. Phytomedicine. 2010;17(8–9):674–8.

23. Skypala IJ, Williams M, Reeves L, Meyer R, Venter C. Sensitivity to food additives, vasoactive amines and salicylates: a review of the evidence. Clin Transl Allergy. 2015;5:34.

24. Mlcek J, Jurikova T, Skrovankova S, Sochor J. Quercetin and its anti-allergic immune response. Molecules (Basel, Switzerland). 2016;21(5):623. https://doi.org/10.3390/molecules21050623.

25. Wood RA. Diagnostic elimination diets and oral food provocation. Chem Immunol Allergy. 2015;101:87–95.

26. IFM. Heal the gut with the IFM elimination diet [Internet]. The Institute for Functional Medicine. 2020 [cited 2021 Mar 9]. Available from: https://www.ifm.org/news-insights/toolkit-heal-microbiome-ifm-elimination-diet/.

27. Virdee K, Musset J, Baral M, Cronin C, Langland J. Food-specific IgG antibody-guided elimination diets followed by resolution of asthma symptoms and reduction in pharmacological interventions in two patients: a case report. Glob Adv Health Med. 2015;4(1):62–6.

28. Genova Diagnostics. IgG food antibodies [Internet]. Genova Diagnostics. 2021 [cited 2021 Feb 28]. Available from: https://www.gdx.net/product/igg-food-antibodies-food-sensitivity-test-blood.

29. Kogan M, Castillo CC, Barber MS. Chronic rhinosinusitis and irritable bowel syndrome: a case report. Integr Med (Encinitas). 2016;15(3):44–54.

30. Vadasz Z, Haj T, Kessel A, Toubi E. Age-related autoimmunity. BMC Med. 2013;11:94.

31. Watad A, Bragazzi NL, Adawi M, Amital H, Toubi E, Porat B-S, et al. Autoimmunity in the elderly: insights from basic science and clinics - a mini-review. Gerontology. 2017;63(6):515–23.

32. Minihane AM, Vinoy S, Russell WR, Baka A, Roche HM, Tuohy KM, et al. Low-grade inflammation, diet composition and health: current research evidence and its translation. Br J Nutr. 2015;114(7):999–1012.

33. Brady D. 30B. An integrative systems-biology approach to autoimmune disease: leaving the era of reaction and entering the new proactive era of prediction. Glob Adv Health Med. 2013;2(1_suppl).:gahmj.2013.097C.

34. Franceschi C, Garagnani P, Morsiani C, Conte M, Santoro A, Grignolio A, et al. The continuum of aging and age-related diseases: common mechanisms but different rates. Front Med (Lausanne). 2018;5:1–23.

35. IFM. Introducing autoimmunity: a functional medicine guide [Internet]. The Institute for Functional Medicine. 2019 [cited 2021 Mar 9]. Available from: https://www.ifm.org/news-insights/introducing-autoimmunity-functional-medicine-guide/.

36. Mayo Clinic. Psoriasis [Internet]. Mayo Clinic. 2020 [cited 2021 Mar 9]. Available from: https://www.mayoclinic.org/diseases-conditions/psoriasis/symptoms-causes/syc-20355840.

37. Mayo Clinic. Inflammatory bowel disease (IBD)- Symptoms and causes [Internet]. Mayo Clinic. 2020 [cited 2021 Mar 9]. Available from: https://www.mayoclinic.org/diseases-conditions/inflammatory-bowel-disease/symptoms-causes/syc-20353315.

38. Mayo Clinic. Celiac disease [Internet]. Mayo Clinic. 2020 [cited 2021 Mar 9]. Available from: https://www.mayoclinic.org/diseases-conditions/celiac-disease/symptoms-causes/syc-20352220.

39. Mayo Clinic. Rheumatoid arthritis - Symptoms and causes [Internet]. Mayo Clinic. 2019 [cited 2021 Mar 9]. Available from: https://www.mayoclinic.org/diseases-conditions/rheumatoid-arthritis/symptoms-causes/syc-20353648.

40. Mayo Clinic. Polymyalgia rheumatica - Symptoms and causes [Internet]. Mayo Clinic. 2020 [cited 2021 Mar 9]. Available from: https://www.mayoclinic.org/diseases-conditions/polymyalgia-rheumatica/symptoms-causes/syc-20376539#:%7E:text=Polymyalgia%20rheumatica%20is%20an%20inflammatory,are%20worse%20in%20the%20morning.

41. Mayo Clinic. Giant cell arteritis- Symptoms and causes [Internet]. Mayo Clinic. 2020 [cited 2021 Mar 9]. Available from: https://www.mayoclinic.org/diseases-conditions/giant-cell-arteritis/symptoms-causes/syc-20372758.

42. Li Y, Yao J, Han C, Yang J, Chaudhry MT, Wang S, et al. Quercetin, inflammation and immunity. Nutrients. 2016;8(3):167.

43. Walker AF, Bundy R, Hicks SM, Middleton RW. Bromelain reduces mild acute knee pain and improves well-being in a dose-dependent fashion in an open study of otherwise healthy adults. Phytomedicine. 2002;9(8):681–6.

44. Siddiqui MZ. Boswellia serrata, a potential antiinflammatory agent: an overview. Indian J Pharm Sci. 2011;73(3):255–61.

45. Nature's Sunshine Products of Australia. Turmeric - Encapsulated Herbal Extract versus Food Grade Turmeric Powder [Internet]. Nature's Sunshine Products of Australia. 2014 [cited 2021 Mar 9]. Available from: https://www.naturessunshine.com.au/blogs/health-articles/147365063-turmeric-encapsulated-herbal-extract-versus-food-grade-turmeric-powder.

46. Hewlings SJ, Kalman DS. Curcumin: a review of its effects on human health. Foods. 2017;6(10)

47. NIH. Vitamin C [Internet]. National Institutes of Health Office of Dietary Supplements. 2020 [cited 2020 Dec 30]. Available from: https://ods.od.nih.gov/factsheets/VitaminC-HealthProfessional/.

48. Hemilä H. Vitamin C and common cold-induced asthma: a systematic review and statistical analysis. Allergy Asthma Clin Immunol. 2013;9(1):46.

49. NIH. Probiotics [Internet]. NIH Office of Dietary Supplements. 2020 [cited 2021 Mar 9]. Available from: https://ods.od.nih.gov/factsheets/Probiotics-HealthProfessional/.

50. Michail S. The role of probiotics in allergic diseases. Allergy Asthma Clin Immunol. 2009;5(1):5.

51. Mirzakhani H, Al-Garawi A, Weiss ST, Litonjua AA. Vitamin D and the development of allergic disease: how important is it? Clin Exp Allergy. 2015;45(1):114–25.

52. Chai SC, Davis K, Zhang Z, Zha L, Kirschner KF. Effects of tart cherry juice on biomarkers of inflammation and oxidative stress in older adults. Nutrients. 2019;11(2):228. https://doi.org/10.3390/nu11020228.

53. Chacko SM, Thambi PT, Kuttan R, Nishigaki I. Beneficial effects of green tea: a literature review. Chin Med. 2010;5:13.

54. Danesi F, Ferguson LR. Could pomegranate juice help in the control of inflammatory diseases? Nutrients. 2017;9(9)

55. Bassiri-Jahromi S. Punica granatum (Pomegranate) activity in health promotion and cancer prevention. Oncol Rev. 2018;12(1):345.

56. Li Y, Mattison CP. Polyphenol-rich pomegranate juice reduces IgE binding to cashew nut allergens. J Sci Food Agric. 2018;98(4):1632–8.

57. NIH. Omega-3 fatty acids [Internet]. NIH Office of Dietary Supplements. 2020 [cited 2021 Mar 4]. Available from: https://ods.od.nih.gov/factsheets/Omega3FattyAcids-HealthProfessional/.

58. Gutiérrez S, Svahn SL, Johansson ME. Effects of Omega-3 fatty acids on immune cells. Int J Mol Sci. 2019;20(20):5028. https://doi.org/10.3390/ijms20205028.

59. Kunisawa J, Arita M, Hayasaka T, Harada T, Iwamoto R, Nagasawa R, et al. Dietary ω3 fatty acid exerts anti-allergic effect through the conversion to 17,18-epoxyeicosatetraenoic acid in the gut. Sci Rep. 2015;5:9750.

60. NIH. Zinc [Internet]. NIH Office of Dietary Supplements. 2020 [cited 2021 Feb 5]. Available from: https://ods.od.nih.gov/factsheets/Zinc-HealthProfessional/.

61. Prasad AS. Zinc is an antioxidant and anti-inflammatory agent: its role in human health. Front Nutr. 2014;1:14.

62. Lang C, Murgia C, Leong M, Tan L-W, Perozzi G, Knight D, et al. Anti-inflammatory effects of zinc and alterations in zinc transporter mRNA in mouse models of allergic inflammation. Am J Physiol Lung Cell Mol Physiol. 2007;292(2):L577–84.

63. Bakhshaee M, Mohammad Pour AH, Esmaeili M, Jabbari Azad F, Alipour Talesh G, Salehi M, et al. Efficacy of supportive therapy of allergic rhinitis by stinging nettle (*Urtica dioica*) root extract: a randomized, double-blind, placebo- controlled, clinical trial. Iran J Pharm Res. 2017;16(Suppl):112–8.

64. Schnedl WJ, Schenk M, Lackner S, Enko D, Mangge H, Forster F. Diamine oxidase supplementation improves symptoms in patients with histamine intolerance. Food Sci Biotechnol. 2019;28(6):1779–84.

65. Yimer EM, Tuem KB, Karim A, Ur-Rehman N, Anwar F. Nigella sativa L. (Black Cumin): a promising natural remedy for wide range of illnesses. Evid Based Complement Alternat Med. 2019;2019:1528635.

66. Ahmad A, Husain A, Mujeeb M, Khan SA, Najmi AK, Siddique NA, et al. A review on therapeutic potential of Nigella sativa: a miracle herb. Asian Pac J Trop Biomed. 2013;3(5):337–52.

67. Ehrlich S. Lemon Balm [Internet]. Penn State Hershey Milton S. Hershey Medical Center. 2015 [cited 2021 Mar 9]. Available from: http://pennstatehershey.adam.com/content.aspx?productid=107&pid=33&gid=000261.

68. Ramanauskienė K, Stelmakiene A, Majienė D. Assessment of lemon balm (Melissa officinalis L.) hydrogels: quality and bioactivity in skin cells. Evid Based Complement Alternat Med. 2015;2015:635975.
69. Miraj S, Rafieian-Kopaei, Kiani S. Melissa officinalis L: a review study with an antioxidant prospective. J Evid Based Complementary Altern Med. 2017;22(3):385–94.
70. Complementary and alternative therapies and the aging population. Editor: Ronald Watson. Elsevier; 2009.
71. Kim Y-J, Lee JY, Kim H-J, Kim D-H, Lee TH, Kang MS, et al. Anti-inflammatory effects of Angelica sinensis (Oliv.) diels water extract on RAW 264.7 induced with lipopolysaccharide. Nutrients. 2018;10(5):647. https://doi.org/10.3390/nu10050647.
72. Mao W-A, Sun Y-Y, Mao J-Y, Wang L, Zhang J, Zhou J, et al. Inhibitory effects of angelica polysaccharide on activation of mast cells. Evid Based Complement Alternat Med. 2016;2016:6063475.
73. Li D, Wu L. Coumarins from the roots of Angelica dahurica cause anti-allergic inflammation. Exp Ther Med. 2017;14(1):874–80.
74. Tattelman E. Health effects of garlic. Am Fam Physician. 2005;72(1):103–6.
75. Schäfer G, Kaschula CH. The immunomodulation and anti-inflammatory effects of garlic organosulfur compounds in cancer chemoprevention. Anti Cancer Agents Med Chem. 2014;14(2):233–40.
76. Zhang Y, Chen X, Yang L, Zu Y, Lu Q. Effects of rosmarinic acid on liver and kidney antioxidant enzymes, lipid peroxidation and tissue ultrastructure in aging mice. Food Funct. 2015;6(3):927–31.
77. Marzocco S, Calabrone L, Adesso S, Larocca M, Franceschelli S, Autore G, et al. Anti-inflammatory activity of horseradish (Armoracia rusticana) root extracts in LPS-stimulated macrophages. Food Funct. 2015;6(12):3778–88.
78. Münstedt K, Männle H. Seasonal allergic rhinitis and the role of apitherapy. Allergol Immunopathol (Madr). 2020;48(6):582–8.
79. Pasupuleti VR, Sammugam L, Ramesh N, Gan SH. Honey, propolis, and royal jelly: a comprehensive review of their biological actions and health benefits. Oxidative Med Cell Longev. 2017;2017:1259510.
80. Samarghandian S, Farkhondeh T, Samini F. Honey and health: a review of recent clinical research. Pharm Res. 2017;9(2):121–7.
81. Asha'ari ZA, Ahmad MZ, Jihan WS, Che CM, Leman I. Ingestion of honey improves the symptoms of allergic rhinitis: evidence from a randomized placebo-controlled trial in the East coast of Peninsular Malaysia. Ann Saudi Med. 2013;33(5):469–75.
82. Tukua D. 6 amazing health benefits of local, raw honey [Internet]. Farmers Almanac. 2020 [cited 2021 Mar 9]. Available from: https://www.farmersalmanac.com/local-raw-honey-22439.
83. Yang C-Y, Leung PSC, Adamopoulos IE, Gershwin ME. The implication of vitamin D and autoimmunity: a comprehensive review. Clin Rev Allergy Immunol. 2013;45(2):217–26.
84. Bener A, Ehlayel MS, Bener HZ, Hamid Q. The impact of Vitamin D deficiency on asthma, allergic rhinitis and wheezing in children: an emerging public health problem. J Family Community Med. 2014;21(3):154–61.
85. IFM. Boosting immunity: functional medicine tips on prevention & optimizing immune function during the COVID-19 (coronavirus) outbreak [Internet]. The Institute for Functional Medicine. 2020 [cited 2021 Mar 9]. Available from: https://www.ifm.org/news-insights/boosting-immunity-functional-medicine-tips-prevention-immunity-boosting-covid-19-coronavirus-outbreak/.
86. IFM. The functional medicine approach to COVID-19: additional research on nutraceuticals and botanicals [Internet]. The Institute for Functional Medicine. 2020 [cited 2021 Mar 9]. Available from: https://www.ifm.org/news-insights/functional-medicine-approach-covid-19-additional-research-nutraceuticals-botanicals/.
87. Poe FL, Corn J. N-acetylcysteine: a potential therapeutic agent for SARS-CoV-2. Med Hypotheses. 2020;143:109862.

88. Polonikov A. Endogenous deficiency of glutathione as the most likely cause of serious manifestations and death in COVID-19 patients. ACS Infect Dis. 2020;6(7):1558–62.

89. Entrenas Castillo M, Entrenas Costa LM, Vaquero Barrios JM, Alcalá Díaz JF, López Miranda J, Bouillon R, et al. Effect of calcifediol treatment and best available therapy versus best available therapy on intensive care unit admission and mortality among patients hospitalized for COVID-19: a pilot randomized clinical study. J Steroid Biochem Mol Biol. 2020;203:105751.

90. Wolowczuk I, Verwaerde C, Viltart O, Delanoye A, Delacre M, Pot B, et al. Feeding our immune system: impact on metabolism. Clin Dev Immunol. 2008;2008:639803.

91. Maggini S, Pierre A, Calder PC. Immune function and micronutrient requirements change over the life course. Nutrients. 2018;10(10):1531. https://doi.org/10.3390/nu10101531.

92. Hoang BX, Shaw G, Fang W, Han B. Possible application of high-dose vitamin C in the prevention and therapy of coronavirus infection. J Glob Antimicrob Resist. 2020;23:256–62.

93. NIH. Vitamin D [Internet]. NIH National Institutes of Health Office of Dietary Suppolements. 2020 [cited 2020 Dec 31]. Available from: https://ods.od.nih.gov/factsheets/VitaminD-HealthProfessional/.

94. Cysteine [Internet]. Restorative medicine. 2020 [cited 2021 Feb 10]. Available from: https://restorativemedicine.org/library/monographs/cysteine/.

95. ClinicalTrials.gov. A study of N-acetylcysteine in patients with COVID-19 infection - full text view [Internet]. ClinicalTrials.gov. 2020 [cited 2021 Mar 9]. Available from: https://clinicaltrials.gov/ct2/show/NCT04374461.

96. Atkuri KR, Mantovani JJ, Herzenberg LA, Herzenberg LA. N-Acetylcysteine – a safe antidote for cysteine/glutathione deficiency. Curr Opin Pharmacol. 2007;7(4):355–9.

97. Rodrigues C, Percival SS. Immunomodulatory effects of glutathione, garlic derivatives, and hydrogen sulfide. Nutrients. 2019;11(2):295. https://doi.org/10.3390/nu11020295.

98. Minich DM, Brown BI. A review of dietary (phyto)nutrients for glutathione support. Nutrients. 2019;11(9):2073. https://doi.org/10.3390/nu11092073.

99. Alschuler L, Weil A, Horwitz R, Stamets P, Chiasson AM, Crocker R, et al. Integrative considerations during the COVID-19 pandemic. Explore (NY). 2020;16(6):354–6.

100. Silverman R. Specialized pro-resolving mediators: a new tool for resolving inflammation [Internet]. The Integrative Practitioner. 2017 [cited 2021 Mar 9]. Available from: https://www.integrativepractitioner.com/about/integrative-healthcare-symposium/specialized-pro-resolving-mediators-new-tool-resolving-inflammation.

101. Spite M, Clària J, Serhan CN. Resolvins, specialized proresolving lipid mediators, and their potential roles in metabolic diseases. Cell Metab. 2014;19(1):21–36.

102. Manoharan Y, Haridas V, Vasanthakumar KC, Muthu S, Thavoorullah FF, Shetty P. Curcumin: a wonder drug as a preventive measure for COVID19 management. Indian J Clin Biochem. 2020;35(3):373–5.

103. Shannon S, Lewis N, Lee H, Hughes S. Cannabidiol in anxiety and sleep: a large case series. Perm J. 2019;23:18–041.

104. Gupta H, Gupta M, Bhargava S. Potential use of turmeric in COVID-19. Clin Exp Dermatol. 2020;45(7):902–3.

105. Meng X, Li Y, Li S, Zhou Y, Gan R-Y, Xu D-P, et al. Dietary sources and bioactivities of melatonin. Nutrients. 2017;9(4):367. https://doi.org/10.3390/nu9040367.

106. Bahrampour Juybari K, Pourhanifeh MH, Hosseinzadeh A, Hemati K, Mehrzadi S. Melatonin potentials against viral infections including COVID-19: current evidence and new findings. Virus Res. 2020;287:198108.

107. Carrillo-Vico A, Lardone PJ, Alvarez-Sánchez N, Rodríguez-Rodríguez A, Guerrero JM. Melatonin: buffering the immune system. Int J Mol Sci. 2013;14(4):8638–83.

108. Cardinali DP, Esquifino AI, Srinivasan V, Pandi-Perumal SR. Melatonin and the immune system in aging. Neuroimmunomodulation. 2008;15(4–6):272–8.

109. NIH. Vitamin A [Internet]. Vitamin A. 2020 [cited 2021 Jan 30]. Available from: https://ods.od.nih.gov/factsheets/VitaminA-HealthProfessional/.

110. NIH. Vitamin E [Internet]. NIH Office of Dietary Supplements. 2020 [cited 2021 Jan 30]. Available from: https://ods.od.nih.gov/factsheets/VitaminE-HealthProfessional/.

111. NIH. Vitamin B6 [Internet]. National Institutes of Health Office of Dietary Supplements. 2020 [cited 2020 Dec 30]. Available from: https://ods.od.nih.gov/factsheets/VitaminB6-HealthProfessional/#:~:text=The%20richest%20sources%20of%20vitamin,1%2C3%2C5%5D.

112. Vitamin B12 [Internet]. NIH National Institutes of Health Office of Dietary Supplements. 2020 [cited 2021 Jan 2]. Available from: https://ods.od.nih.gov/factsheets/VitaminB12-HealthProfessional/.

113. Tamura J, Kubota K, Murakami H, Sawamura M, Matsushima T, Tamura T, et al. Immunomodulation by vitamin B12: augmentation of CD8+ T lymphocytes and natural killer (NK) cell activity in vitamin B12-deficient patients by methyl-B12 treatment. Clin Exp Immunol. 1999;116(1):28–32.

114. NIH. Folate [Internet]. National Institutes of Health Office of Dietary Supplements. 2020 [cited 2020 Dec 30]. Available from: https://ods.od.nih.gov/factsheets/Folate-HealthProfessional/.

115. NIH. Iron [Internet]. NIH Office of Dietary Supplements. 2020 [cited 2021 Mar 5]. Available from: https://ods.od.nih.gov/factsheets/Iron-HealthProfessional/.

116. NIH. Copper [Internet]. NIH Office of Dietary Supplements. 2020 [cited 2021 Mar 9]. Available from: https://ods.od.nih.gov/factsheets/Copper-HealthProfessional/.

117. Percival SS. Copper and immunity. Am J Clin Nutr. 1998;67(5 Suppl):1064S–8S.

118. NIH. Selenium [Internet]. NIH Office of Dietary Supplements. 2020 [cited 2021 Jan 30]. Available from: https://ods.od.nih.gov/factsheets/Selenium-HealthProfessional/.

119. Mereles D, Hunstein W. Epigallocatechin-3-gallate (EGCG) for clinical trials: more pitfalls than promises? Int J Mol Sci. 2011;12(9):5592–603.

120. Chachay VS, Kirkpatrick CMJ, Hickman IJ, Ferguson M, Prins JB, Martin JH. Resveratrol--pills to replace a healthy diet? Br J Clin Pharmacol. 2011;72(1):27–38.

121. Tiralongo E, Wee SS, Lea RA. Elderberry supplementation reduces cold duration and symptoms in air-travellers: a randomized, double-blind placebo-controlled clinical trial. Nutrients. 2016;8(4):182.

122. Ho GT, Wangensteen H, Barsett H. Elderberry and elderflower extracts, phenolic compounds, and metabolites and their effect on complement, RAW 264.7 macrophages and dendritic cells. Int J Mol Sci. 2017;18(3):584. https://doi.org/10.3390/ijms18030584.

123. Petrosino S, Di Marzo V. The pharmacology of palmitoylethanolamide and first data on the therapeutic efficacy of some of its new formulations. Br J Pharmacol. 2017;174(11):1349–65.

124. Hesselink JM, Hekker TA. Therapeutic utility of palmitoylethanolamide in the treatment of neuropathic pain associated with various pathological conditions: a case series. J Pain Res. 2012;437–42. https://doi.org/10.2147/JPR.S32143.

125. Sahebnasagh A, Saghafi F, Avan R, Khoshi A, Khataminia M, Safdari M, et al. The prophylaxis and treatment potential of supplements for COVID-19. Eur J Pharmacol. 2020;887:173530.

126. Pae M, Meydani SN, Wu D. The role of nutrition in enhancing immunity in aging. Aging Dis. 2012;3(1):91–129.

127. Hu X-Y, Wu R-H, Logue M, Blondel C, Lai LYW, Stuart B, et al. Andrographis paniculata (Chuān Xīn Lián) for symptomatic relief of acute respiratory tract infections in adults and children: a systematic review and meta-analysis. PLoS One. 2017;12(8):e0181780.

128. Karsch-Völk M, Barrett B, Kiefer D, Bauer R, Ardjomand-Woelkart K, Linde K. Echinacea for preventing and treating the common cold. Cochrane Database Syst Rev. 2014;(2):CD000530.

129. Allan GM, Arroll B. Prevention and treatment of the common cold: making sense of the evidence. CMAJ. 2014;186(3):190–9.

130. Careddu D, Pettenazzo A. Pelargonium sidoides extract EPs 7630: a review of its clinical efficacy and safety for treating acute respiratory tract infections in children. Int J Gen Med. 2018;11:91–8.

131. Beerepoot M, Geerlings S. Non-antibiotic prophylaxis for urinary tract infections. Pathogens (Basel, Switzerland). 2016;5(2):36. https://doi.org/10.3390/pathogens5020036.

132. Felipe I, Bochio EE, Martins NB, Pacheco C. Inhibition of macrophage phagocytosis of Escherichia coli by mannose and mannan. Braz J Med Biol Res. 1991;24(9):919–24.
133. Hisano M, Bruschini H, Nicodemo AC, Srougi M. Cranberries and lower urinary tract infection prevention. Clinics (Sao Paulo). 2012;67(6):661–8.
134. Akgül T, Karakan T. The role of probiotics in women with recurrent urinary tract infections. Turk J Urol. 2018;44(5):377–83.
135. Orchard A, van Vuuren S. Commercial essential oils as potential antimicrobials to treat skin diseases. Evid Based Complement Alternat Med. 2017;2017:4517971.
136. Lin T-K, Zhong L, Santiago JL. Anti-inflammatory and skin barrier repair effects of topical application of some plant oils. Int J Mol Sci. 2017;19(1):70. https://doi.org/10.3390/ijms19010070.
137. Weil A. Integrative geriatric medicine. Kogan M, editor. Oxford University Press; New York. 2018.
138. Skar GL, Simonsen KA. Lyme disease. StatPearls. Treasure Island (FL): StatPearls Publishing. 2021.
139. Hyman M. 7 strategies to tackle Lyme disease [Internet]. Dr. Mark Hyman. 2019 [cited 2021 Mar 9]. Available from: https://drhyman.com/blog/2015/10/09/7-strategies-to-tackle-lyme-disease/.
140. Kumamoto CA. Inflammation and gastrointestinal Candida colonization. Curr Opin Microbiol. 2011;14(4):386–91.
141. Krasowska A, Murzyn A, Dyjankiewicz A, Łukaszewicz M, Dziadkowiec D. The antagonistic effect of Saccharomyces boulardii on Candida albicans filamentation, adhesion and biofilm formation. FEMS Yeast Res. 2009;9(8):1312–21.
142. Kandola A. Health benefits of olive leaf extract [Internet]. Medical News Today. 2019 [cited 2021 Mar 9]. Available from: https://www.medicalnewstoday.com/articles/324878.
143. Konijeti GG, Kim N, Lewis JD, Groven S, Chandrasekaran A, Grandhe S, et al. Efficacy of the autoimmune protocol diet for inflammatory bowel disease. Inflamm Bowel Dis. 2017;23(11):2054–60.
144. Sears B. Anti-inflammatory diets. J Am Coll Nutr. 2015;34 Suppl 1:14–21.
145. Richards L. The anti-Candida diet: 11 simple rules to follow [internet]. The Candida Diet. 2019 [cited 2021 Mar 9]. Available from: https://www.thecandidadiet.com/anti-candida-diet/.

Chapter 5
Endocrine and Metabolic

Contents

5.1 Cardiovascular Disease

The treatment of cardiovascular disease in the older patient differs from that of younger patients in that most conventional cardiovascular treatments are not treating the symptoms but are decreasing the risk of morbidity and mortality over the course of years and often decades. These common cardiovascular concerns are summarized in Table 5.1. Thus, as the patient enters into the last decades of life, the calculation between costs as measured by negative side effects and the benefits changes. If an older patient does not have a history of cardiovascular disease, stroke,

Table 5.1 Common cardiovascular disease concerns and recommendations

Concern	Diet focus	Supplements
Atrial fibrillation	Ensure adequate hydration (½ weight in ounces/day) Avoid stimulants Avoid blood sugar dysregulation	Magnesium Potassium Motherwort Raspberry leaf Hawthorn *Rhodiola rosea*
Stroke	Avoid red meat and egg Mediterranean diet (oils, whole grains, fruits, vegetables, legumes) Low sodium intake [5]	Beta-carotene Vitamin E Folic acid Niacin Vitamin D [6] Vitamin C Thiamin Vitamin B12 Vitamin D Vitamin K Vitamin B6 Magnesium Manganese Selenium Chromium Calcium Coenzyme Q10 L-carnitine Omega-3 fatty acids [7]
Atherosclerosis	Omega-3 FA Hydroxytyrosol of extra virgin olive oil (EVOO) Lycopene Phytosterols of plants Flavonols of fruits and vegetables [8]	Vitamin C Vitamin E [9] Calendula, elder, and violet Phytoestrogen-rich Karinat (garlic powder, extract of grape seeds, green tea leaves, hop cones, B-carotene, alpha-tocopherol, and ascorbic acid) [10]
Hyperlipidemia	Reduce saturated and trans fats Increasing polyunsaturated and monounsaturated fats Fortifying foods with plant stanols or sterols Add tree nuts Adopt a portfolio, Mediterranean, low-carbohydrate, or low-fat diet Increase intake of soluble fiber and soy protein Eat fatty marine fish [11]	Red yeast rice supplements Omega-3 fatty acid supplements [11] Basil Blueberry Celery Dandelion Dill Eugenol Evening primrose oil Fenugreek Ginger Grape Green tea Nigella Psyllium [12]

Table 5.1 (continued)

Concern	Diet focus	Supplements
Congestive heart failure	Mitochondrial diet (see Appendix) Increase dietary nitrate from beetroot	CoQ10 Magnesium D-ribose L-carnitine Thiamine (subclinical deficiency) Hawthorn

Table 5.2 Cardiovascular medications and associated nutrient depletions [14]

Drug	Associated nutrient depletion
Cardiac glycosides	Calcium, magnesium, phosphorous, and thiamine
Thiazide diuretics	CoQ10, magnesium, phosphorous, potassium, sodium, and zinc
Loop diuretics	Calcium, magnesium, potassium, sodium, thiamine, vitamin B6, vitamin C, and zinc
Potassium-sparing diuretics	Calcium, folic acid, and zinc
HMG-CoA reductase inhibitors	CoQ10, vitamin E, vitamin D, carnitine, omega-3-fatty acids, zinc, selenium, copper, and testosterone
Aspirin	Folic acid, iron, potassium, and sodium

diabetes, or vascular disease, initiating the typical cardiac medications is generally not warranted. Rather, for these patients that may show elevated lipid levels, the use of safe and effective nutritional and supplement choices is our best practice.

Statin medications are heavily overused, specifically in the elderly. For those over 80 years old without a history of cardiovascular disease, statin efficacy is minimal and potentially harmful. The Prospective Study of Pravastatin in the Elderly at Risk (PROSPER) concluded there was no benefit in terms of reduction in total mortality in patients without cardiovascular disease [1]. Compared to younger adults, older adults are at a much higher risk of suffering serious side effects from statin use. Statins can cause muscle pains, aches, and weakness. In older adults, statins can also cause falls, memory loss and confusion, nausea, constipation, and diarrhea. Statins interact with a number of drugs that can lead to even more side effects. They may also increase the risk of type 2 diabetes and cataracts and damage the liver, kidneys, and nerves [2].

For those without a history of cardiovascular disease, the cardiac benefits of statins are offset by the increased frailty, increase in falls, depression, and suicides associated with statin use in the elderly [3]. Target cholesterol levels change; an LDL of 120 probably should be left alone in an 80+-year-old otherwise healthy person as there is not enough evidence for benefits of statins in this population [4].

Statins, along with other cardiovascular medications, are associated with known nutrient deficiencies. Please see Table 5.2 for a summary of these findings.

5.1.1 Hypertension

The best first-line approach to treating hypertension in the older adult is to normalize weight and reduce sodium intake to 2.3 g/day [13]. Table 5.3 provides helpful guidelines as to how to follow an antihypertensive diet. This population is more likely to enjoy the convenience of processed foods which contain copious amounts of salt and can be the most difficult lifestyle change to execute in the older adult. Dietary counseling on low-salt alternatives and beneficial herbs and supplements that fit within the lifestyle of the older patient is critical to a successful intervention. Additionally, as adults age, a slight increase in blood pressure is expected and in and of itself should be considered within normal. Further, the role that stress plays in the blood pressure of aging adults must be considered and addressed as part of a successful integrative approach [14].

When diet and lifestyle fail, medical management is an option. There is continuous controversy about the exact point at which to initiate pharmacological management of HTN in older adults. For younger individuals <50, <130 SBP is ideal. For older adults over 65, this goal can be too aggressive due to increased risk of orthostatic hypertension, trauma, and falls. Thus, for the majority of patients 65+, less aggressive goals SBP 140–150 are more appropriate [15]. Patients and providers should be aware that certain antihypertensives are associated with specific nutrient depletions, as listed in Table 5.4.

> **Sea Salt vs. Iodized Salt**
> The primary differences between sea salt and table salt are in taste, texture, and processing. Sea salt originates from evaporated seawater and is minimally processed, so it often contains trace minerals. These minerals are minor and easily consumed through regular food intake. Iodized table salt comes from salt mines and is processed to eliminate minerals. Iodine is added to prevent goiter, and preservatives are often added to prevent clumping [17]. There are some sea salts with added iodine.

Depending on patient specifics, nutritional and botanical support can be used to supplement antihypertensive treatment. Table 5.5 describes these interventions in detail.

5.1.2 Genetics, Inflammation, and Cardiovascular Disease

Atherosclerosis and associated cardiovascular disease are multifactorial diseases, resulting from a combination of environmental and genetic risk factors. As an emerging science, clinicians must consider not only the change in medical approaches

Table 5.3 Helpful antihypertensive diet guidelines

Foods to seek	Foods to avoid
High-potassium foods such as potato, tomato, beet greens, adzuki and white beans, yogurt, and sweet potato [16]	Caffeine
Plant-based fats such as avocado, olive, nuts, and seeds	Canned soups and prepared foods high in sodium
Fiber-rich foods: fruits, vegetables, and whole grains	Saturated fats
	Refined carbohydrates
	Added salt particularly in processed and convenience foods

Table 5.4 Antihypertensives and associated nutrient depletions [14]

Drug	Associated nutrient depletion
Beta-blockers	CoQ10 and melatonin
ACE (angiotensin-converting enzyme) inhibitors	Zinc and sodium
Calcium channel blockers	Melatonin
Angiotensin receptor	Zinc

Table 5.5 Nutritional and botanical support for hypertension [18]

	Mechanism of action (MOA)	Daily dose	Food sources	Side effects and prescriber notes
Potassium	Potassium is central to changing an electrogenic driving force for Na+ reabsorption in the distal nephron via potassium channels and the NA-K pump [19]	4.7 g [19]	Avocados, beans, bananas, spinach, raisins, dates, and prunes [19]	Potassium chloride and potassium citrate appear equivalent in efficacy [20]
Magnesium	Acts as a natural calcium channel blocker, increases nitric oxide, improves endothelial dysfunction, and induces direct and indirect vasodilation [21]	500–1000 mg [21]	Green leafy vegetables (spinach), legumes, nuts, seeds, and whole grains [22]	Combined increase intake of magnesium and potassium coupled with reduced sodium intake is more effective in reducing BP than single mineral intake and is often as effective as one antihypertensive drug [21]

(continued)

Table 5.5 (continued)

	Mechanism of action (MOA)	Daily dose	Food sources	Side effects and prescriber notes
Calcium	Increases intracellular calcium in vascular smooth muscle cells leading to vasoconstriction and by increasing vascular volume through the renin-angiotensin-aldosterone (RAAS) [23]	1000–1500 mg [24]	Milk, yogurt, cheese, nuts and seeds (almonds, sesame, chia), kale, broccoli, and watercress [25]	Low calcium intake may increase blood pressure through three major mechanisms: parathyroid function, vitamin D, and the RAAS [23]
Vitamin C	Aqueous-phase antioxidant that reduces oxidative stress and enhances endothelial function through effects on nitric oxide production [26]	500 mg [26]	Red pepper, orange, grapefruit, kiwifruit, green pepper, broccoli, and strawberries [27]	Minimum of 8 weeks [26]
Folate	Has been shown to significantly improve endothelial dysfunction [28]	Up to 800–2000 mcg	Beef liver, spinach, black-eyed peas, and breakfast cereals (fortified) [29]	Minimum of 6 weeks [28], biggest benefit more than 12 weeks. Secondary benefit of lowering homocysteine concentrations [30]
B6	Regulates cellular calcium transport through both voltage-mediated and ATP-mediated cellular calcium influx [31]	5 mg/kg [32]	Chickpeas, beef liver, tuna, salmon, and chicken breast [33]	Also protects against ischemia and glutamate-induced neurotoxicity [31]
Omega-3 fats	Modulate ion channel functions in blood vessels; reduce oxidative stress on vasculature [34], leading to vasodilation; and improve arterial compliance [35]	3–4 g [35]	Fish oil, salmon, mackerel, herring, tuna, and sardines [35]	Dietary intake/supplementation of omega-3 polyunsaturated fatty acids (PUFAs) may have a place in the control of patients with mild hypertension before starting drug treatment [35]
L-arginine	Increases nitric oxide production, decreases angiotensin II levels, and reduces oxidative stress, resulting in improved endothelial function and decreased peripheral vascular resistance and blood pressure [36]	1.5–6 g in divided doses 2–3 times daily	Meat, fish, soy, beans, lentils, whole grains, and nuts [36]	Effective in lowering blood pressure in salt-sensitive hypertension but less effective in essential hypertension [36]

Table 5.5 (continued)

	Mechanism of action (MOA)	Daily dose	Food sources	Side effects and prescriber notes
Anti-ACE peptides	Increase phosphorylation of protein kinase B and endothelial nitric oxide synthase and significantly promote nitric oxide production [37]	40 ug/ml [38]	Milk, cheese, egg, spinach, brown cultivar mushroom, macro-algae, rapeseed, canola, sunflower seed protein, soy protein legumes, rice, mung bean, chick beans, [39] olive, and flounder [37]	Could replace conventional synthetic drugs with similar potency and little to no adverse effects [40]
CoQ10	Antioxidant. Acts directly on vascular endothelium to decrease total peripheral resistance. Reduces superoxide synthesis. Possible anti-atherogenic effects as a modular of B-integrin levels on the surface of blood monocytes [41]	100–200 mg [41]	Oily fish (salmon and tuna), liver, and whole grains [42]	Side effects may include diarrhea and rash [42]. 200-mg dose is recommended if patient is on statins
Olive leaf	Antioxidant, anti-inflammatory, reduction in plasma lipids, reduction in blood pressure by vasodilation, and blockade of L-type Ca2+ channels [43]	500 mg twice daily [43]	Source (waste product of olive oil production) [43]	Bioavailability is still uncertain [43]. Also contains antiviral properties
Hawthorn	Antioxidant, vasorelaxation via NO synthesis, vasorelaxant effects of smooth muscles, and weak ACE activity [44]	500 mg [45]	Source (tiny fruits that grow on trees and shrubs belonging to *Crataegus* genus [46]	Concurrent anxiety reduction [45]
Aged garlic	Reduces central blood pressure, pulse wave velocity, pulse pressure, and arterial stiffness. Reduces blood pressure through nitric oxide and hydrogen sulfide production [47]	480–960 mg [48]	Garlic extract, from garlic bulbs that have undergone a natural aging process at room temperature [47]	Rare GI disturbances [48]

(continued)

Table 5.5 (continued)

	Mechanism of action (MOA)	Daily dose	Food sources	Side effects and prescriber notes
Hibiscus	May be due to antioxidant activities, inhibition of α-glucosidase and α-amylase, inhibition of angiotensin-converting enzymes (ACEs), and direct vasorelaxant effect or calcium channel modulation [49]	Tea, 2–3 times per day [1.25 g *H. sabdariffa* (480 mL/d)] every day morning and night] [50]	Dried hibiscus flower. Drink in hibiscus-laded form	
L-citrulline	Increase NO production, promoting vasodilation [51]	3–9 g [51]	Watermelon [51]	Has a synergistic effect when taken with L-arginine [51]

based on a patient's genetic profile but also how environmental factors will impact the expression genetic tendencies to greater or lesser degrees. Of all the environmental factors that exert influence on gene expression – tobacco smoke, physical activity, toxin exposure, nutrient availability, and stress – diet may have the biggest impact on genetic expression as it relates to cardiovascualar disease (CVD) [52]. The confusion in the medical community about which dietary approach is appropriate for CVD may revolve around the bio-individuality related to genetic predispositions. Thus, there is no one diet that research unequivocally supports for prevention or treatment of CVD but rather a diet that will work more or less better for a patient given their genetic makeup.

Because inflammation plays a critical role in atherosclerosis, understanding inflammatory biomarkers associated with cardiovascular disease is an important area of research. A number of epidemiologic studies have identified particular inflammatory biomarkers (such as CRP, ICAM-1, IL-6, and P-selectin) as heritable markers whose levels correlate with increased inflammation and higher cardiovascular disease risk [53].

High levels of inflammation have long been associated with increased risk of heart attacks, strokes, and other consequences of cardiovascular disease. The CANTOS study demonstrated that those who had elevated inflammatory markers despite statin treatment (and a prior heart attack) who were treated with anti-inflammatory interventions reduced their likelihood of subsequent heart attacks or strokes by 15%. Targeting inflammation further decreased the need for major cardiac interventions, such as angioplasty or bypass surgery by 30% [54]. Armed with this knowledge, lifestyle interventions to reduce inflammation such as maintaining healthy weight, increasing activity, and quitting smoking can help reduce the cardiovascular disease burden [55].

Tie is why some people are in a pro-inflammatory state and why those people have to approach diet/lifestyle in a more vigorous way because of predisposition. There cannot be a "one-size-fits-all" approach to dieting.

5.1.3 Nutrigenomics and Cardiovascular Disease

Much progress has been made over the years regarding target genes of interest in cardiovascular health [56]. The study of nutrigenomics allows personalized diets to cater to individual needs based on our understanding of genetic capability [57]. Understanding our genetic makeup and predisposition allows us to manipulate values such as LDL, HDL, BMI, insulin, homocysteine, triglycerides, and blood pressure through diet changes to meet our own personal needs [58]. For examples of nutrigenomics in action, please see ApoE4 callout box below.

At the time of authors writing this book, nutrigenomics is just now entering the field of clinical medicine. The below ApoE4 example shows how lifestyle and diet can be optimized for this specific factor. In the next decade, we anticipate an explosion of this field which will change the practice as we know it.

ApoE4
- Knowing a patient's ApoE4 status can substantially affect clinical care. Basic recommendations (diet, statins, and aspirin (ASA)) with h/o CVD are grossly inadequate. This requires a much more aggressive approach to ward off not just Alzheimer's disease but progression of vascular disease as well:
  - Replacing saturated fats with plant-based unsaturated fats
  - Increase plant antioxidants
- ApoE4 and coconut oil:
  - In some studies, it appears to increase cholesterol and possibly contribute to higher risk of cardiovascular disease [59]. However, when ApoE4 is taken into consideration, this effect disappears. Patients with ApoE4 should be restricting all saturated fats including coconut or medium chain triglycerides (MCT) oils and carefully monitor LDL levels. In these patients, even small amounts of saturated fats can lead to significant LDL elevations.
  - This does not mean that a low-fat diet is recommended, but rather focus should be on matching the type of dietary fat with genomics.

Like all other pathologies discussed in this book, Table 5.6 summarizes known supplements to help treat cardiovascular disease.

Table 5.6 Nutritional and botanical support for cardiovascular disease [60]

	MOA	Daily dose	Food sources	Side effects and prescriber notes
Magnesium	Improves glucose and insulin metabolism, enhances endothelium-dependent vasodilation, and ameliorates lipid profile by actions as an antihypertensive and anti-inflammatory [61]	400–800 mg	Green leafy vegetables (spinach), legumes, nuts, seeds, and whole grains [22]	Avoid citrate or hydroxide forms; these are not well absorbed and cause loose stools. Use with caution when treating patients with kidney disease
CoQ10	Antioxidant, which reduces oxidative stress and lowers risk of cardiovascular disease. Provides mitochondrial support to cardiac muscles. Anti-inflammatory effects through nitric oxide regulation [62]	100–200 mg three times	Oily fish (salmon and tuna), liver, and whole grains [42]	Use with statins. Minor side effects include GI upset and possible rash. Levels are decreased in patients with heart failure, and low correlations correlate with severity and are an independent predictor of mortality [41]
Folate	Lowers blood homocysteine concentration, which reduces atherosclerotic processes and development of CVD [63]	0.5–5 mg [63]	Beef liver, spinach, black-eyed peas, and breakfast cereals (fortified) [29]	Target serum homocysteine under 7.0 uM, consider MTHFR if >8
Vitamin B12	B12 deficiency induces hyperhomocysteinemia. Supplementation can help lower blood homocysteine levels; see above [64]	0.5 mg [65]	Clams, liver, trout, salmon, tuna, and nutritional yeast [66]	If necessary, addition of ~1 mg of B12 to folic acid may help avoid the theoretical risk of neuropathy due to unopposed folic acid therapy in patients deficient in B12 [65]
Vitamin D	May downregulate the RAAS system and have direct effects on cardiac tissue and vasculature or improvement in glycemic control [67]	1000 IU daily [67]	Cod liver oil, trout, salmon, mushrooms, and fortified milk [68]	Supplementation is controversial. Although observational studies have reported an association between low vitamin D levels and elevated risk of CVD, causation cannot be proven because of unmeasured confounding variables [69]

Table 5.6 (continued)

	MOA	Daily dose	Food sources	Side effects and prescriber notes
Potassium	May prevent vascular calcification, thereby reducing atherosclerosis risk. May also prevent calcification of smooth muscle cells [70]	90 mmol (3510 mg) [71]	Avocados, beans, bananas, spinach, raisins, dates, and prunes [19]	Use with caution in patients with kidney disease [72]
Hawthorn	Leaves and flowers contain oligomeric procyanidins (antioxidants) and quercetin (anti-inflammatory) thought to mediate cardiovascular effects	500–750-mg capsules (can also be found in the following forms: powder, paste, and dried berries such as tea)	Source (grow as trees and shrubs belonging to *Crataegus* genus) [46]	Berries have been used as well but thought to be less potent due to lesser concentration of oligomeric procyanidins. Potential side effects: dizziness, nausea, GI disturbance, headache, palpitations, rash, and hypotension
Inorganic nitrates	Reduced to nitric oxide; beneficial vascular effects, reducing smooth muscle contraction and proliferation, reducing platelet adhesion and aggregation, and activity of inflammatory markers [73]	250–500 mL [73]	Beetroot juice (celery, lettuce, radish, arugula, spinach, Swiss chard) [73]	Do not appear to be associated with the formation of N-nitrosamines, a class of carcinogenic substances [73]
L-carnitine	Transports long-chain fatty acids to mitochondria where beta-oxidation and ATP production occur, triggering cardioprotective effects though reduced oxidative stress, inflammation, and necrosis of cardiac myocytes. Regulates calcium influx, endothelial integrity, intracellular enzyme release, and membrane phospholipid content for sustained cellular homeostasis [74]	1–3 g	Beef steak, ground beef, milk, codfish, and chicken breast [75]	No known adverse effects. Some concern that L-carnitine metabolizes into trimethylamine N-oxide (TMAO) by select gut microbes. TMAO concentrations have been associated with higher cardiovascular (CV) events and mortality. Unclear if this is a reflection of cardiovascular safety of carnitine or importance of maintaining gut health
Omega-3	Decreases serum levels of triglycerides, improves endothelial function, decreases resting BP, suppresses acute phase reactants, and resolves inflammation [76]	1–3 g	Fish oil, salmon, mackerel, herring, tuna, and sardines [35]	GI distress

(continued)

Table 5.6 (continued)

	MOA	Daily dose	Food sources	Side effects and prescriber notes
D-ribose	Increases cellular energy levels and improves function following ischemia [77]	5–15 g	Wheat bran, eggs, meat, cheese, and yeast [78]	May induce diarrhea, nausea, hypoglycemia, hyperuricemia, and headache. Avoid individual doses greater than 10 g d/t GI side effects
Red yeast rice	High concentration of monacolin K which can lower blood cholesterol and TG levels [79]	1200–3600 mg	Source	Use with CoQ10. Can be tried as a substitute if patients are unable to tolerate statins [80–82]. Side effects may include abdominal discomfort, heartburn, gas, headache, and dizziness [79]
Motherwort	Reduces platelet aggregation and fibrinogen levels. Potentiates antithrombotic and antiplatelet effects [83]. Antioxidant activity	7.5–15 mg/kg [84]	Source	When taken with benzodiazepines, motherwort can have synergistic sedative effects and may result in coma. Also carries bleeding risk [83]
Raspberry leaf	Antioxidant (high total polyphenol content) [85]	Tea: one cup PO up to 6×/day 1.5-g leaves with 150 mL of water Liquid extract: 4–8 ml PO TID [86]	Raspberry plant	May exhibit estrogenic effects [87]
Rhodiola rosea	Prevents stress-induced catecholamine release and higher cAMP levels in myocardium [88]	50–680 mg [89]	Source	Possible side effects include dizziness, dry mouth, or excessive saliva production [90]
Thiamine	Deficiency in thiamine leads to congestive heart failure [91]	1.1–1.2 mg [91]	Rice, breakfast cereals, egg noodles, pork chop, trout, and black beans [91]	Patients who suffer from chronic alcoholism are at particular risk for thiamine deficiency [91]

Table 5.6 (continued)

	MOA	Daily dose	Food sources	Side effects and prescriber notes
Cocoa	Contains fatty acids, minerals, and polyphenols. Flavanols increase plasma antioxidant activity and improve endothelial wall and platelet function. Reduce nitrogen reactive species. May inhibit ACE. Can inhibit epinephrine-stimulated platelet activation and function [92]	30 g [92]	Dark chocolate best (>85% cacao)	Unclear what percentage of dark chocolate is optimal (white/milk has more dairy and sugar)
Soluble fiber	Increases plasma HDL, decreases plasma homocysteine, and increases glutathione [93]. Reduces LDL, regulates body weight, improves glucose metabolism, controls blood pressure, and reduces inflammation [94]	25–38 g [95]	Whole grains (cereal), legumes, fruits, vegetables, and nuts	Cereal fiber seems to be most strongly associated with decreased cardiovascular risk [94]

5.2 Thyroid Disease

The thyroid gland affects almost every cell in the body as it releases hormones that control the speed at which the body functions, otherwise known as the metabolic rate. Thyroid hormone modulates how much protein tissue makes throughout the body to carry out physiologic needs and how much oxygen cells use [96]. The thyroid is susceptible to both hyperstimulation and hypostimulation, manifesting as hyperthyroidism or hypothyroidism. Just like in other conditions in geriatrics, presentation of thyroid disease may look atypical in older adults. Table 5.7 summarizes these findings.

Overt hypothyroidism occurs in 2–5% of adults over 60 years [97]. Hashimoto's thyroiditis is the most common subtype of hypothyroidism in the United States. Antibodies bind to thyroid stimulating hormone (TSH) receptors, thyroid peroxidase enzyme, and thyroglobulin to inhibit hormone secretion. Patients may present with a constellation of symptoms, including but not limited to depression, dry skin, lethargy, memory problems, hyperlipidemia, weight gain, and slow motility predisposition to SIBO. As Hashimoto's thyroiditis is an autoimmune state, patients see relief with an anti-inflammatory, autoimmune diet. In Hashimoto's, it is believed the prevalence of gluten sensitivity is much higher. Approximately 2% of patients with celiac disease have overt autoimmune hypothyroidism [18]. Gluten elimination in

Table 5.7 Hypothyroidism vs. hyperthyroidism

	Hypothyroidism	Hyperthyroidism
Signs and symptoms	Fatigue, weakness, cold intolerance, dyspnea, weight gain, cognitive dysfunction, constipation, bradycardia, and dry skin [98]	Weight loss, heat intolerance, tremor, palpitations, atrial fibrillation, anxiety, increased frequency of bowel movements, and shortness of breath +/– goiter [99]
Labs	High TSH, low free T4, and normal or low T3 [100]	Low TSH, high or normal free T4, and high T3 [100]

most patients as a trial makes substantial contribution to improvement in biomarkers of autoimmune activity, thyroid peroxidase (TPO) and thyroglobulin (TGA). Hypothyroidism significantly contributes to weight gain and heart disease as the metabolism slows; the thyroid must always be considered when managing these conditions.

For early, mild cases of hypothyroid that are not at the danger of being undertreated (TSH 4–10), one can recommend supplements (see below table) and an elimination diet. Approximately 50% of these patients respond to diet and supplement modifications [18]. Goitrogens can be found in food and the environment and bind to thyroid hormone making it inactive. For a list of sample goitrogenic foods, please see table below. Exercise, in addition to diet modification, stimulates thyroid secretion, increases tissue sensitivity to thyroid hormone, and increases metabolic rate.

Hyperthyroidism is less common than hypothyroidism in the elderly. The prevalence in older adults over 60 years is 0.5–3%, but 10–15% of the hyperthyroid patients are older than 60 years [97]. Hyperthyroidism can cause arrhythmias, as well as weight loss, anxiety, bone loss, etc. Around 85% of hyperthyroidism is attributable to Graves' disease, another autoimmune condition. Hyperthyroidism, like hypothyroidism, can be managed in part with an anti-inflammatory diet. Diets high in calories and supplemented with protein in small, frequent meals can help meet the body's increased metabolic needs.

Both hyperthyroid and hypothyroid patients can be supported with vitamins and supplements. Please see Table 5.8 for a summary of these interventions.

Adrenal Connection

Adrenal disbalances are often contributing to mild cases of hypothyroid disease. Patients who often find a typical thyroid treatment unsatisfactory are the ones most commonly who have this secondary component which, if not treated, will continue to cause disbalance. In such cases, managing mild adrenal disturbances is essential. Often, treatment includes mind-body techniques, graded exercise programs, and botanical adaptogens.

See Appendix for adaptogens. Ref: Kogan Geri Textbook, Endocrine chapter.

Table 5.8 Vitamins and supplements for thyroid health [18]

	MOA	Daily dose	Food sources	Side effects and prescriber notes
Iodine	Thyroid hormones are made from iodine and tyrosine	200–2000 mcg, based on testing. 24-h urine iodine is gold standard	Seaweed	Iodine overdose side effects can cause hyperthyroidism which needs to be monitored (too much iodine inhibits hormone synthesis) Most multivitamins (MTV) have 100–150 mcg iodine
L-tyrosine	Thyroid hormones are made from iodine and tyrosine	500–1500 mg	Soy products, chicken, turkey, fish, peanuts, almonds, avocados, bananas, milk, cheese, yogurt, cottage cheese, lima beans, pumpkin seeds, and sesame seeds [101]	Use with caution in migraines May cause GI disturbance [101]
Zinc	Helps to manufacture thyroid hormone and is a cofactor to convert T4 → T3	5–30 mg	Oysters	GI disturbance [102]
Vitamin E	Helps manufacture thyroid hormone	200–400 IU	Vegetable oils, almonds, peanuts, sunflower seeds, spinach, and broccoli [103]	Very high doses may cause blood thinning (1500 IU) [103]
Vitamin A	Helps manufacture thyroid hormone	25,000 IU [104]	Beef liver, sweet potato, spinach, and carrots [105]	In excess: dizziness, nausea, and headaches [105]
B vitamins	Necessary for thyroid hormone synthesis	Standard B100 complex	Salmon, leafy greens, liver and other organ meats, eggs, milk, beef, oysters, and legumes	In excess: nausea, GI disturbance, hair loss, rashes, and nerve damage [27, 106]
Vitamin C	Necessary for thyroid hormone synthesis	As cofactor, low dose at 100–500 mg daily	Red and green pepper, orange juice, orange, grapefruit juice, kiwifruit, and broccoli [27]	May cause GI disturbance in excess [106]
Selenium	Required cofactor for converting T4 → T3	100–200 mcg	Brazil nuts, tuna, halibut, sardines, ham, and shrimp [107]	Garlic breath, metallic taste, and hair and nail loss [107]

Turmeric	Increase thyroid function	1–2 teaspoons/day or 500–1000 mg of standardized extract	Turmeric (2.5–6% curcumin) and curry [108]	May cause GI disturbance in excess [109]
Ashwagandha, Standardized extract,	Stimulates thyroid activity [110]	100–250 mg	Source	None reported
Foods to avoid with thyroid dysfunction				
Goitrogenic foods and chemicals	Certain foods block iodine use	Avoid	*Brassica* plants (turnips, cabbage, mustard greens, radishes, broccoli, brussels sprouts, kale, rutabagas, cauliflower, horseradishes), cassava root, soybean, peanuts, pine nuts, and millet *Chemicals:* fluoride, mercury, and amiodarone	Very complex topic, for additional reading, recommend https://global.oup.com/academic/product/integrative-environmental-medicine-9780190490911?cc=us&lang=en&

5.3 Type 2 Diabetes Mellitus

For older adults, there is minimal to no evidence that slightly elevated HgA1c (and cholesterol) has any mortality significance. As such, goals of treatments are different. For patients with type 2 diabetes and no other issues, HgA1c of 7.5 is appropriate [111].

Although diet and exercise play key roles in managing diabetes, the quality and quantity of sleep cannot be overlooked. Shorter sleep has been associated with higher BMI, higher dietary fat intake, disturbances in the metabolic hormones leptin and ghrelin, impaired glucose tolerance, and insulin resistance [112]. Beneficial supplements include CoQ10, omega-3 fatty acids and acetyl-L-carnitine, resveratrol, NAC, and vitamin E [113]. For a complete list of supplements, please see Table 5.9.

Exercise has positive impacts individually directly on both sleep and insulin resistance. The relationship between insulin sensitivity and insulin resistance can be directly linked to level of physical activity. Exercise can increase glucose uptake, improve overall glucose tolerance, improve insulin sensitivity, promote weight loss, and reduce inflammation [114]. Obesity-related stress, an imbalance of pro- and antioxidants, has been linked to both metabolic and cardiovascular disease. Exercise helps reduce prooxidants, decrease stress, and reduce inflammation [58].

5.4 Obesity

Going hand in hand with diabetes, obesity creates a conundrum of malnutrition in the context of overnutrition. In short, most obesity is created by people eating too much of the wrong kinds of foods, starving their cells of critical micronutrients while they flood their metabolism with calorie-dense, nutrient-poor food that is engineered in the laboratory to encourage overconsumption and addictive patterns. The concept of weight management being a result of a math equation that takes the number of calories consumed and subtracts the number burned through resting metabolic rate and movement provides a framework but does not address the complete picture of body weight. We must move toward a grander view of nutrition and body composition in order to fully address obesity. The role of toxicity and gut microbiome disturbance in body weight is primary to resolving the issue for most patients that struggle to lose weight and maintain normal body weight. Additionally, screening for thyroid dysfunction is critical and requires a deeper dive than just TSH screen.

Obesity in the older adult leads to decreased physical function and an increase in frailty. The concomitant impact of under- and overnutrition that exists in the aging adult with obesity should be addressed with care when a patient's body mass index (BMI) score is >29.9 or their fat mass is >30% for women or 25% for men. In an

Table 5.9 Nutritional and botanical support for diabetes [115]

	MOA	Daily dose	Food sources	Side effects and prescriber notes
Berberine	Regulates glucose and lipid metabolism [116]	500 mg, 2–3×/day	Main active component of Chinese herb *Coptis chinensis French* [116]	GI disturbance [116]. Also used as antimicrobial to treat dysbiosis
Probiotics	Inhibits glucose spikes in the bloodstream, decreases inflammatory mediator release, and helps reduce BMI, TG, LDL, and total cholesterol and increase HDL [117]	2.5 billion CFU [117]	Yogurt, cultured buttermilk, cheese, miso, tempeh, sauerkraut, beer, sour dough, bread, chocolate, kimchi, olives, pickles, and kefir [118]	*Bifidobacterium bifidum, B. lactis, L. acidophilus, L. brevis, L. casei, L. salivarius, Lactococcus lactis,* and *Lactococcus lactis* [117]
Gymnema sylvestre	Peroxisome proliferator-activated receptor (PPAR) agonist; improves weight, decreases the required insulin dose, and lowers HgA1c; may increase the number of beta cells in the pancreas	200–1000 mg	Source. Vulnerable species is a slow growing, perennial, medicinal woody climber found in central and peninsular India [119]	It is safe at recommended doses; high doses may lead to hypoglycemia, weakness, shakiness, excessive sweating, and muscular dystrophy [120]
Cassia cinnamon	Decreases fatty liver, insulin resistance, lipids, fasting blood sugars, and HgA1c	750 mg	Source (Chinese cinnamon)	Most studies show treatment for at least 4 months to lead to a significant statistical decrease in fasting plasma glucose, along with an improvement in lipid profile [121]
CoQ10	Modest improvements in A1c and fasting blood glucose (FBG). May prevent vascular complications secondary to associated oxidative stress	75–300 mg twice a day or ubiquinol 100–300 mg	Oily fish (salmon and tuna), liver, and whole grains [42]	Minor side effects include GI upset and possible rash. Levels are decreased in patients with heart failure, and low correlations correlate with severity and are an independent predictor of mortality [41]

Table 5.9 (continued)

	MOA	Daily dose	Food sources	Side effects and prescriber notes
L-carnitine	It plays a critical role in energy production. It transports long-chain fatty acids into the mitochondria so they can be oxidized to produce energy. It also transports the toxic compounds generated out of the mitochondria to prevent accumulation. It can help provide energy to failing heart muscles [122]	1–3 g in divided doses	Beef steak, ground beef, milk, codfish, and chicken breast [75]	No known adverse effects. Some concern that L-carnitine metabolizes into trimethylamine N-oxide (TMAO) by select gut microbes. TMAO concentrations have been associated with higher CV events and mortality. Unclear if this is a reflection of cardiovascular safety of carnitine or importance of maintaining gut health
Magnesium	Decreased insulin resistance and decreased FBG	500–1000 mg	Green leafy vegetables (spinach), legumes, nuts, seeds, and whole grains [22]	Avoid citrate or hydroxide forms; these are not well absorbed and cause loose stools. Use caution when treating patients with kidney disease
Chromium	Essential mineral needed for carbohydrate metabolism. Decreases HgA1c and FBG	200–400 mg	Cereal, meat, poultry, and fish [102]	No evidence of effects on body composition in healthy individuals. Long-term toxicity data pending [123]
A. vera juice	Decreases FBG and HgA1c	15–30 ml of juice two or three times	Source	Hypoglycemia [124]
Curcumin	Improved B-cell function, decreased insulin resistance, decreased diabetic nephropathy and retinopathy, and glycemic control	1500 mg to 6 g	Source	Diarrhea, headache, rash, and yellow stool [109]. RCT in prediabetic patients showed prevention of diabetes
Bitter melon	Strong antioxidant and hypoglycemic activities [125]	500–2000 mg [125]	Source. Climbing shrub	Decreases body weight, visceral fat mass, plasma glucose, and Triacylglycerol (TAG) [125]

obese adult, weight loss of just 5–10% will improve markers of metabolic syndrome and systemic inflammation. The impact of aging on the physical body (shrinking height, lower muscle mass) reduces the efficacy of using the traditional tool for assessing obesity, BMI. Better tools for this assessment are the DEXA scan and the bioelectrical impedance measurements. In addition, weight loss over the age of 70 should be undertaken with care. In a 2010 study, adults who were overweight had a 13% lower incidence of death compared to adults considered a normal weight [126].

Considerations for addressing obesity in the aging adult are as follows:

- All calories are not considered equal; encourage the focus on the nutrients foods offer and less on counting the calories. When whole foods are the bulk of the diet, nutrients increase and caloric intake naturally decreases. It's hard to overeat broccoli.
- Focus on the foods that should be in the diet rather than restricting foods that are unhelpful. If the patient can eat 8–10 servings of fruits and vegetables per day (4–6 cups), they are usually too full to grab the calorie-dense, nutrient-poor snacks. See Table 5.10 for recommended supplements.
- The combination of increased exercise and decreased caloric intake equal to about 500 calories per day can promote sustainable weight loss of 1 pound per week and preserve muscle mass.
- Some patients may like to use a tracker for their food such as cronometer or myfitnesspal as it helps them see the nutrient value of the foods they are choosing. Others may not like this option so check in with the patient to be sure it's the right support.

5.5 Therapeutic Diets

5.5.1 Vegan Diet

Vegetarian and vegan diets have shown effectiveness in improving body weight, glycemic control, and cardiovascular risk factors. Vegan diets tend to be lower in harmful factors such as excess energy intake, saturated fat, meat, and heme iron and higher prevalence of protective factors such as fruits, vegetables, and fiber [144]. For further information on a vegan diet, please see Appendix.

5.5.2 Mediterranean Diet

One variation on the Mediterranean diet that has been well studied with respect to hypertension is called the dietary approaches to stop hypertension or DASH diet. Structurally similar to the Mediterranean diet, DASH research has shown the incremental benefit to cardiovascular health from restricting certain foods such as those

Table 5.10 Nutritional and botanical support for obesity [18]

	MOA	Dose	Food sources	Side effects and prescriber notes
5-HTP	Is an appetite modifier and influences postmeal satiety [127]	900 mg [128]	Bananas, plantains, passion fruits, pineapple, pomegranate, strawberry, spinach, tomato, kiwi, green onion, lettuce, paprika, and potato [129]	Caution in use with other drugs that increase serotonin level so as to prevent serotonin syndrome
Medical food powders	Provides prebiotic fiber and complex carbohydrates to support beneficial glucose/insulin response and sustained energy release. Certain formulations can increase GLO-1 levels to stimulate insulin secretion and induce satiety [130]	One serving 1–2 times per day	Often in powder form	Caution in pregnant or nursing women [130]
Fiber	Induces greater satiety, modulates gastric motor function, and blunts postprandial glucose and insulin responses. Postulated effects on gut peptide hormones may prolong meal duration and result in increased mastication [131]	20–35 g [132]	Oat, barley, legumes, peas, beans, broccoli, carrots, root vegetables, and fruits [133]	Minor GI symptoms are flatus, bloating, and abdominal cramping [134]. Insoluble fiber is used as a bulking agent in stool; soluble fiber has favorable effects on glucose and lipid metabolism [131]
Guar gum	Reduces peak postprandial whole blood glucose levels, increases responsiveness to insulin, and reduces total serum cholesterol levels [135]	10 g twice daily [135]	Bread, yogurt, baked goods, and pasta [136]	Improves microbiome as prebiotic fiber [137]
Chromium	Increases insulin sensitivity, can potentiate the actions of insulin at its receptor, can reduce food craving, as well as increases metabolic rate [138]	137–1000 mg [138]	Cereal, meat, poultry, and fish [102]	No evidence of effects on body composition in healthy individuals. Long-term toxicity data pending [123]

(continued)

Table 5.10 (continued)

	MOA	Dose	Food sources	Side effects and prescriber notes
MCT oil	Increases thermogenesis and energy expenditure	1–2 tbsp/day	Source usually derived from coconut or palm oil	Unclear which plays a bigger role, enhanced satiety or enhanced thermic effect of food [139]
Garcinia cambogia	Contrains hydrocitrate, an appetite suppressor	1–2.8 g [140]	Source	GI distress [140]
Meal replacements [18]	Provide high-fiber-meal replacements supporting dietary compliance and convenience	Protein target 2.2 g/kg lean body mass	Numerous, e.g., Medifast	Improvements in body composition, blood pressure, and lean muscle mass and reduction in CRP
Hydroxycitrate (HCA) [18]	Powerful lipogenic inhibitor. Produces a significant reduction in food intake and body weight gain. May be an appetite suppressant	1500 mg TID	Fruit of the Malabar tamarind	Critical that a low-fat diet be maintained because HCA only inhibits conversion of carbohydrates into fat
Fish oil	Reduces expression of adipose inflammatory genes [141]	1.3–4 g [142]	Salmon, sardines, trout, oysters, and sea bass [143]	Significant changes in body composition, more effective in weight loss if combined with dietary interventions [142]

that are fried and high in sodium over some of the more restrictive and therefore difficult to sustain diets, like Dr. Ornish's vegetarian or vegan diet. Please see Table 5.11 for specifics on the DASH diet.

5.5.3 *Mitochondrial Diet*

Mitochondria are the key players in ATP production, energy expenditure, and reduction of reactive oxygen species. Mitochondrial dysfunction consequently negatively impacts lipid and glucose metabolism [145]. To maintain mitochondrial health, decrease toxin exposure, optimize nutrient status that protects mitochondria from oxidative stress, and facilitate ATP production. Therapeutic foods that support healthy mitochondria are high in healthy fats and nutrients needed for mitochondrial function. For more details on the mitochondrial diet, please see Appendix.

Table 5.11 Daily and weekly DASH eating plan goals for a 2000-calorie-a-day diet [148]

Food group	Daily servings
Grains	6–8
Meats, poultry, and fish	6 or less
Vegetables	4–5
Fruit	4–5
Low-fat or fat-free dairy product	2–3
Fats and oils	2–3
Sodium	2300 mg*
	Weekly servings
Nuts, seeds, dry beans, and peas	4–5
Sweets	5 or less

*1,500 milligrams (mg) sodium lowers blood pressure even further than 2,300 mg sodium daily

Table 5.12 Key components of common diets to treat metabolic syndrome

	DASH diet	Plant based	Mediterranean
Stripped carbs			
Intact carbs	X	X	X
Industrial fats	X		
High-quality protein	X	X	X
Low-quality protein	X		
Nutritious fats	X		X

5.5.4 Very-Low-Fat Diet

Reducing the intake of dietary fat can be an effective weight loss strategy, particularly for women which researchers believe may be pursuing this particular diet more due to social conditioning around consumption of fat causing weight gain. The downside to a very-low-fat diet, particularly in older adults, makes this approach a last resort in the eyes of the authors. There are a number of diets known to support metabolic syndrome; there is no one right solution. Please see Table 5.12 for a high-level comparison of the components of each.

Fat: Quality vs. Quantity
More important than "how much" fat one consumes is "what kind" of fat one consumes, quality over quantity. The bulk of one's fat intake should consist of long-chain saturated fats and polyunsaturated fats. Medium-chain triglycerides should be incorporated in moderation, along with omega-3 DHA and EPA. Trans fats should absolutely be avoided. Processed and fried foods contain high amounts of oxycholesterol, which has damaging effects on cells, DNA, and contributes directly to atherosclerosis [146]. Very-low-fat diets can induce hypertriglyceridemia or hyperinsulinemia, so for the elderly, elevated TG levels, decreased HDL levels, and nutritional inadequacy that comes with very-low-fat diets can cause more harm than good [147].

5.5.5 Intermittent Fasting

A key strategy to improve insulin resistance and help prevent onset and progression of metabolic syndrome is weight loss. While regimens such as calorie restriction are common, they are often difficult to maintain. Intermittent fasting has shown promise in achieving weight loss in obese individuals [149]. By reducing energy, amino acids, and carbohydrates, IF (intermittent fasting) has shown to improve cognition and metabolic markers in aging adults [150]. In particular, intermittent fasting has been shown to prompt a "metabolic switch," reducing hepatic glycogen and activating fatty acid mobilization from adipose tissue [151]. As the metabolism is optimized, the patient's weight normalizes while preserving muscle mass, inflammation decreases, and gut microbiome health improves.

5.5.6 Ketogenic Diet

The ketogenic diet has been used successfully in the treatment of obesity and cardiovascular disease. Depending on the genetic makeup of the individual, nutritional ketosis provides an alternative fuel source for cells that no longer respond to the presence of insulin and allows insulin receptors to reset to reduced levels as blood glucose levels decline in the absence of dietary carbohydrates. See Appendix for details on implementing the ketogenic diet.

Table 5.13 summarizes key micronutrients to support endocrine and metabolic health.

5.6 Additional Tools

There are a variety of prognostic tools at a clinician's disposal to help assess a patient's prognosis based on a variety of subjective and objective factors. For a sample of one such calculator (specific for older adults over 70 years old), please see the below link:

E-prognosis calculator:
https://eprognosis.ucsf.edu/calculators/#/

Table 5.13 Micronutrients of primary concern

	MOA	Food sources	RDA for 55+	Side effects/comments for providers
Omega-3	Decreases serum levels of triglycerides, improves endothelial function, decreases resting BP, suppresses acute phase reactants, and resolves inflammation [76]	Flaxseed (oil), chia seeds, walnuts, salmon, canola oil, and sardines	1.6 g M and 1.1 g F (omega-3 fatty acids, 2020)	Preferred source is fatty fish since conversion to EPA/DHA is only 5–8% effective from alpha-linolenic acid which is found in vegetarian sources [152]
B vitamins	Enhances endothelial function	Salmon, leafy greens, liver and other organ meats, eggs, milk, beef, oysters, and legumes	Thiamine, 1 mg Riboflavin, 1.6 mg Niacin, 30 mg Vitamin B6, 3 mg Folate, 400 mcg Vitamin B12, 263 mcg Biotin, 334 mcg Pantothenic acid, 3.3 mg (Lewis, 2013)	Methylated or active forms of B vitamins are preferred for efficacy
Vitamin A	Is an antioxidant, is anti-inflammatory, and supports glucose and insulin homeostasis	Beef liver, sweet potato, spinach, and carrots	700 mcg F and 900 mcg M [105]	In excess: dizziness, nausea, and headaches [105]
Vitamin E	Antioxidant and anti-inflammatory	Red and green pepper, orange juice, orange, grapefruit juice, kiwifruit, and broccoli	200–400 IU [103]	Very high doses may cause blood thinning (1500 IU) [103]
Vitamin K1	Predominant form of vitamin K in diet. Supports endothelial health [153]	Green leafy vegetables	90 mcg F and 120 mcg M [154]	Use with caution with warfarin and similar anticoagulants

(continued)

Table 5.13 (continued)

	MOA	Food sources	RDA for 55+	Side effects/comments for providers
Vitamin K2	Protective mechanisms within CVD, bone development and fractures, chronic kidney disease, and certain cancers [153]	Fermented soy, meat, and dairy produce [153]	180 mcg [155]	MK4 source from gut microbiome, MK7 Not involved in clotting, generally safe for patients on warfarin
Omega-3 fats	Reduces expression of adipose inflammatory genes [141]	Salmon, sardines, trout, oysters, and sea bass [143]	1.3–4 g [142]	Significant changes in body composition, more effective in weight loss if combined with dietary interventions [142]
Fiber	Induces greater satiety, modulates gastric motor function, and blunts postprandial glucose and insulin responses. Postulated effects on gut peptide hormones may prolong meal duration and result in increased mastication [131]	Oat, barley, legumes, peas, beans, broccoli, carrots, root vegetables, and fruits [133]	20–35 g [132]	Minor GI symptoms are flatus, bloating, and abdominal cramping [134]. Insoluble fiber is used as a bulking agent in stool; soluble fiber has favorable effects on glucose and lipid metabolism [131]
Vitamin D	May downregulate the RAAS system and have direct effects on cardiac tissue and vasculature or improvement in glycemic control [67]	Cod liver oil, trout, salmon, mushrooms, and fortified milk [68]	1000 IU daily [67]	Supplementation for cardiovascular disease is controversial. Although observational studies have reported an association between low vitamin D levels and elevated risk of CVD, causation cannot be proven because of unmeasured confounding variables [69]
Vitamin C	Aqueous-phase antioxidant that reduces oxidative stress and enhances endothelial function through effects on nitric oxide production [26]	Red pepper, orange, grapefruit, kiwifruit, green pepper, broccoli, and strawberries [27]	500 mg [26]	Minimum of 8 weeks [26]
Magnesium	Prevents low-grade inflammation and proatherogenic changes [156]	Almonds, spinach, cashews, and peanuts	320 mg F and 420 mg M	May cause anorexia, nausea, vomiting, fatigue, weakness, neurologic changes, arrhythmias, hypocalcemia, and hypokalemia

5.7 Case Studies

5.7.1 Case 1

Steve, a 66-year-old executive with a history of high cholesterol and hypertension, was referred from cardiology after being unable to tolerate three different statins even when administered with coenzyme Q10 200 mg daily. Upon detailed history, the patient was noted to develop hypertension in his mid-50s during a very stressful moment of growth for his company. A year later, he was started on hydrochlorothiazide 25 mg; 2 years later, lisinopril 20 mg was added. Over the last 5 years, he had a gradual increase in LDL. Despite claimed diet change and increased exercise, his LDL has not improved. On presentation, his weight was 194 lbs with height of 6 ft tall, total cholesterol was 245 mg/dl, triglycerides were 174 mg/dl, HDL was 56 mg/dl, and LDL was 154. On review of systems, it was noted that he often has leg cramps, frequent constipation, and trouble falling asleep due to "busy mind."

After detailed lifestyle history, we learned that Steve was not controlling his stress well; he had regular nighttime 2–3 glasses of wine to help him relax after dinner. His diet appeared reasonable, but with detailed discussion, it became clear that he had excess sweets and caffeine, and while his dinners and breakfasts were generally good with the help of his wife, his lunches were often on a go and mostly sandwiches and occasional salads. His exercise was daily 30 min of various *gym* routine but always indoors with little to no daylight exposure, although he was somewhat of a weekend warrior with routine long bike rides on Saturdays or Sundays.

Steve's treatment plan included modification of his diet by decreasing the amount of processed carbohydrates at lunch, choosing salads over sandwiches regularly, and having daily half a cup of organic almonds (part of portfolio diet). He agreed to cut down on alcohol and coffee by 50% and start daily breathing practice at night to help him relax. In addition, we have added red yeast rice 1800 mg in combination with 100 mg of coenzyme Q10 to attempt to bring LDL down. Given elevated triglycerides, we added fish oil 1200 mg of EPA and 500 mg of DHA daily. Given possible subtle signs of magnesium deficiency (leg cramps, constipation, sleep disturbances), we added magnesium citrate 300 mg at bedtime. We also added *Rhodiola* extract 300 mg twice daily 5 days/week during workdays to help Steve handle stress better.

At 3-month follow-up, Steve reported 5-lbs weight loss without trying, resolution of constipation, leg cramps, and much better sleep, but also he has noted that his blood pressure became rather low, and he stopped hydrochlorothiazide after contacting his cardiologist. This is a rather common effect of magnesium deficiency being addressed effectively bringing blood pressure down. His repeat cholesterol revealed total cholesterol of 187 mg/dl, triglycerides of 96 mg/dl, HDL of 52 mg/dl, and LDL of 115.

5.7.2 Case 2

Kate, a 68-year-old retired nurse, self-referred herself to our integrative medicine practice for better management of type 2 diabetes, obesity, hypertension, and anxiety. Kate had diabetes for over 5 years and recently was started on insulin due to persistently high HbA1c over 8.0%. This was a wake-up call for her and she decided to take matters in her hand. On our intake form, she wrote the following in the personal goal section: "to improve diet, supplements to lose weight and get off insulin." Kate expressed frustration that all her prior attempts at managing diabetes without insulin failed; she also grew tired of taking so many supplements and wanted to simplify the regimen.

On presentation, Kate's medication regimen was metformin 1000 mg twice daily, Lantus 24 U at bedtime, ASA 81 mg, losartan 100 mg daily, simvastatin 40 mg, and citalopram 20 mg. Lantus was started 3 months ago and her HgbA1c improved from 8.3% to 6.2%. Her diet consisted of oatmeal with milk and honey for breakfast and salad bowl for lunch, and dinner was lean animal protein mostly from fish or poultry with vegetables, rice, potatoes, or sweet potatoes. She did not snack much but craved sweets with lunch and dinner and usually had dark chocolate after lunch and a piece of fruit before bedtime. She did not drink coffee or soft drinks and had aversion to most spices. Her exercise routine consisted of twice-daily walking her dog for 30 min each time and yoga class for 60 min twice weekly. She also tried to go to the swimming pool weekly for a 60-min slow swim. She volunteered at her church 3 times/week and stated that her life since retirement has been very enjoyable and not stressed. After her own research, she had self-formulated the following supplements and herbs: berberine 200 mg twice daily, cinnamon 500 mg once daily, bitter melon 1000 mg once daily (capsules), gymnema capsules 400 mg once daily, chromium 500 mg once daily, B complex, and coenzyme Q10 100 mg.

On the exam, Kate appeared obese with BMI over 33, and her blood pressure was 150/78. Our initial plan concentrated on diet and optimizing her supplements. We changed Kate's breakfast by increasing protein, rotating breakfast meats/fish, and having Greek or regular yogurt and eggs, when taking oatmeal, adding whey or pea protein powder. We also added regular garlic and broccoli (at least 3 times/week), substituted half of fruits/day with berries, and added beets at least 3 times/week. We asked her to stop bitter melon supplement and instead added it as food as part of salads 2–3 times/week. We consolidated her supplements into one high-quality specially designed multivitamin with B complex and high dose of chromium. We changed her cinnamon from capsules to 1 teaspoon daily mixed with oatmeal, drinks, or any other foods. We increased her berberine to 1 gm twice daily and changed gymnema from capsules to liquid tincture to take 1 ml mixed with water and take with meals. Gymnema makes sweet taste less pleasant and helps to decrease cravings. We also asked her to add matcha green tea ½ teaspoon twice daily and 1 teaspoon of turmeric daily.

Three months later, Kate came back smiling; she was able to cut her insulin dose down to 16 IU and noticed slow but steady weight loss of about 10 lbs. We continued her on this regimen and in addition asked her to purchase a 14-day continuous glucose monitor that identified that rice, sweet potatoes, and regular potatoes that she still had in small amounts have triggered substantial sugar spikes 1–2 h after meals. She subsequently cut those out. Three months later, Kate lost an additional 7 lbs and went off insulin completely. Twelve months later, Kate's BMI was 28 and HgbA1c was 6.7% without the use of insulin.

5.7.3 Case 3

Stan, a 71-year-old photographer, spent most of his retired days traveling the world doing advanced photography, often presenting his art at different shows. Being a perfect picture of health until late 60s, he fully enjoyed his retirement. Despite an excellent lifestyle with little stress, exceptionally balanced diet, and at least 1 h of daily exercise or movement such as photographing nature on foot or kayaking, swimming, and doing the daily Tai Chi routine that he learned over 20 years ago, he developed hypertension. While amlodipine 10 mg controlled his blood pressure well, he wanted to try a more natural approach. On his own accord, he started magnesium oxide 400 mg daily and coenzyme Q10 100 mg but has not noticed any significant changes in his blood pressure that, with amlodipine, stayed mostly around 140 mmHg systolic.

After reviewing his diet, the only change we recommended is to increase his fiber given that he often had days without bowel movements; we also had him change his regular salt to potassium salt with half less sodium. We also asked him to add hibiscus tea and hawthorn tea. The directions were to have 1 glass of each or mixed together 2–3 times/day.

We also changed his magnesium oxide to magnesium citrate which helps to maintain more regular bowel movements.

At follow-up, Stan reported that his blood pressure has been mostly under 130 mmHg systolic and he wanted to try to cut down on amlodipine. Eight weeks later, his blood pressure remained in 130–140 mmHg systolic despite cutting dose of amlodipine in half down to 5 mg. At the next follow-up, Stan wanted to try an even more aggressive approach to see if he can stop amlodipine all together. To attempt this, we added powdered L-arginine 3 gm and L-citrulline 3 gm mixed together with hibiscus or hawthorn teas 2–3 times/day. This further lowered blood pressure down to under 130 mmHg systolic, and in 3 months despite being off amlodipine, Stan's blood pressure maintained steady under 140 mmHg systolic, considered at goal for his age. Readers may question the complexity of this treatment and concern of cost and needing to take several different powders and supplements. However, this regimen completely resolved Stan's slow bowel movements and was an important personal achievement for him.

References

1. Ayan M, Pothineni NV, Siraj A, Mehta JL. Cardiac drug therapy-considerations in the elderly. J Geriatr Cardiol. 2016;13(12):992–7.
2. Cholesterol drugs for people 75 and older [Internet]. Choosing Wisely. 2014 [cited 2021 Jan 16]. Available from: https://www.choosingwisely.org/patient-resources/cholesterol-drugs-for-people-75-and-older/.
3. May Clinic Staff. Statin side effects: weigh the benefits and risks [Internet]. May Clini. 2020 [cited 2021 Jan 16]. Available from: https://www.mayoclinic.org/diseases-conditions/high-blood-cholesterol/in-depth/statin-side-effects/art-20046013.
4. Félix-Redondo FJ, Grau M, Fernández-Bergés D. Cholesterol and cardiovascular disease in the elderly. Facts and gaps. Aging Dis. 2013;4(3):154–69.
5. Spence JD. Diet for stroke prevention. Stroke Vasc Neurol. 2018;3(2):44–50.
6. Hankey GJ. Vitamin supplementation and stroke prevention. Stroke. 2012;43(10):2814–8.
7. Benzie IFF. Cardiovascular disease. In: Wachtel-Galor S, editor. Herbal medicine: biomolecular and clinical aspects. 2nd ed. Boca Raton; Taylor and Francis Group, LLC. 2011.
8. Casas R, Estruch R, Sacanella E. Influence of bioactive nutrients on the atherosclerotic process: a review. Nutrients. 2018;10(11):1630. https://doi.org/10.3390/nu10111630.
9. Moss JWE, Ramji DP. Nutraceutical therapies for atherosclerosis. Nat Rev Cardiol. 2016;13(9):513–32.
10. Orekhov AN, Sobenin IA, Korneev NV, Kirichenko TV, Myasoedova VA, Melnichenko AA, et al. Anti-atherosclerotic therapy based on botanicals. Recent Pat Cardiovasc Drug Discov. 2013;8(1):56–66.
11. Kelly RB. Diet and exercise in the management of hyperlipidemia. Am Fam Physician. 2010;81(9):1097–102.
12. Rouhi-Boroujeni H, Rouhi-Boroujeni H, Heidarian E, Mohammadizadeh F, Rafieian-Kopaei M. Herbs with anti-lipid effects and their interactions with statins as a chemical anti- hyperlipidemia group drugs: a systematic review. ARYA Atheroscler. 2015;11(4):244–51.
13. Whelton PK, Carey RM, Aronow WS, Casey DE, Collins KJ, Dennison Himmelfarb C, et al. 2017 ACC/AHA/AAPA/ABC/ACPM/AGS/APHA/ASH/ASPC/NMA/PCNA guideline for the prevention, detection, evaluation, and management of high blood pressure in adults: a report of the American College of Cardiology/American Heart Association task force on clinical practice guidelines. Hypertension. 2018;71(6):1269–1324. https://doi.org/10.1161/HYP.0000000000000066.
14. Kogan M, Weil A. Cardiovascular disease. In: Wiley, editor. Integrative geriatric medicine; Oxford University Press. New York. 2017. p. 228.
15. Agarwala A. Older adults and hypertension: beyond the 2017 guideline for prevention, detection, evaluation, and management of high blood pressure in adults [Internet]. American College of Cardiology. 2020 [cited 2021 Jan 13]. Available from: https://www.acc.org/latest-in-cardiology/articles/2020/02/26/06/24/older-adults-and-hypertension.
16. USDA. Dietary guide for Americans [Internet]. US Department of Health and Human Services. 2020 [cited 2021 Jan 1]. Available from: https://health.gov/our-work/food-nutrition/previous-dietary-guidelines/2015.
17. Wergin A. Is sea salt healthier than table salt? [Internet]. Mayo Clinic Health System. 2015 [cited 2021 Jan 17]. Available from: https://www.mayoclinichealthsystem.org/hometown-health/speaking-of-health/is-sea-salt-healthier-than-table-salt#:~:text=The%20main%20differences%20between%20sea,from%20which%20it%20is%20evaporated.
18. Pizzorno NDJE Jr, Murphy NDMT, Joiner-Bey NDH. The Clinician's Handbook of Natural Medicine. 3rd ed. Elsevier; St Louis, Missouri. 2016.
19. Staruschenko A. Beneficial effects of high potassium. Hypertension. 2018;71(6):1015–22.
20. He FJ, Markandu ND, Coltart R, Barron J, MacGregor GA. Effect of short-term supplementation of potassium chloride and potassium citrate on blood pressure in hypertensives. Hypertension. 2005;45(4):571–4.

21. Houston M. The role of magnesium in hypertension and cardiovascular disease. J Clin Hypertens (Greenwich). 2011;13(11):843–7.
22. NIH. Magnesium [Internet]. National Institutes of Health Office of Dietary Supplements. 2020 [cited 2020 Dec 30]. Available from: https://ods.od.nih.gov/factsheets/Magnesium-HealthProfessional/#:~:text=Magnesium%20is%20widely%20distributed%20in,cereals%20and%20other%20fortified%20foods.
23. Villa-Etchegoyen C, Lombarte M, Matamoros N, Belizán JM, Cormick G. Mechanisms involved in the relationship between low calcium intake and high blood pressure. Nutrients. 2019;11(5):1112. https://doi.org/10.3390/nu11051112.
24. Cormick G, Ciapponi A, Cafferata M, Belizan JM. Extra Calcium to prevent high blood pressure. Cochrane Libr [Internet]. 2015 Jun 30 [cited 2020 Dec 30]; Available from: https://www.cochrane.org/CD010037/HTN_extra-calcium-to-prevent-high-blood-pressure.
25. Cormick G, Belizán JM. Calcium intake and health. Nutrients. 2019;11(7):1606. https://doi.org/10.3390/nu11071606.
26. Juraschek SP, Guallar E, Appel LJ, Miller ER. Effects of vitamin C supplementation on blood pressure: a meta-analysis of randomized controlled trials. Am J Clin Nutr. 2012;95(5):1079–88.
27. NIH. Vitamin C [Internet]. National Institutes of Health Office of Dietary Supplements. 2020 [cited 2020 Dec 30]. Available from: https://ods.od.nih.gov/factsheets/VitaminC-HealthProfessional/.
28. McRae MP. High-dose folic acid supplementation effects on endothelial function and blood pressure in hypertensive patients: a meta-analysis of randomized controlled clinical trials. J Chiropr Med. 2009;8(1):15–24.
29. NIH. Folate [Internet]. National Institutes of Health Office of Dietary Supplements. 2020 [cited 2020 Dec 30]. Available from: https://ods.od.nih.gov/factsheets/Folate-HealthProfessional/.
30. Wang W-W, Wang X-S, Zhang Z-R, He J-C, Xie C-L. A meta-analysis of folic acid in combination with anti-hypertension drugs in patients with hypertension and hyperhomocysteinemia. Front Pharmacol. 2017;8:585.
31. Dakshinamurti S, Dakshinamurti K. Antihypertensive and neuroprotective actions of pyridoxine and its derivatives. Can J Physiol Pharmacol. 2015;93(12):1083–90.
32. Aybak M, Sermet A, Ayyildiz MO, Karakilçik AZ. Effect of oral pyridoxine hydrochloride supplementation on arterial blood pressure in patients with essential hypertension. Arzneimittelforschung. 1995;45(12):1271–3.
33. NIH. Vitamin B6 [Internet]. National Institutes of Health Office of Dietary Supplements. 2020 [cited 2020 Dec 30]. Available from: https://ods.od.nih.gov/factsheets/VitaminB6-HealthProfessional/#:~:text=The%20richest%20sources%20of%20vitamin,1%2C3%2C5%5D.
34. Cabo J, Alonso R, Mata P. Omega-3 fatty acids and blood pressure. Br J Nutr. 2012;107 Suppl 2:S195–200.
35. Filipovic MG, Aeschbacher S, Reiner MF, Stivala S, Gobbato S, Bonetti N, et al. Whole blood omega-3 fatty acid concentrations are inversely associated with blood pressure in young, healthy adults. J Hypertens. 2018;36(7):1548–54.
36. Vasdev S, Gill V. The antihypertensive effect of arginine. Int J Angiol. 2008;17(1):7–22.
37. Oh J-Y, Je J-G, Lee H-G, Kim E-A, Kang SI, Lee J-S, et al. Anti-hypertensive activity of novel peptides identified from olive flounder (Paralichthys olivaceus) surimi. Foods. 2020;9(5):647. https://doi.org/10.3390/foods9050647.
38. Ibrahim HR, Ahmed AS, Miyata T. Novel angiotensin-converting enzyme inhibitory peptides from caseins and whey proteins of goat milk. J Adv Res. 2017;8(1):63–71.
39. Miguel M, Aleixandre A. Antihypertensive peptides derived from egg proteins. J Nutr. 2006;136(6):1457–60. https://doi.org/10.1093/jn/136.6.1457.
40. Abachi S, Bazinet L, Beaulieu L. Antihypertensive and angiotensin-I-converting enzyme (ACE)-inhibitory peptides from fish as potential cardioprotective compounds. Mar Drugs. 2019;17(11):613. https://doi.org/10.3390/md17110613.

41. Ho MJ, Li ECK, Wright JM. Blood pressure lowering efficacy of coenzyme Q10 for primary hypertension. Cochrane Database Syst Rev. 2016;3:CD007435.
42. Saini R. Coenzyme Q10: the essential nutrient. J Pharm Bioallied Sci. 2011;3(3):466–7.
43. Lockyer S, Yaqoob P, Spencer JPE, Rowland I. Olive leaf phenolics and cardiovascular risk reduction: physiological effects and mechanisms of action. NUA. 2012;1(2):125–40.
44. Tassell MC, Kingston R, Gilroy D, Lehane M, Furey A. Hawthorn (Crataegus spp.) in the treatment of cardiovascular disease. Pharmacogn Rev. 2010;4(7):32–41.
45. Walker AF, Marakis G, Morris AP, Robinson PA. Promising hypotensive effect of hawthorn extract: a randomized double-blind pilot study of mild, essential hypertension. Phytother Res. 2002;16(1):48–54.
46. NIH. Hawthorn [Internet]. NIH National Center for Complementary and Integrative Health. 2020 [cited 2020 Dec 31]. Available from: https://www.nccih.nih.gov/health/hawthorn.
47. Ried K, Travica N, Sali A. The effect of kyolic aged garlic extract on gut microbiota, inflammation, and cardiovascular markers in hypertensives: the gargic trial. Front Nutr. 2018;5:122.
48. Ried K, Frank OR, Stocks NP. Aged garlic extract reduces blood pressure in hypertensives: a dose-response trial. Eur J Clin Nutr. 2013;67(1):64–70.
49. Da-Costa-Rocha I, Bonnlaender B, Sievers H, Pischel I, Heinrich M. Hibiscus sabdariffa L. - a phytochemical and pharmacological review. Food Chem. 2014;165:424–43.
50. Jalalyazdi M, Ramezani J, Izadi-Moud A, Madani-Sani F, Shahlaei S, Ghiasi SS. Effect of hibiscus sabdariffa on blood pressure in patients with stage 1 hypertension. J Adv Pharm Technol Res. 2019;10(3):107–11.
51. Khalaf D, Krüger M, Wehland M, Infanger M, Grimm D. The effects of oral l-arginine and l-citrulline supplementation on blood pressure. Nutrients. 2019;11(7):1679. https://doi.org/10.3390/nu11071679.
52. Corella D, Ordovas JM. Nutrigenomics in cardiovascular medicine. Circ Cardiovasc Genet. 2009;2(6):637–51.
53. Raman K, Chong M, Akhtar-Danesh G-G, D'Mello M, Hasso R, Ross S, et al. Genetic markers of inflammation and their role in cardiovascular disease. Can J Cardiol. 2013;29(1):67–74.
54. Aday AW, Ridker PM. Antiinflammatory therapy in clinical care: the CANTOS trial and beyond. Front Cardiovasc Med. 2018;5:62.
55. Johns Hopkins Medicine. Fight inflammation to help prevent heart disease [Internet]. Hopkins Medicine. 2021 [cited 2021 Jan 17]. Available from: https://www.hopkinsmedicine.org/health/wellness-and-prevention/fight-inflammation-to-help-prevent-heart-disease.
56. Ordovas JM, Ferguson LR, Tai ES, Mathers JC. Personalised nutrition and health. BMJ. 2018;361:bmj.k2173.
57. Merched AJ, Chan L. Nutrigenetics and nutrigenomics of atherosclerosis. Curr Atheroscler Rep. 2013;15(6):328.
58. Huang C-J, McAllister MJ, Slusher AL, Webb HE, Mock JT, Acevedo EO. Obesity-related oxidative stress: the impact of physical activity and diet manipulation. Sports Med Open. 2015;1(1):32.
59. Neelakantan N, Seah JYH, van Dam RM. The effect of coconut oil consumption on cardiovascular risk factors: a systematic review and meta-analysis of clinical trials. Circulation. 2020;141(10):803–14.
60. Weil A, Kogan M. Cardiovascular disease. In: Integrative geriatric nutrition; Oxford University Press. New York. 2017. p. 229–30.
61. Rosique-Esteban N, Guasch-Ferré M, Hernández-Alonso P, Salas-Salvadó J. Dietary magnesium and cardiovascular disease: a review with emphasis in epidemiological studies. Nutrients. 2018;10(2):168. https://doi.org/10.3390/nu10020168.
62. Zozina VI, Covantev S, Goroshko OA, Krasnykh LM, Kukes VG. Coenzyme Q10 in cardiovascular and metabolic diseases: current state of the problem. Curr Cardiol Rev. 2018;14(3):164–74.
63. Li Y, Huang T, Zheng Y, Muka T, Troup J, Hu FB. Folic acid supplementation and the risk of cardiovascular diseases: a meta-analysis of randomized controlled trials. J Am Heart Assoc. 2016;5(8): e003768. https://doi.org/10.1161/JAHA.116.003768.

64. Pawlak R. Is vitamin B12 deficiency a risk factor for cardiovascular disease in vegetarians? Am J Prev Med. 2015;48(6):e11–26.

65. Collaboration HLT. Lowering blood homocysteine with folic acid based supplements: meta-analysis of randomised trials. BMJ. 1998;316(7135):894–8.

66. Vitamin B12 [Internet]. NIH National Institutes of Health Office of Dietary Supplements. 2020 [cited 2021 Jan 2]. Available from: https://ods.od.nih.gov/factsheets/VitaminB12-HealthProfessional/.

67. Judd SE, Tangpricha V. Vitamin D deficiency and risk for cardiovascular disease. Am J Med Sci. 2009;338(1):40–4.

68. NIH. Vitamin D [Internet]. NIH National Institutes of Health Office of Dietary Suppolements. 2020 [cited 2020 Dec 31]. Available from: https://ods.od.nih.gov/factsheets/VitaminD-HealthProfessional/.

69. Barbarawi M, Kheiri B, Zayed Y, Barbarawi O, Dhillon H, Swaid B, et al. Vitamin D supplementation and cardiovascular disease risks in more than 83 000 individuals in 21 randomized clinical trials: a meta-analysis. JAMA Cardiol. 2019;4(8):765–76.

70. Piazza G. How too little potassium may contribute to cardiovascular disease [Internet]. NIH National Institues of Health. 2017 [cited 2021 Jan 2]. Available from: https://www.nih.gov/news-events/nih-research-matters/how-too-little-potassium-may-contribute-cardiovascular-disease.

71. WHO. Increasing potassium intake to reduce blood pressure and risk of cardiovascular diseases in adults [Internet]. World Health Organization. 2019 [cited 2021 Jan 1]. Available from: https://www.who.int/elena/titles/potassium_cvd_adults/en/#:~:text=WHO%20recommends%20an%20increase%20in,mg%2Fday)%20for%20adults.

72. Aburto NJ, Hanson S, Gutierrez H, Hooper L, Elliott P, Cappuccio FP. Effect of increased potassium intake on cardiovascular risk factors and disease: systematic review and meta-analyses. BMJ. 2013;346:f1378.

73. Machha A, Schechter AN. Inorganic nitrate: a major player in the cardiovascular health benefits of vegetables? Nutr Rev. 2012;70(6):367–72.

74. Wang Z-Y, Liu Y-Y, Liu G-H, Lu H-B, Mao C-Y. l-Carnitine and heart disease. Life Sci. 2018;194:88–97.

75. NIH. Carnitine [Internet]. NIH National Institutes of Health Office of Dietary Supplements. 2017 [cited 2021 Jan 2]. Available from: https://ods.od.nih.gov/factsheets/Carnitine-HealthProfessional/.

76. Mohebi-Nejad A, Bikdeli B. Omega-3 supplements and cardiovascular diseases. Tanaffos. 2014;13(1):6–14.

77. Shecterle LM, Terry KR, St Cyr JA. Potential clinical benefits of D-ribose in ischemic cardiovascular disease. Cureus. 2018;10(3):e2291.

78. Wu B, Wei Y, Wang Y, Su T, Zhou L, Liu Y, et al. Gavage of D-Ribose induces Aβ-like deposits, Tau hyperphosphorylation as well as memory loss and anxiety-like behavior in mice. Oncotarget. 2015;6(33):34128–42.

79. Mayo Clinic Staff. Red yeast rice [Internet]. Mayo Clinic. 2020 [cited 2021 Jan 1]. Available from: https://www.mayoclinic.org/drugs-supplements-red-yeast-rice/art-20363074.

80. Roth EM, Moriarty P, Li S, Duan Z, Guo S, Liu P, et al. Abstract 11306: red yeast rice extract shows equivalency to statins. Circulation. 2018;128. https://www.ahajournals.org / https://doi.org/10.1161/circ.128.suppl_22.A11306.

81. Li Y, Jiang L, Jia Z, Xin W, Yang S, Yang Q, et al. A meta-analysis of red yeast rice: an effective and relatively safe alternative approach for dyslipidemia. PLoS One. 2014;9(6):e98611.

82. Iskandar I, Harahap Y, Wijayanti TR, Sandra M, Prasaja B, Cahyaningsih P. Efficacy and tolerability of a nutraceutical combination of red yeast rice, guggulipid, and chromium picolinate evaluated in a randomized, placebo-controlled, double-blind study. Complement Ther Med. 2020;48:102282.

83. Gersh BJ. Use of herbal products and potential interactions in patients with cardiovascular diseases. Yearbook of Cardiology. 2012;2012:282–4.

84. Wojtyniak K, Szymański M, Matławska I. Leonurus cardiaca L. (motherwort): a review of its phytochemistry and pharmacology. Phytother Res. 2013;27(8):1115–20.

85. Dudzińska D, Boncler M, Watala C. The cardioprotective power of leaves. Arch Med Sci. 2015;11(4):819–39.

86. Raspberryleaf(Herb/Supplement)[Internet].Medscape.2021[cited2021Jan16].Availablefrom: https://reference.medscape.com/drug/red-raspberry-rubus-idaeus-raspberry-leaf-344515.

87. Greenfield R. Red raspberry leaf [Internet]. Andrew Weil, MD. 2016 [cited 2021 Jan 16]. Available from: https://www.drweil.com/vitamins-supplements-herbs/herbs/red-raspberry-leaf/.

88. Maslova LV, Kondrat'ev BI, Maslov LN, Lishmanov IB. [The cardioprotective and antiadrenergic activity of an extract of Rhodiola rosea in stress]. Eksp Klin Farmakol. 1994;57(6):61–3.

89. What is Rhodiola Rosea? [Internet]. Examine. 2021 [cited 2021 Jan 16]. Available from: https://examine.com/supplements/rhodiola-rosea/.

90. NIH. Rhodiola [Internet]. NIH Nataionl Center for Complementary and Integrative Health. 2020 [cited 2021 Jan 16]. Available from: https://www.nccih.nih.gov/health/rhodiola.

91. NIH. Thiamin [Internet]. National Institues of Health Office of Dietary Supplements. 2020 [cited 2021 Jan 16]. Available from: https://ods.od.nih.gov/factsheets/Thiamin-HealthProfessional/#:~:text=Food%20sources%20of%20thiamin%20include,major%20source%20of%20the%20vitamin.

92. Saunders PR. Cocoa drink improves walking distance in those with peripheral artery disease . Natural Medicine Journal [Internet]. 2020 Jun [cited 2021 Feb 4];12(6). Available from: https://www.naturalmedicinejournal.com/journal/2020-06/cocoa-drink-improves-walking-distance-those-peripheral-artery-disease.

93. Mietus-Snyder ML, Shigenaga MK, Suh JH, Shenvi SV, Lal A, McHugh T, et al. A nutrient-dense, high-fiber, fruit-based supplement bar increases HDL cholesterol, particularly large HDL, lowers homocysteine, and raises glutathione in a 2-wk trial. FASEB J. 2012;26(8):3515–27.

94. Satija A, Hu FB. Cardiovascular benefits of dietary fiber. Curr Atheroscler Rep. 2012;14(6):505–14.

95. McRae MP. Dietary fiber is beneficial for the prevention of cardiovascular disease: an umbrella review of meta-analyses. J Chiropr Med. 2017;16(4):289–99.

96. Hershman J. Overview of the thyroid gland [Internet]. Merck Mnual Consumer Version. 2020 [cited 2021 Jan 31]. Available from: https://www.merckmanuals.com/home/hormonal-and-metabolic-disorders/thyroid-gland-disorders/overview-of-the-thyroid-gland#:~:text=The%20thyroid%20gland%20secretes%20thyroid,of%20oxygen%20that%20cells%20use.

97. Ajish TP, Jayakumar RV. Geriatric thyroidology: an update. Indian J Endocrinol Metab. 2012;16(4):542–7.

98. Surks M. Clinical manifestations of hypothyroidism [Internet]. UpToDate. 2020 [cited 2021 Feb 3]. Available from: https://www.uptodate.com/contents/clinical-manifestations-of-hypothyroidism?search=hypothyroid&source=search_result&selectedTitle=3~150&usage_type=default&display_rank=3#H1.

99. Ross MD DS. Overview of the clinical manifestations of hyperthyroid in adults [Internet]. UpToDate. 2020 [cited 2021 Feb 3]. Available from: https://www.uptodate.com/contents/overview-of-the-clinical-manifestations-of-hyperthyroidism-in-adults?search=hyperthyroid%20hypothyroid&source=search_result&selectedTitle=1~150&usage_type=default&display_rank=1#H17.

100. Ross D. Laboratory assessment of thyroid function [Internet]. UpToDate. 2019 [cited 2021 Feb 3]. Available from: https://www.uptodate.com/contents/laboratory-assessment-of-thyroid-function?search=hyperthyroid%20hypothyroid&source=search_result&selectedTitle=5~150&usage_type=default&display_rank=5.

101. Mount Sinai. Tyrosine [Internet]. Mount Sinai Health Library. 2021 [cited 2021 Jan 30]. Available from: https://www.mountsinai.org/health-library/supplement/tyrosine#:~:text=Dietary%20Sources,pumpkin%20seeds%2C%20and%20sesame%20seeds..

102. Institute of Medicine (US) Panel on Micronutrients. Dietary reference intakes for vitamin a, vitamin K, arsenic, boron, chromium, copper, iodine, iron, manganese, molybdenum, nickel, silicon, vanadium, and zinc. Washington (DC): National Academies Press (US); 2001.

103. NIH. Vitamin E [Internet]. NIH Office of Dietary Supplements. 2020 [cited 2021 Jan 30]. Available from: https://ods.od.nih.gov/factsheets/VitaminE-HealthProfessional/.

104. Farhangi MA, Keshavarz SA, Eshraghian M, Ostadrahimi A, Saboor-Yaraghi AA. The effect of vitamin A supplementation on thyroid function in premenopausal women. J Am Coll Nutr. 2012;31(4):268–74.

105. NIH. Vitamin A [Internet]. Vitamin A. 2020 [cited 2021 Jan 30]. Available from: https://ods.od.nih.gov/factsheets/VitaminA-HealthProfessional/.

106. Kennedy DO. B vitamins and the brain: mechanisms, dose and efficacy – a review. Nutrients. 2016;8(2):68.

107. NIH. Selenium [Internet]. NIH Office of Dietary Supplements. 2020 [cited 2021 Jan 30]. Available from: https://ods.od.nih.gov/factsheets/Selenium-HealthProfessional/.

108. Lee W-H, Loo C-Y, Bebawy M, Luk F, Mason RS, Rohanizadeh R. Curcumin and its derivatives: their application in neuropharmacology and neuroscience in the 21st century. Curr Neuropharmacol. 2013;11(4):338–78.

109. Hewlings SJ, Kalman DS. Curcumin: a review of its effects on human health. Foods (Basel, Switzerland). 2017;6(10):92. https://doi.org/10.3390/foods6100092.

110. Panda S, Kar A. Changes in thyroid hormone concentrations after administration of ashwagandha root extract to adult male mice. J Pharm Pharmacol. 1998;50(9):1065–8.

111. Leung E, Wongrakpanich S, Munshi MN. Diabetes management in the elderly. Diabetes Spectr. 2018;31(3):245–53.

112. Grandner MA, Patel NP, Perlis ML, Gehrman PR, Xie D, Sha D, et al. Obesity, diabetes, and exercise associated with sleep-related complaints in the American population. Z Gesundh Wiss. 2011;19(5):463–74.

113. Pizzorno J. Mitochondria-fundamental to life and health. Integr Med (Encinitas). 2014;13(2):8–15.

114. Venkatasamy VV, Pericherla S, Manthuruthil S, Mishra S, Hanno R. Effect of physical activity on insulin resistance, inflammation and oxidative stress in diabetes mellitus. J Clin Diagn Res. 2013;7(8):1764–6.

115. Weil A. Endocrine disorders. Integrative geriatric medicine. Oxford; Oxford University Press. 2017. p. 254.

116. Yin J, Xing H, Ye J. Efficacy of berberine in patients with type 2 diabetes mellitus. Metab Clin Exp. 2008;57(5):712–7.

117. Kesika P, Sivamaruthi BS, Chaiyasut C. Do probiotics improve the health status of individuals with diabetes mellitus? A review on outcomes of clinical trials. Biomed Res Int. 2019;2019:1531567.

118. Syngai GG, Gopi R, Bharali R, Dey S, Lakshmanan GMA, Ahmed G. Probiotics - the versatile functional food ingredients. J Food Sci Technol. 2016;53(2):921–33.

119. Kanetkar P, Singhal R, Kamat M. Gymnema sylvestre: a memoir. J Clin Biochem Nutr. 2007;41(2):77–81.

120. Tiwari P, Mishra BN, Sangwan NS. Phytochemical and pharmacological properties of Gymnema sylvestre: an important medicinal plant. Biomed Res Int. 2014;2014:830285.

121. Kawatra P, Rajagopalan R. Cinnamon: mystic powers of a minute ingredient. Pharm Res. 2015;7(Suppl 1):S1–6.

122. NIH. Carnitine [Internet]. NIH Office of Dietary Supplements. 2017 [cited 2021 Jan 29]. Available from: https://ods.od.nih.gov/factsheets/Carnitine-HealthProfessional/#:~:text=Carnitine%20plays%20a%20critical%20role,organelle%20to%20prevent%20their%20accumulation.

123. Maret W. Chromium supplementation in human health, metabolic syndrome, and diabetes. Met Ions Life Sci. 2019;19. /books/9783110527872/9783110527872-015/9783110527872-015.xml. https://doi.org/10.1515/9783110527872-015.

124. Yagi A, Hegazy S, Kabbash A, Wahab EA-E. Possible hypoglycemic effect of Aloe vera L. high molecular weight fractions on type 2 diabetic patients. Saudi Pharm J. 2009;17(3):209–15.
125. Alam MA, Uddin R, Subhan N, Rahman MM, Jain P, Reza HM. Beneficial role of bitter melon supplementation in obesity and related complications in metabolic syndrome. J Lipids. 2015;2015:496169.
126. Flicker L, McCaul KA, Hankey GJ, Jamrozik K, Brown WJ, Byles JE, et al. Body mass index and survival in men and women aged 70 to 75. J Am Geriatr Soc. 2010;58(2):234–41.
127. Halford JCG, Harrold JA, Lawton CL, Blundell JE. Serotonin (5-HT) drugs: effects on appetite expression and use for the treatment of obesity. Curr Drug Targets. 2005;6(2):201–13.
128. Cangiano C, Ceci F, Cascino A, Del Ben M, Laviano A, Muscaritoli M, et al. Eating behavior and adherence to dietary prescriptions in obese adult subjects treated with 5-hydroxytryptophan. Am J Clin Nutr. 1992;56(5):863–7.
129. Briguglio M, Dell'Osso B, Panzica G, Malgaroli A, Banfi G, Zanaboni Dina C, et al. Dietary neurotransmitters: a narrative review on current knowledge. Nutrients. 2018;10(5):591. https://doi.org/10.3390/nu10050591.
130. Metagenics. Ultra glucose control: support for the nutritional management of glucose response [Internet]. Metagenics. 2021 [cited 2021 Jan 4]. Available from: https://www.metagenics.com/ultra-glucose-control.
131. Papathanasopoulos A, Camilleri M. Dietary fiber supplements: effects in obesity and metabolic syndrome and relationship to gastrointestinal functions. Gastroenterology. 2010;138(1):65–72.e1.
132. Lyon MR, Kacinik V. Is there a place for dietary fiber supplements in weight management? Curr Obes Rep. 2012;1(2):59–67.
133. Akbar A, Shreenath AP. High Fiber diet. StatPearls. Treasure Island (FL): StatPearls Publishing; 2020.
134. Bliss DZ, Savik K, Jung H-JG, Whitebird R, Lowry A. Symptoms associated with dietary fiber supplementation over time in individuals with fecal incontinence. Nurs Res. 2011;60(3 Suppl):S58–67.
135. Krotkiewski M. Effect of guar gum on body-weight, hunger ratings and metabolism in obese subjects. Br J Nutr. 1984;52(1):97–105.
136. Mudgil D, Barak S, Khatkar BS. Guar gum: processing, properties and food applications-a review. J Food Sci Technol. 2014;51(3):409–18.
137. Yasukawa Z, Inoue R, Ozeki M, Okubo T, Takagi T, Honda A, et al. Effect of repeated consumption of partially hydrolyzed guar gum on fecal characteristics and gut microbiota: a randomized, double-blind, placebo-controlled, and parallel-group clinical trial. Nutrients. 2019;11(9):2170. https://doi.org/10.3390/nu11092170.
138. Onakpoya I, Posadzki P, Ernst E. Chromium supplementation in overweight and obesity: a systematic review and meta-analysis of randomized clinical trials. Obes Rev. 2013;14(6):496–507.
139. St-Onge M-P, Bosarge A. Weight-loss diet that includes consumption of medium-chain triacylglycerol oil leads to a greater rate of weight and fat mass loss than does olive oil. Am J Clin Nutr. 2008;87(3):621–6.
140. Onakpoya I, Hung SK, Perry R, Wider B, Ernst E. The use of garcinia extract (hydroxycitric acid) as a weight loss supplement: a systematic review and meta-analysis of randomised clinical trials. J Obes. 2011;2011:509038.
141. Maggio M, Artoni A, Lauretani F, Borghi L, Nouvenne A, Valenti G, et al. The impact of omega-3 fatty acids on osteoporosis. Curr Pharm Des. 2009;15(36):4157–64.
142. Albracht-Schulte K, Kalupahana NS, Ramalingam L, Wang S, Rahman SM, Robert-McComb J, et al. Omega-3 fatty acids in obesity and metabolic syndrome: a mechanistic update. J Nutr Biochem. 2018;58:1–16.
143. NIH. Omega-3 fatty acids [Internet]. NIH Office of Dietary Supplements. 2020 [cited 2021 Mar 4]. Available from: https://ods.od.nih.gov/factsheets/Omega3FattyAcids-HealthProfessional/.

144. Turner-McGrievy G, Harris M. Key elements of plant-based diets associated with reduced risk of metabolic syndrome. Curr Diab Rep. 2014;14(9):524.
145. Bournat JC, Brown CW. Mitochondrial dysfunction in obesity. Curr Opin Endocrinol Diabetes Obes. 2010;17(5):446–52.
146. Sampson MT. Little known type of cholesterol may pose the greatest heart disease risk [Internet]. ACS. 2009 [cited 2021 Feb 4]. Available from: https://www.acs.org/content/acs/en/pressroom/newsreleases/2009/august/little-known-type-of-cholesterol-may-pose-the-greatest-heart-disease-risk.html.
147. Lichtenstein AH, Van Horn L. Very low fat diets. Circulation. 1998;98(9):935–9.
148. NIH. DASH Eating Plan [Internet]. NIH National Heart, Lung, and Blood Institute. 2020 [cited 2020 Dec 31]. Available from: https://www.nhlbi.nih.gov/health-topics/dash-eating-plan.
149. Welton S, Minty R, O'Driscoll T, Willms H, Poirier D, Madden S, et al. Intermittent fasting and weight loss: systematic review. Can Fam Physician. 2020;66(2):117–25.
150. Ooi TC, Meramat A, Rajab NF, Shahar S, Ismail IS, Azam AA, et al. Intermittent fasting enhanced the cognitive function in older adults with mild cognitive impairment by inducing biochemical and metabolic changes: a 3-year progressive study. Nutrients. 2020;12(9):2644. https://doi.org/10.3390/nu12092644.
151. Anton SD, Moehl K, Donahoo WT, Marosi K, Lee SA, Mainous AG, et al. Flipping the metabolic switch: understanding and applying the health benefits of fasting. Obesity (Silver Spring). 2018;26(2):254–68.
152. Nettleton JA. Omega-3 fatty acids: comparison of plant and seafood sources in human nutrition. J Am Diet Assoc. 1991;91(3):331–7.
153. Rynders CA, Thomas EA, Zaman A, Pan Z, Catenacci VA, Melanson EL. Effectiveness of intermittent fasting and time-restricted feeding compared to continuous energy restriction for weight loss. Nutrients. 2019;11(10):2442. https://doi.org/10.3390/nu11102442.
154. Schwalfenberg GK. Vitamins K1 and K2: the emerging group of vitamins required for human health. J Nutr Metab. 2017;2017:6254836.
155. Patti AM, Al-Rasadi K, Giglio RV, Nikolic D, Mannina C, Castellino G, et al. Natural approaches in metabolic syndrome management. Arch Med Sci. 2018;14(2):422–41.
156. Dibaba DT, Xun P, Fly AD, Yokota K, He K. Dietary magnesium intake and risk of metabolic syndrome: a meta-analysis. Diabet Med. 2014;31(11):1301–9.

Chapter 6
Skin, Lung, Eyes, and Hair

Contents

6.1 Skin

The relationship between gut health and skin health is seen clinically as gut-healing efforts are manifested in improvements in skin health. Thus, all efforts to heal the skin must include attention to the gut, even in the absence of gastrointestinal symptoms. Additionally, observations of skin health can be a reliable nutritional evaluation tool as outlined in Table 6.1:

Table 6.1 Common skin conditions and associated nutritional status [1]

Indication	Nutrition deficiency	Nutritional approach	Comments
Tongue (inflamed, coated, bald, slick, red)	Niacin, digestive enzymes, probiotics, fiber, B vitamins, iron, and folate	Brewer's yeast, rice, and wheat bran, liver, peanuts, sesame and sunflower seeds, oysters, white beans, dark chocolate, lentils, breakfast cereals, spinach, black-eyed peas, asparagus, clams, trout, salmon, tuna, nutritional yeast, and chicken	Glossitis is generally benign, with any identifiable causes reversible with appropriate nutritional supplementation. If there is any question of malignancy, area should be biopsied so as not to delay treatment [2]. Consider Crohn's
Mouth (cheilosis)	Riboflavin, iron, niacin, and pyridoxine	Oysters, white beans, dark chocolate, beef liver, lentils, spinach, tofu, brewer's yeast, almonds, wheat germ, rice, breakfast cereals, and chicken	Especially likely in older individuals wearing dentures [3]
Ears (hard earwax, vertical lobe crease, sound sensitivity, and tinnitus)	Omega-3, magnesium, B complex, CoQ10, zinc, niacinamide, and pyridoxine	Fatty fish, leafy greens, oysters, nuts, pumpkin seeds, ginger, kelp, molasses, buckwheat, wheat, clams, liver, trout, salmon, tuna, nutritional yeast, beef, crab, flaxseed, and chia	Allergies, cardiovascular risk [4], and TMJ disorder
Eyes (burning, itching, bloodshot, dry, soft cornea, xerosis, eyelid pallor, copper ring of iris, vision dysfunction)	Riboflavin, vitamin A, zinc, iron, omega-3, thiamine, folate, B12, and niacin	Liver, chili peppers, dandelion root, carrots, dried apricots, leafy greens, breakfast cereals, oysters, white beans, chocolate, beef liver, spinach, black-eyed peas, asparagus, clams, trout, salmon, tuna, nutritional yeast, chicken, beef, crab, flaxseed, chia, walnuts, and salmon	Excess copper: Wilson's disease and hypoadrenalism [1]
Hair (lackluster, thinning/loss)	Protein, zinc, biotin, linoleic acid, copper, vitamin C, selenium, and B12	HCl acid to support protein digestion, brewer's yeast, liver, soy, rice, peanuts, nuts, fatty fish, flaxseed, chia, oysters, red peppers, orange juice, orange, grapefruit juice, clams, liver, trout, salmon, tuna, nutritional yeast, beef, crab, Greek yogurt, and beans	Check for hypothyroidism and excess vitamin A [1]

Table 6.1 (continued)

Indication	Nutrition deficiency	Nutritional approach	Comments
Nail (white spots, pale nail beds)	Zinc, calcium, iron, vitamin A, and vitamin C	Oysters, pumpkin seeds, ginger, pecans, split peas, Brazil nuts, wheat, rye, oats, red peppers, orange juice, orange, grapefruit juice, breakfast cereals, white beans, chocolate, beef, crab, and liver	Zn and Ca deficiencies may create white lines (*transverse leukonychia*), which run horizontally across the nail. Malnutrition or low protein can create parallel white lines called *Muehrcke's lines* which often occur in roughly the same position in different nails. Fe deficiencies cause white vertical ridges/grooves [5]
Skin (acne, peeling hands/feet, rosacea)	Vitamin D, niacin, B6, selenium, magnesium, and B12	Clams, liver, trout, salmon, tuna, nutritional yeast, chicken, Brazil nuts, green leafy vegetables, legumes, nuts, and seeds	Consider dairy sensitivity [1]
Skin (poor wound healing, pressure ulcers)	Protein, vitamin C, and zinc	Meats, Greek yogurt, beans, nuts, red peppers, orange juice, orange, grapefruit juice, oysters, beef, and crab	Consider poor vascular perfusion [1]
Skin (fine lines, shedding, scales/plaques)	Vitamin A and omega-3	Flaxseed, chia, nuts, salmon, liver, and breakfast cereals	Consider environmental or hygiene factors [1]
Skin (dermatitis)	Niacin, tryptophan, zinc, and omega-3	Liver, chicken, dairy, fruits, seeds, oysters, beef, crab, flaxseed, chia, nuts, and salmon	Consider thermal, sun, and chemical burns, Addison's disease, and allergies [1]
Skin (pallor)	Iron, folic acid, and B12	Breakfast cereals, oysters, white beans, chocolate, beef liver, spinach, black-eyed peas, asparagus, clams, trout, salmon, trout, tuna, and nutritional yeast	Consider other skin pigmentation disorders, hemorrhage, and low volume/perfusion [1]
Skin (petechiae, ecchymoses)	Vitamins K and C	Collards, turnips, spinach, kale, broccoli, red peppers, orange juice, orange, and grapefruit juice	Consider ASA overdose, liver disease, and trauma [1]
Sinusitis	Vitamins C, A, and B5, zinc, quercetin, and beta-carotene	Acerola, chili peppers, guavas, sweet peppers, leafy greens, onions, apples, and pomegranate	Consider allergies, especially dairy [1]

Table 6.1 (continued)

Indication	Nutrition deficiency	Nutritional approach	Comments
Decreased taste and/or smell	Zn, Cu, and vitamins A, B6, and B12	Oysters, beef liver, baking chocolate, potatoes, mushrooms, chickpeas, chicken breast, clams, trout, salmon, tuna fish, nutritional yeast, sweet potato, spinach, and carrots	Use zinc tally test to assess zinc sufficiency Consider medications that influence zinc status Numerous toxins block zinc [6]
Metallic taste	B12	Clams, beef liver, trout, salmon, tuna fish, and nutritional yeast	Consider excess zinc toxic metals. Eating cold foods tends to be helpful [7]

6.1.1 Xerosis

Upward of 56% of older adults experience some degree of xerosis, most of which occur in women [8]. Hydration status and fatty acid deficiency are the primary targets of the nutritional approach to addressing this common concern. Most older adults experience dehydration from one of many causes: medication side effects (diuretics), low fluid intake, or dry indoor air [9]. Given the importance of hydration for skin health, patients should be advised to drink half of their weight in ounces per day of water or herbal tea. If there are diuretics or polypharmacy present, the patient may need to drink more than that. Additionally, the intake of healthy fats in the diet should be assessed, particularly with the older adult who may have come of age in the era of the demonization of dietary fats, to ensure proper building blocks for the cellular membrane. Further, many patients lack the ability to efficiently convert linoleic acid from vegetables and seeds into the essential omega-6 fat, gamma linoleic acid (GLA) which is otherwise difficult to obtain in a normal diet. Functional nutritional testing can help assess the enzyme deficiency, and supplementation with GLA directly is advised. For full nutritional and botanical support recommendations, please see Table 6.2.

6.1.2 Psoriasis

Psoriasis is the end result of a complex and partially unknown cascade of events that arise out of an autoimmune reaction. Breaking down the component parts of the psoriatic process allows us to identify nutritional opportunities to interrupt the inflammatory cascade that results in the classic skin lesions. From the perspective of the autoimmune process, integrative medicine looks to identify a trigger, heal the

Table 6.2 Nutritional and botanical support for xerosis

	MOA	Dose	Food sources	Side effects and prescriber notes
Essential fatty acids	Supplements the stratum corneum to improve function and resistance [10]	30 mcg [11]	Fish oil, salmon, mackerel, herring, tuna, and sardines [12]	Promotes wound healing. Consider following order of potency: omega-9 > omega-6 > omega-3 [13]
GLA	Supplies hydrolipids required to maintain membrane integrity and function [14]	0.5–2 g GLA	Evening primrose, borage, and black currant seed	The human skin cannot synthesize GLA from natural precursors [15]
Vitamin A	Plays critical role in retinal photoreceptor function, epithelial proliferation, and keratinization [16]	700–900 mcg [16]	Beef liver, sweet potato, spinach, and carrots [17]	Xerosis is often a presenting symptom of vitamin A deficiency. Often due to malabsorption or bariatric surgery
Zinc	Necessary for the normal cell growth, proliferation, and regeneration [18]	3 mg [19]	Oysters	Zinc deficiency can often lead to xerosis

leaky gut that invariably exists, and support the genetic tendencies that create the misfiring of the immune system. Refer to the digestive chapter for complete guidance on gut-healing support and consider advanced functional stool testing to assess digestion, microbial balance, and inflammation as a starting point for the patient.

Diet recommendations are as follows:

- Increase fiber.
- Increase cold-water fish (salmon, mackerel, anchovies].
- Eliminate gluten, sugar, animal fats, alcohol, and dairy.
- Focus on whole, unprocessed foods that do not contain the inflammatory industrial seed oils.

For complete nutritional and botanical support recommendations, please see Table 6.3.

Topical Cannabinoids
- Endocannabinoids play an important role in modulating skin health.
- Alterations in the endocannabinoid system due to hormonal changes, diet, toxins, etc. can manifest on the skin.
- By stimulating endocannabinoid receptors, topical cannabinoids can help treat a number of skin conditions, including acne, eczema, psoriasis, herpes, and skin cancer [20].

Table 6.3 Nutritional and botanical support for psoriasis [21]

	MOA	Daily dose	Food sources	Side effects and prescriber notes
Topical cannabinoids	Reduces inflammation by shifting pro-inflammatory Th1 response to anti-inflammatory Th2 response [22]. Cannabis helps reduce inflammation, itching, and even stress [23]. It also slows the growth and helps prevent buildup of new skin cells [24]	THC distillate cream. Recommend to start low and increase slowly	Cannabis	Useful in cream or paste form by combining with oils such as olive oil, shea butter, beeswax, and jojoba oil. Very helpful in treating painful symptoms of psoriasis, the cracked and bleeding skin [25]
Vitamin D	Antiproliferative and prodifferentiating actions on keratinocytes mediate expression of pro-inflammatory proteins	2000 IU	Cod liver oil, trout, salmon, mushrooms, and fortified milk [26]	Rare and only in gross excess
Flaxseed oil	Increases anti-inflammatory cascade	1 tbsp	Source	Rich source of ALA (alpha-lipoic acid) [27]
Vitamin E	Increases selenium and increases glutathione [28]	400 IU	Vegetable oils, almonds, peanuts, sunflower seeds, spinach, and broccoli [29]	Very high doses may cause blood thinning (1500 IU) [29]
Chromium	Increases insulin receptor sensitivity	400 IU	Ham, beef, Turkey, lettuce, green beans, apples, and bananas [30]	Psoriatics tend to have increased serum insulin and glucose
Vitamin A	Integral to skin integrity	50,000 IU	Beef liver, sweet potato, spinach, and carrots [17]	In excess: dizziness, nausea, and headaches [17]
Selenium	Influence immune response by changing the expression of cytokines and their receptors or by making immune cells more resistant to oxidative stress [31]	200 mg	Brazil nuts, tuna, halibut, sardines, ham, and shrimp [32]	Garlic breath, metallic taste, and hair and nail loss with toxicity [32]
Zinc	Integral to skin integrity	30 mg	Oysters	In excess: dizziness, nausea, and headaches with toxicity [17]

	MOA	Daily dose	Food sources	Side effects and prescriber notes
Goldenseal, standardized extract	Inhibits hyperproliferation [33]	Dried root 1–4 g and 1:1 extract 2–4 mL	Source (plant)	Consider if associated impaired digestion or liver function
Milk thistle	Anti-inflammatory and antioxidant	70–210 mg TID	Silymarin found primarily in fruits but also found in leaves and seeds [34]	Consider if associated impaired digestion or liver function

6.1.3 Eczema

Atopic dermatitis, or eczema, often surfaces in the older adult with a medical history of environmental allergies. The integrative approach to resolving eczema targets food and environmental reactivity and systemic inflammatory responses. It can be difficult to connect the dots between triggers and skin eruptions; thus, food sensitivity testing may be extremely helpful. The most likely contributors to eczema and the accompanying environmental allergies are as follows:

(a) Food sensitivities: different from food allergies, food sensitivities create a delayed response in body systems, usually outside of the gut such as brain fog, pain, eczema, and fatigue. An elimination diet that excludes the six most common food sensitivity triggers (gluten, dairy, corn, eggs, peanuts, and soy) for 6 weeks followed by a systematic reintroduction of each type of food can help identify the triggers. This is also a perfect situation for food sensitivity testing to personalize the elimination diet.

(b) Candida overgrowth is symptomatic of dysbiosis in the gut microbiome that allows this normal resident of the gut to increase in number and become a source of endotoxins. Fed by consumption of carbohydrates, elimination of all refined carbohydrates and restriction of high-carbohydrate foods such as fruits and starchy vegetables can help reduce the overgrowth and support a beneficial microbial balance in the gut. This beneficial balance improves the health of the gut and the skin and reduces reactivity to food triggers that results in resolution of eczema.

(c) Histamine reactivity can drive eczema breakouts. In the dysbiotic gut, the balance between internal production of histamine, consumption of foods high in histamine, and enzymatic breakdown of histamine sets the stage for reactivity that leads to eczema. To understand histamine intolerance more, refer to the immune chapter.

For a complete list of nutritional and botanical support recommended for eczema, please see Table 6.4.

Table 6.4 Nutritional and botanical support for eczema

	MOA	Dose	Food sources	Side effects and prescriber notes
Vitamin A	Plays a regulatory role in immune functions and skin integrity [35]	50,000 IU	Beef liver, sweet potato, spinach, and carrots [17]	Vitamin A and vitamin D co-deficiency may exacerbate eczema symptoms [35]
Vitamin E	Is an antioxidant and reduces IgE antibodies [36]	400 IU [36]	Vegetable oils, almonds, peanuts, sunflower seeds, spinach, and broccoli [29]	Patients receiving anticoagulant or those with vitamin K deficiency and who are at increased risk of bleeding should be under direct supervision for receiving vitamin E [36]
Zinc	Is an anti-inflammatory and antioxidant and increases reepithelialization [37]	Topical formulations are most well studied (zinc sulfate, 2.5%) [37]	Oysters, beef chuck roast, crab, beef patty, and lobster [38]	Zinc oxide and zinc sulfate paste are both efficacious [37]
Quercetin	Is immune modulating and anti-inflammatory (inhibits mast cell secretions and production of Th2 cytokines) and reduces flare-ups [39]	5–40 mg [40]	Apples, berries, brassica vegetables, capers, grapes, onions, and shallots [41]	No significant side effects
Probiotics	Promote local and systemic immunity [42]	Mixture of different bacterial species or *Lactobacillus* species [42]	Fermented milks, cheese, buttermilk, yogurts, miso, tempeh, sauerkraut, kimchi, and kefir [43]	Limited side effects
GLA	Corrects deficiencies in skin lipids which improves a dysregulated inflammatory and immune system [44]	220 mg [44]	Human milk, organ meats, primrose, black currant, borage, and fungal oil	No known side effects
Coleus forskohlii	Anti-inflammatory [45]	10% extract [45]	Source, plant native to India [46]	May decrease blood pressure [47]
Glycyrrhiza glabra	Is anti-inflammatory and reinforces cortisol's inhibition of antibody formation, stress reaction, and inflammation [48]	2% extract [48]	Dried roots from licorice plant [48]	Most successful when used in combination with improved skin care and exclusion of exacerbating factors [48]
Topical cannabinoids	Anti-inflammatory, antimicrobial, and anti-pruritus [49]	Topical full-spectrum 1:1 THC/CBD or triple topical THC/CBD/CBDa (CBDa is a potent anti-inflammatory and analgesic)	Source	In addition to topical cannabis, dietary hempseed oil can also be helpful in reducing skin dryness and itchiness [50]

6.1.4 Chronic Obstructive Pulmonary Disease (COPD)

The integrative approach to asthma, bronchitis, and COPD is fundamentally the same which is to avoid triggers such as inhaled toxins and irritants that set the underlying inflammation in motion. For more specific details about the treatment approach for asthma, consult the immune chapter.

Nutritional considerations for the older adult experiencing COPD should be made in the context of deficiencies in caloric balance as well as nutrition due to the likely increase in energy spent breathing and the impact of the difficulty in breathing on food intake.

Considerations for diet and lifestyle support of COPD include the following:

- Small, frequent meals:

  - Eating 5–6 small meals per day helps conserve energy, as smaller meals require less effort to eat [51].
  - Full stomachs can put pressure on the lungs and breathing muscles, making it more difficult to breathe [51].

- Elimination of food allergens and sensitivities:

  - Allergen triggers can make COPD worse [52].

- Avoidance of toxins, particularly inhalants:

  - Key offenders include outdoor and indoor air pollution, occupational hazards, infections, tobacco, and secondhand smoke [53].

- Tai Chi:

  - Enhances quality of life, psychosocial function, and possibly exercise capacity
  - Encourages patients to move fluidly, with less strain, safe in the deconditioned
  - Safe adjunct or alternative to conventional exercise training [54]

- Breath work such as the Buteyko method and *Breath* by James Nestor:

  - Buteyko method: switching from mouth to nose breathing on a permanent basis, helping breathing become more efficient and reducing the feeling of breathlessness, coughing, wheezing, and chest tightness [55].
  - "Slow and low" breaths through the nose can help relieve stress and reduce blood pressure [56].

- See Table 6.5 for nutritional and botanical support recommendations.

- Honey for Wound Healing [69]
- Honey has rich antioxidant, antibacterial, and anti-inflammatory properties.
- It can be used directly as a wound dressing to improve healing.
- Honey also has high acidity, high osmotic effect, and high hydrogen peroxide content.
- It supplies pain relief in burns.

Table 6.5 Nutritional and botanical support for COPD [57]

	MOA	Daily dose	Food sources	Side effects and prescriber notes
Inhaled glutathione	Is an antioxidant and replenishes glutathione stores which is the first line of defense against oxidative stress in the lower respiratory tract [58]	600 mg [58]	Meat, fish, broccoli, cabbage, garlic, onions, cereals, and dairy products [59]	Urine should be tested for sulfites. If positive, glutathione is contraindicated [58]
Resolvins	Inhibits cigarette smoke-induced pro-inflammatory response in human lung cells by activating anti-inflammatory pathways [53]	1–2 gm [60]	Omega-3-rich foods (fatty fish, flax-/hemp-/chia seeds)	Resolvin D1 derived from DHA [53]
N-Acetyl cysteine	Protects the lungs against toxins by increasing pulmonary defense mechanisms through its direct antioxidant properties and its indirect role as a precursor of GSH synthesis [61]	600 mg [61]	Broccoli, brussels sprouts, egg yolks, garlic, oats, onions, poultry, red bell peppers, wheat germ, and yeast [62]	Especially beneficial for those patients not on inhaled steroids [61]
Magnesium [63]	Is anti-inflammatory and prevents bronchoconstriction [53]	300 mg [64]	Pumpkin seeds, chia seeds, almonds, spinach, cashews, and peanuts [65]	Particularly useful in exacerbations
Potassium	While potassium-wasting diuretics are the preferred agents for treating hypertension in patients with COPD, they may worsen carbon dioxide retention in hypoventilating patients and potentiate hypokalemia in those receiving corticosteroids	200–1000 mg titrated based on personal demand	Potato, tomato, beet greens, adzuki and white beans, yogurt, and sweet potato [66]	In addition, β-agonists may substantially lower serum potassium levels in patients already rendered hypokalemic by diuretics. Must have normal kidney function to supplement
EFA	Metabolism produces eicosanoids, potent mediators of inflammation, thrombosis, and vaso- and bronchoconstriction [53]	1200 mg ALA, 700 mg EPA, and 340 mg DHA [53]	Fish oil, salmon, mackerel, herring, tuna, and sardines [12]	Additionally reverses muscle wasting and improves functional capacity [53]
Vitamin C	Hydrophilic antioxidant [53]	100 mg [67]	Red and green pepper, orange juice, orange, grapefruit juice, kiwifruit, and broccoli [68]	Protective independent of smoking history [67]

6.1.5   Age-Related Macular Degeneration (AMD) [70]

Oxidative damage is a key driver of AMD. Nutritional targets to reduce this oxidative stress include high antioxidant dietary intake and the avoidance of foods containing oxidized fats such as the refined vegetable oils found in processed foods. AMD affects over 10% of adults over 65 and 30% of adults over 75 years old [1]. A seminal study, AREDS2, identified key nutritional supports that slow the progression of AMD: vitamins C and E, beta-carotene, and zinc. Further, other research shows that people who consume DHA in the form of cold-water fish at least weekly were half as likely to experience AMD as those who consumed DHA less frequently [71, 72].

Diet recommendations are as follows:

- Focus on an anti-inflammatory, antioxidant-rich diet of whole foods, colorful fruits and vegetables, and healthy fats.
- Reduce animal fats and processed baked goods.
- Encourage a high intake of red/purple foods including wine, grapes, onion, and berries.
- See Table 6.6 for nutritional and botanical support recommendations.

6.1.6   Alopecia

Excluding male pattern baldness, hair can reveal much about a patient's underlying health status. Diffuse alopecia can be related to stress and nutritional deficiencies and a result of chemotherapy. Alopecia areata is an autoimmune disease that integrative medicine views as an imbalance which can be remedied when the root cause is adequately addressed. Autoimmune diseases stem from the confluence of three conditions: genetic predisposition, intestinal permeability, and environmental triggers. Nutritional targets around healing intestinal permeability, or leaky gut, and identifying triggers often result in remission of the autoimmune process.

Common triggers for alopecia (diffuse and areata) include the following:

- Stress
- Nutritional deficiencies: protein, zinc, iron, and EFA
- Food sensitivities:

  - *Gluten:* some studies show patients with celiac disease have a higher risk of alopecia areata [88]. The prevalence of gliadin antibody (celiac) in patients with alopecia areata is about 1 in 116, or 18 in 100 [89, 90]. Alopecia can be a skin manifestation of celiac disease.
  - *Dairy:* milk protein, casein, can irritate immune system and worsen alopecia [91].
  - *Corn:* it is a common immune system irritant; avoiding corn can help keep the immune system in check [92].

Table 6.6 Nutritional and botanical support for macular degeneration [21]

	MOA	Dose	Food sources	Side effects and prescriber notes
Alpha-lipoic acid (ALA)	Is an antioxidant, supports glutathione synthesis, acts as free radical scavenger, chelates transition metal ions, and elevates SOD activity [73]	0.2 g [73]	Flaxseed, soybean, chia seeds, hemp seeds, and avocados	Improves visual quality of dry AMD patients [73]
Arginine	Nitric oxide precursor. There is less NO in acute macular degeneration eyes. This could be associated with neuronal degeneration in the retina and vasoconstriction and hemodynamic changes in AMD choroid [74]	3–5 grams	Legumes, nuts, and meats	Abnormalities of the choroidal circulation have been hypothesized to contribute to the development of age-related macular degeneration (AMD) [75]
Beta-carotene	Provitamin A activity	15 mg	Carrots, sweet potatoes, winter squash, spinach, kale, and cantaloupe	Reduces visual acuity loss
Choline	Precursor to phosphatidylcholine, largest fraction of phospholipids that make cell membrane [76]	550 mg [77]	Fish, beef, poultry, and eggs	Choline is neuroprotective; in the eyes, neurodegeneration occurs with degeneration of retinal ganglion cells and optic nerve fibers [78]
Copper	Is an antioxidant and encourages the development of flexible connective tissue for proper eye structure [79]	2 mg [70]	Shellfish, seeds, nuts, organ meats, wheat-bran cereals, whole-grain products, and chocolate	Binds with zinc and should be supplemented together [79]
DHA	Major lipid component of retinal photoreceptor outer segment membranes. Anti-inflammatory and antiangiogenic properties [80]	At least 350 mg [80]	Salmon, tuna, trout, oysters, clams, and crab	Not corroborated by AREDS2 study, results mixed [80]
Lutein	Antioxidant and chemoprotective [81]	10 mg	Egg yolks, green leafy vegetables, kale, avocado, and maize	Antioxidant combinations are more effective than single
Zeaxanthin	Protective effect on UV damage in retinal pigment epithelial cells [81]	1–2 mg	Green leafy vegetables, kale, avocado, and maize	Similar effects are seen with 3-O-glucoside and luteins [81]
Lycopene	Antioxidant	30 mg [82]	Tomatoes, watermelon, and grapefruit	Most abundant carotenoid in serum [83]

Table 6.6 (continued)

	MOA	Dose	Food sources	Side effects and prescriber notes
Zinc	Essential for metabolism of the retina	80 mg	Oysters, crab, and lobsters	Elderly are at high risk for Zn deficiency
Vitamin C	Antioxidant	500 mg	Red and green pepper, orange juice, orange, grapefruit juice, kiwifruit, and broccoli [68]	Best results when combined with vitamins A and E
Vitamin E	Antioxidant	400 IU	Vegetable oils, almonds, peanuts, sunflower seeds, spinach, and broccoli [29]	Best results when combined with vitamins A and C
Taurine	Prevents retinal degenerations that proceed with photoreceptor and prevents drusen buildup	50 mg [84]	Shellfish and dark meat	Supplement with vitamin D
Selenium	Antioxidant	200 mcg	Brazil nuts, tuna, halibut, sardines, ham, and shrimp [32]	Low intake of selenium known to cause a reduction of total polyunsaturated fatty acids in the retinal pigment epithelium [85]
Glutathione	Antioxidant	250–500 mg	Broccoli, cauliflower, brussels sprouts, kale, watercress, mustard greens, garlic, onions, shallots, avocado, spinach, okra, and whey	Oxidative damage and free radicals are most prominent in the outer retina, specifically on the photoreceptor cells, the retinal pigment epithelium, and the choriocapillaris [86]
Melatonin	Controls eye pigmentation, regulating the amount of light reaching the photoreceptors, to scavenge hydroxyradicals and to protect retinal pigment epithelium (RPE) cells from oxidative damage [87]	3 mg [87]	Tart cherries, goji berries, eggs, milk, fish, and nuts	Physiologic decrease in melatonin in the elderly [87]
Vitamin A	Essential role in human retinal pigment epithelial cells [85]	700 mcg for men and 600 mcg for women	Carrots, broccoli, cantaloupe, and squash	Toxic if consumed in excess. Best results with vitamins C and E

- *Eggs:* these are a common allergen; one can consider eliminating and reintroducing once symptoms reside.
- *Peanuts:* allergies to peanuts may instigate an increased immune response, causing the scalp to become inflamed, constricting blood flow to hair follicles [93].
- *Soy:* thought to be due to phytoestrogens [94].

See Table 6.7 for recommended nutritional and botanical support for alopecia.

Table 6.7 Nutritional and botanical support for alopecia [63]

	MOA	Dose	Food sources	Side effects and prescriber notes
Zinc	Essential cofactor for multiple enzymes and functional activities in the hair follicle. Zinc is a potent inhibitor of hair follicle regression and it accelerates hair follicle recovery [95]	50 mg [95]	Oysters, crab, and lobsters	Better results with mild alopecia. Side effects include mild nausea [95]
Biotin	Coenzyme for numerous metabolic pathways. More promising roles in genetic and epigenetic regulation [96]	30 mcg [97]	Nuts, legumes, whole grains, unpolished rice, and egg yolk [96]	Excess in the body is rare, as biotin is water soluble. Most beneficial in pathologic brittle hair syndrome or uncombable hair syndrome [96]
Vitamin A	Can cause alopecia areata in excess [98]	400 mcg [99]	Carrots, broccoli, cantaloupe, and squash	Should also avoid gluten and dairy when able [99]
Iron	Is a cofactor for DNA synthesis and has an important role in tissues with high cellular turnover [100]	72 mg	Lean meat, seafood, poultry, iron-fortified breakfast cereals, beans, spinach, peas, nuts, and dried fruits	Insufficient evidence to recommend giving iron supplementation therapy to patients with alopecia and iron deficiency in the absence of iron deficiency anemia [101]
EFA	Anti-inflammatory	410 mg	Fish oil, salmon, mackerel, herring, tuna, and sardines [12]	High doses (>1000 mg) can cause GI distress
Folate	Contributes to nucleic acid production and has important role in highly proliferative hair follicle [98]	400–1000 mcg [98]	Dark leafy green vegetables, asparagus, brussels sprouts, beans, peanuts, and sunflower seeds	Folate deficiency can cause hair, skin, and nail changes [98]

Table 6.7 (continued)

	MOA	Dose	Food sources	Side effects and prescriber notes
Vitamin B6	It plays a key role in skin development and maintenance, and more importantly, it contributes in cysteine incorporation in hair cells [102]	1.7 mg M and 1.5 mg F [103]	Chickpeas, beef liver, tuna, salmon, and chicken	Results improved when supplemented with L-cysteine [102]
Vitamin B12	Necessary for DNA synthesis and important for highly proliferative hair follicles [98]	2.4 mcg [98]	Clams, beef liver, trout, salmon, and tuna	Low potential for toxicity
Amino acids	Cystine: supports hair strength and rigidity Lysine: supports iron absorption [104]	Cystine (70 mg) Lysine (1.5 mg) [104]	Lysine: meat and eggs Cystine: chicken, turkey, yogurt, cheese, eggs, and sunflower seeds	All amino acid studies must be combined with other supplements [104]
Taurine	Is an antioxidant and inhibits pro-inflammatory mediators [105]	150 mg [105]	Shellfish and dark meat	Not only shields catabolic effects of TGF-B1 but promotes hair survival [105]
Glutathione	Antioxidant	500 mg twice	Broccoli, cauliflower, brussels sprouts, kale, watercress, mustard greens, garlic, onions, shallots, avocado, spinach, okra, and whey	Potential role of oxygen free radicals in pathogenesis. Use extra caution in sun
Selenium	Is an antioxidant and maintains immunological competence [106]	55 mcg	Brazil nuts, tuna, halibut, sardines, ham, and shrimp [32]	Increased demands for Se in alopecia patches [106]
Melatonin	Antioxidant [107]	3 mg every other day [107]	Tart cherries, goji berries, eggs, milk, fish, and nuts	Potential role of oxygen free radicals in pathogenesis [107]

6.1.7   Therapeutic Diets

Elimination Diet   An elimination diet is a key part of resolving concerns around the skin, hair, and lung tissue due to the impact that inflammation in the gut has on the epithelial tissue. Research shows that when food sensitivities are resolved, the reduction in SIgG levels measured in the gut correlates with a reduction of eczema [108].

Mediterranean Diet   In and of itself, the Mediterranean diet will eliminate many inflammatory foods from the patient's diet that can improve concerns with the skin, lungs, and hair particularly if the patient has been following a standard American diet. Around 78% of people on the Mediterranean diet showed improvement in asthma after switching to this eating pattern [109]. For more details on the Mediterranean diet, please refer to the Appendix.

Anti-candida Diet   The relationship between dysbiosis (a microbiome imbalance where some microbes have high elevated concentrations and others have depleted) and skin health is established in research. Often, a normal resident of our microbiome, *Candida albicans*, takes advantage of the dysbiotic environment, and a diet that is rich in refined carbohydrates creates a toxic environment within the gut that manifests in genetically predisposed patients as concerns with hair, skin, and lung tissue [110]. For more information on the anti-candida diet, please see the Appendix.

Table 6.8 summarizes the key nutrients of primary concern for health of the skin, lungs, eyes, and hair.

Table 6.8 Micronutrients of primary concern

	MOA	Food sources	RDA for 55+	Side effects/ comments for providers
EFA (GLA)	Anti-inflammatory	Flaxseed oil, chia seeds, walnuts, and salmon	1.6 g M and 1.1 g F	Dry skin and eczema
Zinc	Is anti-inflammatory and antioxidant and increases reepithelialization [37]	Oysters, crab, and lobsters	11 g M and 8 g F	Mild nausea
Vitamin A	Essential role in human retinal pigment epithelial cells [85]	Carrots, broccoli, cantaloupe, and squash	900 mcg M and 700 mcg F	Toxic if consumed in excess
Vitamin E	Anti-inflammatory	Vegetable oils, almonds, peanuts, sunflower seeds, spinach, and broccoli [29]	15 mg	Very high doses may cause blood thinning (1500 IU) [29]

6.2 Case Studies

6.2.1 Case 1

Kate, a 67-year-old retired teacher, presented with years of chronic dry skin. For years, she tried different topical products and had seen countless dermatologists, and while a number of topical moisturizers did help her, she was convinced that there was another way of dealing with the problem, and she was tired of frequent daily applications of creams over large areas of her body. While generally healthy, Kate had a history of severe menstrual cramps decades ago, she also had a history of recurrent breast pain that got better after menopause. None of these symptoms had been addressed well in the past and Kate learned to live with them. Her other problems were well-controlled hypertension and occasional bouts of diarrhea that were diagnosed as irritable bowel syndrome and managed by taking occasional Imodium. On exam, Kate's skin was not just dry but was closer to eczematous with some patches of frank eczema over arms and legs. Given her health history, we decided to do a comprehensive nutritional analysis that includes a detailed omega-3 fatty acid test. The result is shown in Fig. 6.1.

Essential and Metabolic Fatty Acids Markers (RBCs)

Omega 3 Fatty Acids

Analyte (cold water fish, flax, walnut)	Value	Reference Range
α-Linoleni (ALA) 18:3 n3	0.06	>= 0.09 wt %
Eicosapentaenoic (EPA) 20:5 n3	0.74	>= 0.16 wt %
Docosapentaenoic (DPA) 22:5 n3	1.90	>= 1.14 wt %
Docosahexaenoic (DHA) 22:6 n3	4.3	>= 2.1 wt %
% Omega 3s	8.0	>= 3.8

Omega 9 Fatty Acids

Analyte (olive oil)	Value	Reference Range
Oleic 18:1 n9	13	10-13 wt %
Nervonic 24:1 n9	4.3	2.1-3.5 wt %
% Omega 9s	17.5	13.3-16.6

Saturated Fatty Acids

Analyte (meat, dairy, coconuts, palm oil)	Value	Reference Range
Palmitic C16:0	21	18-23 wt %
Stearic C18:0	19	14-17 wt %
Arachidie C20:0	0.27	0.22-0.35 wt %
Behenic C22:0	0.91	0.92-1.68 wt %
Tricosanoic C23:0	0.25	0.12-0.18 wt %
Lignoceric C24:0	2.5	2,1-3,8 wt %
Pentadecanoic C15:0	0.15	0.07-0.15 wt %
Margaric C17:0	0.38	0.22-0.37 wt %
% Saturated Fats	44.3	39.8-43.6

Omega 6 Fatty Acids

Analyte (vegetable oil, gains, most meats, dairy)	Value	Reference Range
Linoleic (LA) 18:2 n6	10.2	10.5-16.9 wt %
γ-Linoleic (GLA) 18:3 n6	0.05	0.03-0.13 wt %
Dihomo-γ-Linoleic (DGLA) 20:3 n6	0.73	>= 1.19 wt %
Arachidonic (AA) 20:4 n6	16	15-1-21 wt %
Docosatetraenoic (DTA) 22:4 n6	1.49	1.50-4.20 wt %
Eicosadienoic 20:2 n6	0.10	<= 0,26 wt %
% Omega 6s	29.0	30.5-39.7

Monounsaturated Fats

Omega 7 Fats	Value	Reference Range
Palmitoleic 16:1 n7	0.23	<= 0.64 wt %
Vaccenic 18:1 n7	0.83	<= 1.13 wt %

Trans Fat	Value	Reference Range
Elaidic 18:1 n9t	0.19	<= 0.59 wt %

Delta -6 Desaturase Activity
Upregulated Functional Impaired

	Value	Reference Range
Linoleic DGLA 18:2 n6 / 20:3 n6	14.0	6.0-12.3

Cardiovascular Risk

Analyte	Value	Reference Range
Omega 6s / Omega 3s	3.6	3.4-10.7
AA / EPA 20:4 n6 / 20:5 n3	9	12-125
Omega 3 Index	6.0	>= 4.0

Fig. 6.1 Essential and metabolic fatty acids markers (RBCs) [111]

Upon reviewing this result with the patient, we started her on GLA oil derived from borage oil at a dose of 1 gm twice daily for 4 weeks and decreasing dose to 500 mg twice daily after. In addition to balancing fatty acids, we also suggested that she further increase her omega-3 intake by supplementing with fish oil despite normal test results. At 3 months of follow-up, the patient reported that her dry skin had dramatically improved and also that her periodic diarrhea completely resolved.

The repeat fatty acid test revealed that her GLA increased significantly despite gamma GLA not increasing much. At 6 months of follow-up, the patient maintained nearly complete resolution of dry skin and periodic diarrhea. The follow-up test result was obtained to decide on long-term supplementation. See result below (Fig. 6.2). Given that her gamma GLA had only increased by about 20% despite GLA increasing more than twofold, it was decided that she will continue long-term fatty acid supplementation with 2 gm of combined 1:1 EPA/DHA and 1 gm of GLA daily.

6.2.2 Case 2

Steve, a 82-year-old retired diplomat, had chronic leg eczema for decades. After finishing distinguished diplomatic career, he decided to concentrate on optimizing his health and quality of life and eventually found his way to see us. He had a number of medical problems including hypertension, high cholesterol, coronary artery disease with history of myocardial infarction when he had several stents placed, well-controlled diabetes type 2, and chronic eczema. While his doctors always spent most of the time talking to him about management of his diabetes, hypertension, and heart disease, it was eczema that affected his quality of life the most. Being an avid golfer, he despised the appearance of his legs as it required covering legs and

Essential and Metabolic Fatty Acids Markers (RBCs)

Omega 3 Fatty Acids		
Analyte (cold water fish, flax, walnut)		Reference Range
α-Linolenic (ALA) 18:3 n3	0.27	>= 0.09 wt %
Eicosapentaenoic (EPA) 20:5 n3	4.88	>= 0.16 wt %
Docosapentaenoic (DPA) 22:5 n3	2.34	>= 1.14 wt %
Docosahexaenoic (DHA) 22:6 n3	5.6	>= 2.1 wt %
% Omega 3s	13.1	>= 3.8

Omega 6 Fatty Acids		
Analyte (vegetable oil, grains, most meats, dairy)		Reference Range
Linoleic (LA) 18:2 n6	17.0	10.5-16.9 wt %
γ-Linolenic (GLA) 18:3 n6	0.12	0.03-0.13 wt %
Dihomo-γ-linolenic (DGLA) 20:3 n6	0.91	>= 1.19 wt %
Arachidonic (AA) 20:4 n6	10	15-21 wt %
Docosatetraenoic (DTA) 22:4 n6	0.49	1.50-4.20 wt %
Eicosadienoic 20:2 n6	0.18	<= 0.26 wt %
% Omega 6s	28.3	30.5-39.7

Omega 9 Fatty Acids		
Analyte (olive oil)		Reference Range
Oleic 18:1 n9	13	10-13 wt %
Nervonic 24:1 n9	2.8	2.1-3.5 wt %
% Omega 9s	15.7	13.3-16.6

Monounsaturated Fats		
Omega 7 Fats		Reference Range
Palmitoleic 16:1 n7	0.38	<= 0.64 wt %
Vaccenic 18:1 n7	0.85	<= 1.13 wt %

Fig. 6.2 Essential and metabolic fatty acids markers (RBCs) [111]

his legs were hurting after being on his feet too long. Moreover, the day after golf-
ing, his leg eczema would usually get worse causing increased pain and swelling
requiring spending time in chart with legs elevated. The use of topical steroids as
main treatment had some benefits but never improved the issue enough to not impact
Steve's quality of life.

Since eczema was his main problem, we decided to concentrate on this issue
first. Upon reviewing his diet and supplements, it was felt that he had an excellent
nutritional status. While some of his medications including statin and hydrochlorothiazide were known to decrease the number of nutrients, his prior nutritionist had
thought of this and added coenzyme Q10 and minerals to his daily regimen. But
when we discussed his history more, few additional important issues came up.
When Steve was growing up, he had asthma that he "outgrew" when he moved from
New York to Europe with his parents who were also diplomats. In midlife, he had a
number of skin reactions that were all thought to be allergies but never severe
enough to cause him to address it in any regularity. He remembered simply taking
antihistamine medications that would help. Upon hearing this story, we decided to
obtain a food allergy test concentrating on IgG reactions rather than IgE. The initial
result had demonstrated multiple high and moderate food reactions. See Fig. 6.3.

After reviewing the result, the patient had several visits with a nutritionist to
proceed with a comprehensive elimination diet. We also decided to try topical 1:1
THC/CBD full-spectrum medical cannabis oil applied to affected areas twice daily.
At 6 months of follow-up, the patient had near-complete resolution of his eczema.
He was also pleased that he had more energy and noted more regular bowel movements. Also as seen from Fig. 6.3, he had resolution of multiple food allergies on the
food IgG assessment.

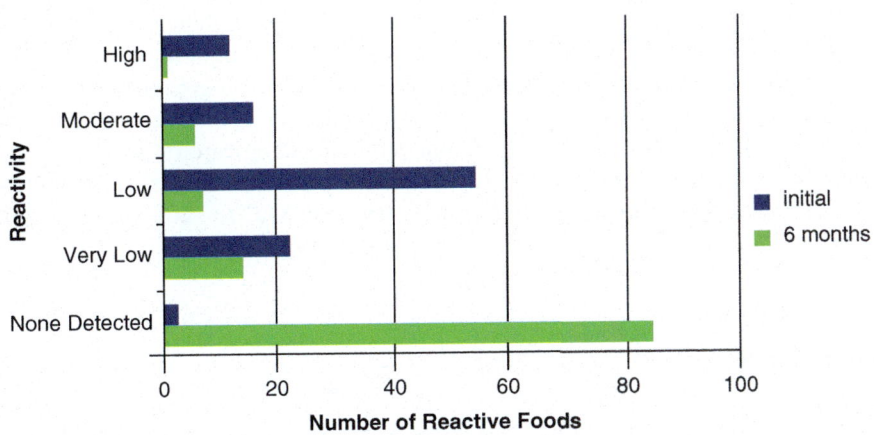

Abbreviation: IgG, immunoglobulin G.

Fig. 6.3 IgG food antibody assessment 6 months apart [112]. Abbreviation: IgG immunoglobulin G

6.2.3   Case 3

Sam, a 69-year-old farmer, presented to our clinic to support his progressing COPD. He was diagnosed with emphysema years ago but despite quitting smoking his disease progressed. Sam's love for horses, raising them, riding them, and running small horseback riding business with his wife Judy was what he wanted to do for the rest of his life. Unfortunately, progressive breathing difficulties began to interfere with horse riding and taking care of horses. His wife has read that inhaled glutathione can be helpful and wanted to try it.

Despite 40-pack-year history of smoking, frequent constipation managed with Colace and senna, and high cholesterol well managed with a low-dose statin, Sam was very healthy. He did like to take few drinks daily and occasionally more on weekend. Judy cooked most of their meals, and since diagnosis of COPD, Sam underwent major diet change from more or less standard American diet to mostly plant-based, nearly all organic meal plan on which his cholesterol went down so much that his primary care doctor suggested discontinuing the statin.

In addition to decreasing amount of alcohol that is known to decrease glutathione production and checking food allergies, which Sam did not have, we recommended complex regimen of inhaled glutathione 200 mg twice daily via standard commercial nebulizer, oral NAC 600 mg twice daily, and magnesium citrate 300 mg taken at bedtime. Earlier in life, Sam enjoyed karate and got rather interested in trying Tai Chi. We also recommended that he starts practicing Buteyko breathing techniques daily for 20–30 min. In 3 months, Sam reported that while his breathing did not get much better, he felt that he could do most of his activities including taking care of horses better. There was energy improvement, and his constipation resolved (likely due to addition of magnesium citrate). He really enjoyed his daily Tai Chi practice and Judy joined him to keep company. At 12 months of follow-up, Sam reported that his breathing definitely improved significantly and even though his pulmonologist reported that pulmonary function tests revealed very slight improvement, Sam felt the improvement was very significant as he no longer was getting short of breath with his regular activities and although he still could not jog or do continuous heavy activities, he was very happy as he could continue taking care of horses. Of note, inhaled glutathione is rather expensive treatment, and due to this, we decided to discontinue doing it at 12 months but increased oral NAC to 1200 mg twice daily. Despite this change, Sam has been doing well several years later.

References

1. Weil A. Integrative geriatric medicine. Kogan M, editor. Oxford University Press; 2018.
2. Sharabi AF, Winters R. Glossitis. StatPearls. Treasure Island: StatPearls Publishing; 2020.
3. Bhutta BS, Hafsi W. Cheilitis. StatPearls. Treasure Island: StatPearls Publishing; 2020.
4. Agouridis AP, Elisaf MS, Nair DR, Mikhailidis DP. Ear lobe crease: a marker of coronary artery disease? Arch Med Sci. 2015;11(6):1145–55.

5. Lama SC. Vitamin deficiencies and spots on finger nails I Livestrong.com [Internet]. Livestrong.com. 2019 [cited 2021 Feb 9]. Available from: https://www.livestrong.com/article/528741-vitamin-deficiencies-spots-on-finger-nails/.

6. Bromley SM. Smell and taste disorders: a primary care approach. Am Fam Physician [Internet]. 2000 Jan 15 [cited 2021 Feb 9];61(2):427–36. Available from: https://www.aafp.org/afp/2000/0115/p427.html.

7. Rehwaldt M, Wickham R, Purl S, Tariman J, Blendowski C, Shott S, et al. Self-care strategies to cope with taste changes after chemotherapy. Oncol Nurs Forum. 2009;36(2):E47–56.

8. Paul C, Maumus-Robert S, Mazereeuw-Hautier J, Guyen CN, Saudez X, Schmitt AM. Prevalence and risk factors for xerosis in the elderly: a cross-sectional epidemiological study in primary care. Dermatology (Basel). 2011;223(3):260–5.

9. Taylor K, Jones EB. Adult dehydration. StatPearls; 2020 Apr 22.

10. Conti A, Rogers J, Verdejo P, Harding CR, Rawlings AV. Seasonal influences on stratum corneum ceramide 1 fatty acids and the influence of topical essential fatty acids. Int J Cosmet Sci. 1996;18(1):1–12.

11. Moore EM, Wagner C, Komarnytsky S. The enigma of bioactivity and toxicity of botanical oils for skin care. Front Pharmacol. 2020;11:785.

12. Filipovic MG, Aeschbacher S, Reiner MF, Stivala S, Gobbato S, Bonetti N, et al. Whole blood omega-3 fatty acid concentrations are inversely associated with blood pressure in young, healthy adults. J Hypertens. 2018;36(7):1548–54.

13. Cardoso CRB, Souza MA, Ferro EAV, Favoreto S, Pena JDO. Influence of topical administration of n-3 and n-6 essential and n-9 nonessential fatty acids on the healing of cutaneous wounds. Wound Repair Regen. 2004;12(2):235–43.

14. Augustin M, Wilsmann-Theis D, Körber A, Kerscher M, Itschert G, Dippel M, et al. Diagnosis and treatment of xerosis cutis - a position paper. J Dtsch Dermatol Ges. 2019;17 Suppl 7:3–33.

15. Brosche T, Platt D. Effect of borage oil consumption on fatty acid metabolism, transepidermal water loss and skin parameters in elderly people. Arch Gerontol Geriatr. 2000;30(2):139–50.

16. Phanachet P, Shantavasinkul PC, Chantrathammachart P, Rattanakaemakorn P, Jayanama K, Komindr S, et al. Unusual manifestation of vitamin A deficiency presenting with generalized xerosis without night blindness. Clin Case Rep. 2018;6(5):878–82.

17. NIH. Vitamin A [Internet]. Vitamin A. 2020 [cited 2021 Jan 30]. Available from: https://ods.od.nih.gov/factsheets/VitaminA-HealthProfessional/.

18. Kim JE, Yoo SR, Jeong MG, Ko JY, Ro YS. Hair zinc levels and the efficacy of oral zinc supplementation in patients with atopic dermatitis. Acta Derm Venereol. 2014;94(5):558–62.

19. Bolke L, Schlippe G, Gerß J, Voss W. A collagen supplement improves skin hydration, elasticity, roughness, and density: results of a randomized, placebo-controlled, blind study. Nutrients. 2019;11(10):2494.

20. Eagleston L, Kalani NK, Patel RR, Flaten HK, Dunnick CA, Dellavalle RP. Cannabinoids in dermatology: a scoping review. Dermatol. Online J. 2018;24(6):13030/qt7pn8c0sb.

21. Pizzorno JE Jr, Murphy MT, Joiner-Bey H. The clinician's handbook of natural medicine. 3rd ed. St. Louis: Elsevier; 2016.

22. Friedman A, Momeni K, Kogan M. Topical cannabinoids for the management of psoriasis vulgaris: report of a case and review of the literature. J Drugs Dermatol. 2020;19(8):795.

23. Wilson, PhD DR. Can cannabis help treat psoriasis? [Internet]. Medical News Today. 2018 [cited 2021 Jan 31]. Available from: https://www.medicalnewstoday.com/articles/320086.

24. Wilkinson JD, Williamson EM. Cannabinoids inhibit human keratinocyte proliferation through a non-CB1/CB2 mechanism and have a potential therapeutic value in the treatment of psoriasis. J Dermatol Sci. 2007;45(2):87–92.

25. Li S-S, Wang L-L, Liu M, Jiang S-K, Zhang M, Tian Z-L, et al. Cannabinoid CB_2 receptors are involved in the regulation of fibrogenesis during skin wound repair in mice. Mol Med Rep. 2016;13(4):3441–50.

26. NIH. Vitamin D [Internet]. NIH National Institutes of Health Office of Dietary Supplements. 2020 [cited 2020 Dec 31]. Available from: https://ods.od.nih.gov/factsheets/VitaminD-HealthProfessional/.

27. Goyal A, Sharma V, Upadhyay N, Gill S, Sihag M. Flax and flaxseed oil: an ancient medicine & modern functional food. J Food Sci Technol. 2014;51(9):1633–53.

28. Fairris GM, Lloyd B, Hinks L, Perkins PJ, Clayton BE. The effect of supplementation with selenium and vitamin E in psoriasis. Ann Clin Biochem. 1989;26(Pt 1):83–8.

29. NIH. Vitamin E [Internet]. NIH Office of Dietary Supplements. 2020 [cited 2021 Jan 30]. Available from: https://ods.od.nih.gov/factsheets/VitaminE-HealthProfessional/.

30. NIH. Chromium [Internet]. NIH Office of Dietary Supplements. 2020 [cited 2021 Jan 31]. Available from: https://ods.od.nih.gov/factsheets/chromium-Consumer/.

31. Nazıroğlu M, Yıldız K, Tamtürk B, Erturan İ, Flores-Arce M. Selenium and psoriasis. Biol Trace Elem Res. 2012;150(1–3):3–9.

32. NIH. Selenium [Internet]. NIH Office of Dietary Supplements. 2020 [cited 2021 Jan 30]. Available from: https://ods.od.nih.gov/factsheets/Selenium-HealthProfessional/.

33. Neag MA, Mocan A, Echeverría J, Pop RM, Bocsan CI, Crişan G, et al. Berberine: botanical occurrence, traditional uses, extraction methods, and relevance in cardiovascular, metabolic, hepatic, and renal disorders. Front Pharmacol. 2018;9:557.

34. Silybum marianum (milk thistle). Altern Med Rev. 1999;4(4):272–4.

35. Xiang J, Wang H, Li T. Comorbidity of vitamin A and vitamin D deficiency exacerbates the severity of atopic dermatitis in children. Dermatology (Basel). 2019;235(3):196–204.

36. Jaffary F, Faghihi G, Mokhtarian A, Hosseini SM. Effects of oral vitamin E on treatment of atopic dermatitis: a randomized controlled trial. J Res Med Sci. 2015;20(11):1053–7.

37. Gupta M, Mahajan VK, Mehta KS, Chauhan PS. Zinc therapy in dermatology: a review. Dermatol Res Pract. 2014;2014:709152.

38. NIH. Zinc [Internet]. NIH Office of Dietary Supplements. 2020 [cited 2021 Feb 5]. Available from: https://ods.od.nih.gov/factsheets/Zinc-HealthProfessional/.

39. Choopani R, Mehrbani M, Fekri A, Mehrabani M. Treatment of atopic dermatitis from the perspective of traditional Persian medicine: presentation of a novel therapeutic approach. J Evid Based Complement Altern Med. 2017;22(1):5–11.

40. Jafarinia M, Sadat Hosseini M, Kasiri N, Fazel N, Fathi F, Ganjalikhani Hakemi M, et al. Quercetin with the potential effect on allergic diseases. Allergy Asthma Clin Immunol. 2020;16:36.

41. Li Y, Yao J, Han C, Yang J, Chaudhry MT, Wang S, et al. Quercetin, inflammation and immunity. Nutrients. 2016;8(3):167.

42. Schlichte MJ, Vandersall A, Katta R. Diet and eczema: a review of dietary supplements for the treatment of atopic dermatitis. Dermatol Pract Concept. 2016;6(3):23–9.

43. Syngai GG, Gopi R, Bharali R, Dey S, Lakshmanan GMA, Ahmed G. Probiotics - the versatile functional food ingredients. J Food Sci Technol. 2016;53(2):921–33.

44. Kawamura A, Ooyama K, Kojima K, Kachi H, Abe T, Amano K, et al. Dietary supplementation of gamma-linolenic acid improves skin parameters in subjects with dry skin and mild atopic dermatitis. J Oleo Sci. 2011;60(12):597–607.

45. Hebbani Nagarajappa S, Pandit S, Divanji M, Mariyanna B, Kumar P, Godavarthi A. Effect of Coleus forskohlii and its major constituents on cytochrome P450 induction. J Tradit Complement Med. 2016;6(1):130–3.

46. Henderson S, Magu B, Rasmussen C, Lancaster S, Kerksick C, Smith P, et al. Effects of coleus forskohlii supplementation on body composition and hematological profiles in mildly overweight women. J Int Soc Sports Nutr. 2005;2:54–62.

47. Coleus [Internet]. emedicinehealth. 2019 [cited 2021 Feb 8]. Available from: https://www.emedicinehealth.com/coleus/vitamins-supplements.htm.

48. Saeedi M, Morteza-Semnani K, Ghoreishi MR. The treatment of atopic dermatitis with licorice gel. J Dermatolog Treat. 2003;14(3):153–7.

49. Mounessa JS, Siegel JA, Dunnick CA, Dellavalle RP. The role of cannabinoids in dermatology. J Am Acad Dermatol. 2017;77(1):188–90.

50. Friedman A, Marks D. The therapeutic potential of cannabinoids in dermatology [Internet]. Skin Therapy Letter. 2018 [cited 2021 Feb 10]. Available from: https://www.skintherapyletter.com/dermatology/cannabinoids-potential/.

51. Nicholson A. Meal planning [Internet]. COPD. 2015 [cited 2021 Feb 10]. Available from: https://copd.net/living-with-copd/pulmonary-rehab/weight-management/meal-planning/#:~:text=COPD%20patients%20are%20also%20usually,make%20it%20harder%20to%20breathe.

52. Asthma-COPD Overlap [Internet]. American College of Allergy, Asthma and immunology. 2014 [cited 2021 Feb 10]. Available from: https://acaai.org/asthma/types-asthma/asthma-copd-overlap.

53. Scoditti E, Massaro M, Garbarino S, Toraldo DM. Role of diet in chronic obstructive pulmonary disease prevention and treatment. Nutrients. 2019;11(6):1357.

54. Yeh GY, Roberts DH, Wayne PM, Davis RB, Quilty MT, Phillips RS. Tai chi exercise for patients with chronic obstructive pulmonary disease: a pilot study. Respir Care. 2010;55(11):1475–82.

55. Buteyko Clinic. COPD and the Buteyko method [Internet]. Buteyko Clinic International. 2019 [cited 2021 Feb 10]. Available from: https://buteykoclinic.com/copd/.

56. Nestor J. Breath: the new science of a lost art. Riverhead Books: New York; 2020.

57. Raymond J, Morrow K. Medical nutrition therapy for pulmonary disease. In: Krause and Mahan's food & the nutrition care process. 15th ed. St. Louis: Elsevier; 2021. p. 716.

58. Prousky J. The treatment of pulmonary diseases and respiratory-related conditions with inhaled (nebulized or aerosolized) glutathione. Evid Based Complement Alternat Med. 2008;5(1):27–35.

59. Rodrigues C, Percival SS. Immunomodulatory effects of glutathione, garlic derivatives, and hydrogen sulfide. Nutrients. 2019;11(2):295.

60. Metagenics. SPM active [Internet]. Metagenics. 2021 [cited 2021 Feb 21]. Available from: https://www.metagenics.com/spm-active.

61. Dekhuijzen PNR, van Beurden WJC. The role for N-acetylcysteine in the management of COPD. Int J Chron Obstruct Pulmon Dis. 2006;1(2):99–106.

62. Cysteine [Internet]. Restorative medicine. 2020 [cited 2021 Feb 10]. Available from: https://restorativemedicine.org/library/monographs/cysteine/.

63. Gaby A. Nutritional medicine. 2nd ed. Concord, NH: Fritz Perlberg Publishing; 2017.

64. Sergi G. Effect of Magnesium Supplementation in COPD; 2016.

65. NIH. Magnesium [Internet]. National Institutes of Health Office of Dietary Supplements. 2020 [cited 2020 Dec 30]. Available from: https://ods.od.nih.gov/factsheets/Magnesium-HealthProfessional/#:~:text=Magnesium%20is%20widely%20distributed%20in,cereals%20and%20other%20fortified%20foods.

66. USDA. Dietary guide for Americans [Internet]. US Department of Health and Human Services. 2020 [cited 2021 Jan 1]. Available from: https://health.gov/our-work/food-nutrition/previous-dietary-guidelines/2015.

67. Park HJ, Byun MK, Kim HJ, Kim JY, Kim Y-I, Yoo K-H, et al. Dietary vitamin C intake protects against COPD: the Korea National Health and Nutrition Examination Survey in 2012. Int J Chron Obstruct Pulmon Dis. 2016;11:2721–8.

68. NIH. Vitamin C [Internet]. National Institutes of Health Office of Dietary Supplements. 2020 [cited 2020 Dec 30]. Available from: https://ods.od.nih.gov/factsheets/VitaminC-HealthProfessional/.

69. Yaghoobi R, Kazerouni A, Kazerouni O. Evidence for clinical use of honey in wound healing as an anti-bacterial, anti-inflammatory anti-oxidant and anti-viral agent: a review. Jundishapur J Nat Pharm Prod. 2013;8(3):100–4.

70. AREDS2 Research Group, Chew EY, Clemons T, SanGiovanni JP, Danis R, Domalpally A, et al. The age-related eye disease study 2 (AREDS2): study design and baseline characteristics (AREDS2 report number 1). Ophthalmology. 2012;119(11):2282–9.

71. Smith W, Mitchell P, Leeder SR. Dietary fat and fish intake and age-related maculopathy. Arch Ophthalmol. 2000;118(3):401–4.

72. Augood C, Chakravarthy U, Young I, Vioque J, de Jong PTVM, Bentham G, et al. Oily fish consumption, dietary docosahexaenoic acid and eicosapentaenoic acid intakes, and associations with neovascular age-related macular degeneration. Am J Clin Nutr. 2008;88(2):398–406.

73. Tao Y, Jiang P, Wei Y, Wang P, Sun X, Wang H. α-lipoic acid treatment improves vision-related quality of life in patients with dry age-related macular degeneration. Tohoku J Exp Med. 2016;240(3):209–14.

74. Bhutto IA, Baba T, Merges C, McLeod DS, Lutty GA. Low nitric oxide synthases (NOSs) in eyes with age-related macular degeneration (AMD). Exp Eye Res. 2010;90(1):155–67.

75. Grunwald JE, Hariprasad SM, DuPont J. Effect of aging on foveolar choroidal circulation. Arch Ophthalmol. 1998;116(2):150–4.

76. BodyBio. Phosphatidylcholine and vision: will the real PC please stand up? [Internet]. Body Bio. 2014 [cited 2021 Feb 12]. Available from: https://bodybio.com/blogs/blog/phosphatidylcholine-and-vision-will-the-real-pc-please-stand-up.

77. Druke T. Choline builds healthy eyes [Internet]. Natural products insider. 2017 [cited 2021 Feb 12]. Available from: https://www.naturalproductsinsider.com/womens-health/choline-builds-healthy-eyes.

78. Brisco E, Gazella K. Optimizing eye health with citicoline. Nat Med J. 2019;1–4. https://www.naturalmedicinejournal.com/sites/default/files/uploads/white_paper_citicoline.pdf

79. Macular degeneration vitamins. Copper [Internet]. Macular degeneration vitamins. [cited 2021 Feb 12]. Available from: https://macular-degeneration-vitamins.com/copper-to-prevent-zinc-anemia/.

80. Wu J, Cho E, Giovannucci EL, Rosner BA, Sastry SM, Willett WC, et al. Dietary intakes of eicosapentaenoic acid and docosahexaenoic acid and risk of age-related macular degeneration. Ophthalmology. 2017;124(5):634–43.

81. Silván JM, Reguero M, de Pascual-Teresa S. A protective effect of anthocyanins and xanthophylls on UVB-induced damage in retinal pigment epithelial cells. Food Funct. 2016;7(2):1067–76.

82. Devaraj S, Mathur S, Basu A, Aung HH, Vasu VT, Meyers S, et al. A dose-response study on the effects of purified lycopene supplementation on biomarkers of oxidative stress. J Am Coll Nutr. 2008;27(2):267–73.

83. Mac RN. Lycopene and macular degeneration [Internet]. Lycopene and macular degeneration. 2021 [cited 2021 Feb 12]. Available from: https://www.webrn-maculardegeneration.com/lycopene.html.

84. Campbell P. Vitamin D and homotaurine show potential benefit for macular degeneration [Internet]. HCP. 2020 [cited 2021 Feb 11]. Available from: https://www.hcplive.com/view/vitamin-d-and-homotaurine-potential-benefit-for-macular-degeneration.

85. Khoo HE, Ng HS, Yap W-S, Goh HJH, Yim HS. Nutrients for prevention of macular degeneration and eye-related diseases. Antioxidants (Basel). 2019;8(4):85.

86. Winkler BS, Boulton ME, Gottsch JD, Sternberg P. Oxidative damage and age-related macular degeneration. Mol Vis. 1999;5:32.

87. Yi C, Pan X, Yan H, Guo M, Pierpaoli W. Effects of melatonin in age-related macular degeneration. Ann N Y Acad Sci. 2005;1057:384–92.

88. Mokhtari F, Panjehpour T, Naeini FF, Hosseini SM, Nilforoushzadeh MA, Matin M. The frequency distribution of celiac autoantibodies in alopecia areata. Int J Prev Med. 2016;7:109.

89. Volta U, Bardazzi F, Zauli D, DeFranceschi L, Tosti A, Molinaro N, et al. Serological screening for coeliac disease in vitiligo and alopecia areata. Br J Dermatol. 1997;136(5):801–2.

90. Hallaji Z, Akhyani M, Ehsani AH, Noormohammadpour P, Gholamali F, Bagheri M, et al. Prevalence of anti-gliadin antibody in patients with alopecia areata: a case-control study. Tehran Univ Med J. 2011;68(12):738–42.

91. Kakar P. Alopecia areata - here's everything you should know about it [Internet]. Skin Kraft Laboratories. 2020 [cited 2021 Feb 16]. Available from: https://skinkraft.com/blogs/articles/alopecia-areata.

92. Ibrahim O, Bergfeld WF, Piliang M. Eosinophilic esophagitis: another atopy-related alopecia areata trigger? J Investig Dermatol Symp Proc. 2015;17(2):58–60.

93. 4 foods that could be causing hair loss [Internet]. Ottawa Life Magazine. 2017 [cited 2021 Feb 16]. Available from: https://www.ottawalife.com/article/4-foods-that-could-be-causing-hair-loss?c=6.

94. Pratt CH, King LE, Messenger AG, Christiano AM, Sundberg JP. Alopecia areata. Nat Rev Dis Primers. 2017;3:17011.

95. Park H, Kim CW, Kim SS, Park CW. The therapeutic effect and the changed serum zinc level after zinc supplementation in alopecia areata patients who had a low serum zinc level. Ann Dermatol. 2009;21(2):142–6.

96. Bistas KG, Tadi P. Biotin [Internet]. 2020 [cited 2021 Feb 12]. Available from: https://www.ncbi.nlm.nih.gov/books/NBK554493/.

97. NIH. Biotin [Internet]. NIH Office of Dietary Supplements. 2020 [cited 2021 Feb 12]. Available from: https://ods.od.nih.gov/factsheets/Biotin-HealthProfessional/.

98. Almohanna HM, Ahmed AA, Tsatalis JP, Tosti A. The role of vitamins and minerals in hair loss: a review. Dermatol Ther (Heidelb). 2019;9(1):51–70.

99. Harvey CJ. Combined diet and supplementation therapy resolves alopecia areata in a paediatric patient: a case study [Internet]. Cureus. 2020 [cited 2021 Feb 12]. Available from: https://www.cureus.com/articles/42894-combined-diet-and-supplementation-therapy-resolves-alopecia-areata-in-a-paediatric-patient-a-case-study.

100. Thompson JM, Mirza MA, Park MK, Qureshi AA, Cho E. The role of micronutrients in alopecia areata: a review. Am J Clin Dermatol. 2017;18(5):663–79.

101. Trost LB, Bergfeld WF, Calogeras E. The diagnosis and treatment of iron deficiency and its potential relationship to hair loss. J Am Acad Dermatol. 2006;54(5):824–44.

102. Labrozzi A. Nutrients in hair supplements: evaluation of their function in hair loss treatment. Hair Ther Transplant. 2020;10(1):1–6.

103. NIH. Vitamin B6 [Internet]. National Institutes of Health Office of Dietary Supplements. 2020 [cited 2020 Dec 30]. Available from: https://ods.od.nih.gov/factsheets/VitaminB6-HealthProfessional/#:~:text=The%20richest%20sources%20of%20vitamin,1%2C3%2C5%5D.

104. Hosking A-M, Juhasz M, Atanaskova MN. Complementary and alternative treatments for alopecia: a comprehensive review. Skin Appendage Disord. 2019;5(2):72–89.

105. MPB Research. Taurine, anti-aging and hair growth benefits [Internet]. MPB Research. 2016 [cited 2021 Feb 12]. Available from: https://www.hairloss-research.org/UpdateTaurineAnti-agingandHairGrowthBenefits8-16.html#:~:text=Numerous%20studies%20have%20shown%20Taurine,and%20other%20auto%2Dimmune%20disorders.

106. El-Tahlwai SM, El-Ramly AZ, El-Nabarawy E, El-Ghaffar N, Nagwa A, Emam H, et al. Serum selenium levels in alopecia areata. J Egypt Women Dermatol Soc. 2012;9(3):174–7.

107. Al-Gaff AN, Humadi S, Wohaieb SA. Effect of melatonin on oxidative stress markers in patients with alopecia areata. Iraqi J Pharm. 2005;5(1):33–9.

108. Nosrati A, Afifi L, Danesh MJ, Lee K, Yan D, Beroukhim K, et al. Dietary modifications in atopic dermatitis: patient-reported outcomes. J Dermatolog Treat. 2017;28(6):523–38.

109. Lv N, Xiao L, Ma J. Dietary pattern and asthma: a systematic review and meta-analysis. J Asthma Allergy. 2014;7:105–21.

110. Jeziorek M, Frej-Mądrzak M, Choroszy-Król I. The influence of diet on gastrointestinal Candida spp. colonization and the susceptibility of Candida spp. to antifungal drugs. Rocz Panstw Zakl Hig. 2019;70(2):195–200.

111. Genova Diagnostics. Essential & metabolic fatty acids analysis (EMFA) [Internet]. Genova Diagnostics. 2021 [cited 2021 Mar 9]. Available from: https://www.gdx.net/product/essential-metabolic-fatty-acids-analysis-nutritional-test-blood.

112. Kogan M, Castillo CC, Barber MS. Chronic rhinosinusitis and irritable bowel syndrome: a case report. Integr Med (Encinitas). 2016;15(3):44–54.

Chapter 7
Musculoskeletal

Contents

The human body is built to move, and as we consider the nutritional support for the physical body, we must acknowledge the importance of movement in achieving optimal physical well-being. Exercise and movement are foundational to all aspects of health but none more directly than our physical body. Research suggests that regular physical movement slows the decline in functional capacity and increases healthy life span by 7 years [2]. Thus all recommendations for support should recognize the need for a personalized movement plan.

7.1 Muscle and Joint Pain

Discomfort in the skeletal muscle and joints has a myriad of causes which can be exacerbated by unidentified food sensitivities, malnutrition, and inflammatory foods. Food sensitivity testing may be indicated to help identify foods since triggers can be healthy foods which individually do not work for the patient. In addition, the five most common foods that cause sensitivities are gluten, dairy, corn, soy, and eggs, and this can be a reasonable place to start in order to test for symptom improvement in 4–6 weeks. Table 7.1 summarizes key herbal and supplemental support for muscle and joint pain.

J. Wendt et al., *Integrative Geriatric Nutrition*,
https://doi.org/10.1007/978-3-030-81758-9_7

Table 7.1 Herbal and supplemental support for muscle and joint pain [3]

	MOA	Daily dose	Food sources
Curcumin	Anti-inflammatory	1000 mg [7]	Turmeric
A. montana (homeopathic and herbal)	Improves symptoms as effectively as a gel containing NSAID, but with no better adverse event profile [3]	Variable as needed	Herbal and homeopathic
Glucosamine	Protects chondrocytes. Superior to placebo in treatment of pain and functional impairment resulting from symptomatic osteoarthritis [3]	1500 mg [8]	Shellfish (shrimp, lobster, crab)
Chondroitin	Works well in combination with glucosamine. Protects chondrocytes. Lowers risk of serious adverse events compared to control	800–1200 mg [9]	Cow, pig, fish, shark, and bird
SAMe	Unclear. May reduce inflammation, increase proteoglycan synthesis, or have analgesic effect [10]	800–1200 mg [11] *Warning: possibility of manic episodes with high doses (>400 mg)*	Turkey, beef, fish, pork, tofu, milk, cheese, nuts, beans, and quinoa
EGCG	Chondroprotective, anti-inflammatory, and palliative [12]	400–1200 mg [13]	Green tea
EPA/DHA	Analgesic and anti-inflammatory [14]	Ratio beneficial when >1.5, ~2.6 g total [14]	Salmon, sardines, trout, oysters, sea bass/flaxseed (oil), chia seeds, English walnuts, canola oil, salmon, and soybean oil [15]
Resveratrol	Antioxidant and anti-inflammatory [16]	500 mg [16]	Grapes, wine, peanuts, and soy [17]
Avocado soybean unsaponifiables (ASU)	Anti-catabolic properties prevent cartilage degradation and inhibit fibrinolysis and anabolic properties stimulating collagen and aggrecan synthesis [18]	300 mg [18]	Avocado and soybean oil
Topical or systemic cannabinoids	Cannabinoid receptor agonists block but acute and chronic pain and attenuate inflammation [19]	Varies	Source
MSM	Anti-inflammatory	3 g BID [20]	Fruits, vegetables, grains, beer, port wine, coffee, tea, and cow's milk [20]

Table 7.1 (continued)

	MOA	Daily dose	Food sources
Tart cherries	Anti-inflammatory	480 ml [21]	Source
Quercetin	Anti-inflammatory, antioxidant, and antinociceptive [22]	500 mg	Onions, apples, grapes, berries, pomegranate, broccoli, and tea [23]
Bromelain	Anti-inflammatory, analgesic, anti-edematous, antithrombotic, and fibrinolytic [24]	540 mg [24]	Pineapple
Vitamin B12	Analgesic, mechanism poorly understood [25]	1000 μg	Clams, beef liver, trout, salmon, tuna fish, and nutritional yeast [26]
Methylfolate	Analgesic	1–15 mg *Warning: high doses can cause severe irritability and anxiety due to hypermethylation*	Spinach, asparagus, romaine, turnips, cauliflower, and broccoli

- *Arthritis:*

  - Osteoarthritis:

    Anti-inflammatory diet.
    Specific trial elimination of nightshades (tomato, potato, pepper, eggplant) and gluten for 6 weeks. If symptoms improve, reintroduce each food separately (two servings daily), waiting 4 days before adding in a different food.

  - Rheumatoid arthritis:

    Autoimmune diet protocols are relevant.
    Vegan diet.
    Elimination diet focused on eliminating gluten, dairy, and sugar.
    Gut health support including probiotic-rich foods. See the gut Chap. 3 for specific details.

- *Gout:*

  - *Reduce or eliminate* [3]:

    Fructose in the diet from soft drinks and sweetened beverages as well as other processed sweets.
    Purine-rich animal foods and seafood.
    Beer, spirits, and wine.
    Synthetic vitamin A derivatives.
    High-dose niacin (>50 mg q.d.) is contraindicated [4].

– *Increase or maintain* [3]:

> Low-fat dairy consumption is recommended.
> Healthy weight.
> One serving of cherries (½ cup) per day reduced gout attacks by 35% [5].
> Vegetables, oatmeal, legumes, and mushrooms.
> Coffee intake four or more cups per day reduced serum uric acid levels.
> EPA.
> Vitamin C 500 mg/day [6].
> Anti-inflammatory foods such as B-carotene, omega-3 fatty acids, luteolin-rich foods (celery, green peppers), and rutin–/quercetin-rich foods.

7.2   Anorexia of Aging

Weight loss and frailty in the aging adult have unfortunately become an expected outcome of the aging process and are often overlooked by providers. Rather than normalize the loss of weight, specific nutritional interventions can be recommended that arrest the physical and biochemical processes that cause poor health outcomes.

Key interventions to interrupt the anorexia of aging cycle are as follows:

- Assess for protein-energy malnutrition. Goal protein intake = 1.0–1.2 g per kilogram of body weight.
- Address other causes of loss of appetite such as ill-fitting dentures or damaged teeth, unmanaged stress, slowed digestion and dysbiosis, and difficulty in preparing and acquiring food.
- Screen patients using a validated assessment tool such as the Simplified Nutritional Assessment Questionnaire (SNAQ) or Mini Nutritional Assessment (MNA).

7.3   Sarcopenia

Age-related loss of muscle mass and function increases risk of falls and decreases quality of life. Early screening and prevention are critical to preventing the associated decline in functional capacity and frailty [27]. Ensuring adequate protein intake, addressing achlorhydria, and well-rounded exercise routine will reduce the natural process of decreasing muscle mass with age.

7.4   Osteopenia/Osteoporosis [28]

Since bone density is established in young adulthood and gradually decreases through older age, the aging adult faces the implications of diminishing bone density and is often looking for answers on how to stop and reverse bone loss.

Key nutritional interventions include the following:

- Adequate intake of calcium from food and supplements combined which requires a dietary assessment in order to understand what, if any, supplemental needs a person has.
- Patients avoiding dairy need to pay extra attention to dietary sources of calcium and most often will need a calcium supplement.
- Physical movement provides signals to the body to use nutrients to build bone mass.
- High-protein diets are associated with bone mineral density.
- Caffeine intake is associated with lower bone mass density.
- Vitamin K2 supplementation when necessary. See Table 7.2 for distinction between vitamins K1 and K2.
- Table 7.3 outlines herbal and botanical support for bone health.

Secondary risk factors [30] are as follows:

- Hormonal imbalance [31].
- Dysfunction in vitamin D metabolism [32].
- Chronic renal failure [33].
- Medication such as corticosteroids and proton pump inhibitors [34].
- Blood sugar imbalance [35].
- Oxidative stress and systemic inflammation [36].

Therapeutic diets are as follows:

- Mediterranean diet: following this dietary pattern is associated with a decrease in hip fractures [51] related to these key attributes:
  - Fruits, vegetables, and legumes are the foundation of the diet, accounting for 80% of intake.
  - Adequate calcium intake from regular dairy intake.
  - Variety of protein sources including meat, poultry, fish, soy, and legumes.

Table 7.2 Vitamin K1 vs. K2 [29]

	Vitamin K1	Vitamin K2 and menaquinone-4 (MK4)	Vitamin K2 and menaquinone-7 (MK7)
Function	Participates in blood clotting and is cofactor for carboxylation	Osteocalcin (synthesized in the bone) serves as matrix GLA protein, involved in calcium transport, and helps improve bone density	As for MK4 but long-chain form with longer half-life
Source	Green leafy vegetables and some plant oils	Butter, eggs, yolks, lard, and animal-based foods. Synthesized by bacteria in intestinal tract	Fermented foods and some cheese
Dose	100–500 µg *Must be avoided if warfarin is co-administered*	15–45 mg *Caution is advised with warfarin; check INR within 2 weeks after initiating*	50–500 µg *Caution is advised with warfarin; check INR within 2 weeks after initiating*

Table 7.3 Herbal and botanical support for bone health [37]

	MOA	Daily dose	Food sources
Calcium	Essential for healthy bones. Important to consider dietary calcium intake from both dairy and nondairy sources [37]	600–1200 mg/day, divided [37] Best to split up into 300–400 mg TID dosing. Possible increase in cardiac risks with once-daily dosing of over 500 mg [38]	Dairy, leafy greens, fish with bones, red pepper, fortified orange juice, grapefruit juice, and kiwi
Vitamin D	Essential for calcium absorption. May help prevent falls in elderly by improving skeletal muscles and increasing strength and balance [37]	2000 IU/day [37]	Cod liver oil, trout, sockeye salmon, mushrooms, and milk [39]
Vitamin K2 Menaquinones [4 or 7]	Is involved in calcium transport, preventing calcium deposition in the lining of blood vessel walls, and helps improve bone density [40]	45 mg MK4 100–500 µg MK7	Fermented *natto* soy foods (MK7) Animal sources such as egg yolk (MK4) Generally very small amounts of vitamin K2 can be found in food. Human intestinal flora is a major producer of vitamin MK7 but not MK4
Green tea	Anti-inflammatory [37]	1–3 cups [41]	Source
Black cohosh [37]	Supports bone turnover and remodeling [42]	40 mg [42]	Source
Astragalus membranaceus [37]	Supports chondrocyte proliferation [43]	1.3 g	*Astragalus* root
Curcumin [37]	Inhibits osteoporosis by inhibiting osteoclasts [44]	200 mg [45]	Turmeric
Walnut extract [37]	Anti-inflammatory	Varies	Walnut
Magnesium	Supports bone crystal formation [46]	300–600 mg/day	Almonds, spinach, cashews, and peanuts
Omega-3	Effect on calcium balance, osteoblastogenesis and osteoblast activity, change of membrane function, decrease in inflammatory cytokines, and modulation of peroxisome proliferators [47]	ALA dose: 3000–5000 mg EPA/DHA: 1500–3000 mg	Fatty fish and flax–/hemp–/chia seeds [15]

Table 7.3 (continued)

	MOA	Daily dose	Food sources
Collagen calcium chelate	Improves bone mineral density and bone turnover and reduces bone loss [48]	500 mg elemental calcium 200 IU vitamin D [48]	Cod liver oil, trout, salmon, mushrooms, milk, yogurt, orange juice, cheese, and sardines [39, 49]
Copper	Copper deficiency can block normal collagen production	0.5–2 mg *Monitor serum levels throughout therapy. High levels are known to be associated with increased risk of Alzheimer's disease* [50]	Nuts and seeds
Zinc	Enhances calcium absorption and vitamin D metabolism	5–30 mg [50]	Oysters

- Anti-inflammatory diet: focusing on anti-inflammatory foods such as colorful fruits and vegetables, healthy fats, whole grains, nuts and seeds, and fatty fish is associated with increased bone density:

  - Actively avoiding oxidants from the diet such as fried foods, processed foods with chemical additives, and foods high in refined carbohydrates.

  Table 7.4 highlights key micronutrients for musculoskeletal health.

7.5   Case Studies

7.5.1   *Osteoarthritis*

John, a 69-year-old woodworker, presented a few months after he had renal failure from regular intake of NSAIDs (mostly ibuprofen) for several years. His renal failure improved after all NSAIDs were discontinued, but his chronic osteoarthritis that affected his fingers, wrists, knees, and lower back got a lot worse. Over his years, he built a successful boutique furniture business and had no interest in stopping making his own furniture. Acetaminophen was barely helpful, and opioids caused too many side effects including constipation and nausea. John had tried acupuncture with some improvement but did not continue it due to minimal benefit. His other issues include chronic mild constipation, frequent cramps, and seasonal affective disorder. He was noted to have mildly elevated blood pressure on multiple different doctor's visits, but he never took

Table 7.4 Micronutrients of primary concern

	MOA	Food sources	RDA for 55+	Side effects/comments for providers
Omega-3	Effect on calcium balance, osteoblastogenesis and osteoblast activity, change of membrane function, decrease in inflammatory cytokines, and modulation of peroxisome proliferators [47]	Flaxseed (oil), chia seeds, walnuts, salmon, anchovies, herring, mackerel, canola oil, and sardines [15]	1.6 g M and 1.1 g F [15]	Preferred source is fatty fish since conversion to EPA/DHA is only 5–8% effective from alpha-linolenic acid which is found in vegetarian sources [52]
Calcium	Key role in skeleton mineralization and required for normal growth, development, and bone strength [53]	Milk, cheese, yogurt, fortified orange juice, and sardines with bones [49]	500 mg [54]	Very high levels of supplementation can increase risk of kidney stones and myocardial infarction [54]
Magnesium	Increases bone mineral density [54]	Pumpkin seeds, chia seeds, almonds, spinach, cashews, and peanuts [55]	250–350 mg [54]	Rare. Excess magnesium may cause diarrhea, nausea, and abdominal cramping [55]
Vitamin D	Essential for calcium absorption and bone mineralization, positively associated with bone mineral density and immunoregulation [56]	Liver, egg yolk, saltwater fish, and sun [39]	400–1000 IU [54]	Requires sufficient calcium intake [57]
Vitamin K2	Improves bone properties that increase bone strength without increasing mineral content [54]	Fermented soy, meat, and dairy produce [58]	50–150 µg [54]	MK4 source from gut microbiome, MK7 Not involved in clotting and generally safe for patients on warfarin
Boron	Improves calcium and magnesium retention. Increases bone strength [54]	Coffee, milk, apples, dried and cooked beans, and potatoes [59]	1–3 mg [54]	No toxicity reported and rapidly excreted in urine [54]
Silicon	Supports collagen synthesis and/or its stabilization and matrix mineralization [60]	Cereals, grains, some fruits, and vegetables [60]	3–12 mg [60]	Oral ingestion of crystalline or amorphous silica/silicates may cause toxicity, particularly renal toxicity [60]

Table 7.4 (continued)

	MOA	Food sources	RDA for 55+	Side effects/comments for providers
Strontium	Elevates bone mineral density and reduces fragility fractures [61]	Seafood, whole milk, wheat bran, meat, poultry, and root vegetables	680 mg [61]	Excessive strontium ultimately results in decreased bone calcium content, dissolution of mineralized bone, disruption of bone architecture, and lower bone mineral density [61]
Vitamin C	Essential for forming collagen and fracture healing [54]	Red pepper, orange, grapefruit, kiwifruit, green pepper, broccoli, and strawberries [62]	500– 100 mg [54]	Side effects are rare except in extreme overdose. May cause headache, GI symptoms, and insomnia [63]
Manganese	Cofactor in the formation of bone cartilage and collagen, as well as in bone mineralization [64]	Cereals, nuts, pineapples, beans, mollusks, dark chocolate, cinnamon, and tea [64]	1.8– 2.3 mg [54]	Is rare except for extreme overdose and causes Parkinson syndrome [65]
CoQ10	Promotes osteoblast proliferation and differentiation [66]	Oily fish (salmon and tuna), liver, and whole grains	20 mg/kg [66]	Low toxicity and no serious adverse effects reported in humans [67]
Creatine	Enhances bone mineral properties and decreases bone resorption [68]	Red meat, seafood, and poultry [68]	5–8 g [68]	Results mixed, most positive when combined with resistance training [68]
Protein	Increases insulin-like growth factor 1, key mediator in bone health, increases intestinal calcium absorption, suppresses parathyroid hormone, and improves muscle strength and mass, all of which may benefit the skeleton [29]	Meat and meat products, cereals, milk, and many vegetables [69]	0.8 g/kg [70]	Beneficial with adequate calcium intake [29]
B complex	May support bone health and possibly reduce fracture risk as cofactors for enzymes involved in a variety of energy producing pathways [71]	Leafy greens. However, patients with MTHFR variants may need methylated vitamins as enzyme conversion is inhibited	One per day, in the morning	There are several possible mechanisms, but randomized clinical trials have rarely shown protective effects [71]

any medications or had any treatment for this. He did not have any special diet but often ate late due to his work schedule. His diet contained a high amount of starches and grains as well as animal protein and fat. While his wife tried to have him eat greens and vegetables, he often left those untouched on the plate. He did not usually snack on foods often being consumed by his work. He never exercised, but his work was very physically demanding with often lifting heavy pieces of wood and furniture. Despite having successful business and number of people working for him, he still preferred to do lots of manual work himself, and when his wife got him Fitbit for one of his birthdays, it showed that he often clocked over 15,000 steps daily. John was not taking any medications, but his wife made him take multivitamin with 800 IU of vitamin D.

On exam, John appeared well built and overall healthy, but he is found to be borderline hypertensive with BP 145/85. His skin is somewhat dry and flaky. His blood work confirmed our suspicion of magnesium deficiency with RBC magnesium at 4.0 mg/dL (normal range 4.2–6.8 mg/dL). Blood work also revealed mildly elevated total cholesterol at 230 mg/dL, LDL at 135 mg/dL, mildly elevated cardiac C-reactive protein at 3.5 mg/L, and low vitamin D 25OH at 11.5 ng/mL.

Given resistance to dietary changes, we referred John to a nutritional health coach after prescribing Mediterranean diet with nighttime fasting between 7 PM and 9 AM. Given his laboratory findings, we prescribed 400 mg of magnesium citrate at bedtime to both replete magnesium and also improve constipation and cramps. We have changed his multivitamin to much-higher-potency one with high-dose B vitamins including 1000 μg of folate and methylcobalamin. We also prescribed him high-dose fish oil of 3000 mg daily of combined EPA and DHA, glucosamine sulfate 1500 mg in combination with chondroitin sulfate 1200 mg and MSM 900 mg, and vitamin D3 5000 units daily with 100 μg of vitamin K2 (MK7). Given seasonal affective disorder and osteoarthritis, we also decided to start him on 200 mg of SAMe and over 4 weeks increase dose to 800 mg once daily. John was resistant to any idea of medical cannabis but was open to try hemp-based CBD and CBDa products. Additionally, we added CBDa soft gels 20 mg twice daily and recommended that he use topical high-potency CBD and/or CBDa creams as needed in addition or instead of Tylenol.

3 months later, John's wife called to express her immense gratitude. John was able to change his diet and take all supplements as recommended. He specifically liked CBDa capsules and CBDa cream that improved his pain significantly and within a short time. Not only John had dramatic improvement in his osteoarthritis and rarely needed any Tylenol, but his blood pressure normalized and constipation improved. On follow-up blood work 6 months later, his cholesterol improved to 205 mg/dL with LDL of 116 mg/dL, cardiac C-reactive protein decreased to 1.2 mg/L, and vitamin D normalized to 37 ng/mL and his home BPs were all under 135 systolic.

7.5.2 Weight Loss and Sarcopenia

Carolyn, an 83-year-old woman with multiple medical problems, suffered a stroke 6 months before coming to the clinic. Prior to stroke, she had high blood pressure, diabetes, atrial fibrillation, and remote history of breast cancer in remission. While she did not have any focal neurologic deficits, she became very fatigued and weak, and despite physical therapy, good diet, and outstanding home support, she was slowly losing weight and became deeply demoralized and often talked about not wanting to be a burden to her children. She denied depression, but she was missing many of her prior activities like daily walks with dogs, going to dance social events with her friends, and doing grocery shopping and taking care of the house. While her goals of care included avoiding any life-prolonging treatments in case of terminal illness, she clearly expressed interest in feeling better and trying to walk again. Her diet had good amount of complex carbohydrate, fruits, vegetables, and greens. Upon advice of her cardiologist, she was on low-salt diet and did not eat any red meat and eggs and stayed away from most saturated foods. Carolyn was on complex medical regimen including diabetic regimen with metformin, hypertension with lisinopril and metoprolol, atrial fibrillation with apixaban, and stroke with high-dose rosuvastatin. In addition, she was taking multivitamin, 1000 mg of fish oil, and vitamin D 1000 units. On exam, her vitals showed heart rate in low 50s and were irregular, and her blood pressure was 100/60. She appeared thin and frail. Her mood was depressed but she was engaging and motivated to get better. Her basic blood work was normal; however, her total cholesterol was noted to be 116 mg/dL and LDL at 32 mg/dL.

Before proceeding to discuss changes in her diet, it is essential to mention that part of this case was difficult conversation with her cardiologist, neurologist, the patient, and her family about the fact that she was overtreated with medications. While it is routine that after stroke patients are often put on maximum dose of high-potency statins, total cholesterol of 110 mg/dL and LDL of 35 mg/dL are not normal and simply too low. Same was true of her blood pressure routinely being 100/60. After multiple conversations, we decided to discontinue metoprolol and decrease rosuvastatin to ¼ of presenting dose. Additionally, we recommended she stops low-salt diet and adds cup of bone broth daily, as well as 20 gm of plant-based protein powder. In addition, we added 3 grams of L-carnitine and ubiquinol (biologically active form of CoQ10) 200 mg daily and increased her fish oil intake to 3000 mg. Given severe fatigue, we also decided to try high-dose nicotinamide riboside at 500 mg twice daily. In 4 weeks, Carolyn felt that her energy improved enough to start working with physical therapy and begin walking out of house with walker. By 3 months, she was able to walk slowly with cane 3–4 blocks without getting short of breath. At 6 months of follow-up, she walked into the office smiling saying that she has not felt this good even before the stroke. Her home blood pressure remained under 130 systolic, while heart rate increased to 70–80s but not above 100. While her cholesterol increased significantly to total 184 mg/dL and LDL at 69 mg/dL, it was still in good range despite significantly lower dose of rosuvastatin.

7.5.3   Osteoporosis

Mary, a 72-year-old woman, came to see us after she developed osteoporosis. Highly active and otherwise basically healthy Mary, an avid horse rider, was afraid of fractures, especially given more than average risk of falls. Her primary care doctor recommended starting oral alendronate, but after reading side effects, she decided to try nutritional approach. After careful review of her diet, we learned that Mary was pescatarian and ate no dairy and very little grains. She was not open to adding any meat or bone broth. However, she agreed to add at least once weekly canned sardines, specifically ones that had their bones not removed; she also did not consume regular soy foods and was interested in adding more tofu and miso soup at least 2–3 times/week. She was already taking multivitamins with minerals and separate calcium 1000 mg daily. Her other supplements included glucosamine for joints and biotin for thinning hair. We have changed her supplements to specialized bone multivitamin that had 800 mg of calcium and 400 mg of magnesium, both in organic chelated form for best absorption. Additionally, same formula contained all

Bone Density Exams Results:

Region	Age	BMD	T-score	BMD Change	BMD Change
Exam Date		g/cm2		vs Baseline	vs Previous

Total Hip (Left) Statistically no significant change from previous scan.

05/10/2016	72	0.690	-2.1	-0.060(-8.0%)*	0.007(1.0%)
08/25/2014	71	0.683	-2.1	-0.067(-8.9%)*	-0.039(-5.5%)*
08/21/2013	70	0.723	-1.8	-0.027(-3.6%)	-0.037(-4.9%)*
08/15/2012	69	0.760	-1.5	0.010(1.3%)	-0.001(-0.1%)
08/08/2011	68	0.760	-1.5	0.010(1.4%)	0.009(1.2%)
07/28/2010	67	0.751	-1.6	0.010(0.2%)	0.005(0.7%)
07/16/2009	66	0.746	-1.6	-0.004(-0.5%)	-0.004(-0.5%)
07/13/2007	64	0.750	-1.6		

*Denotes significance at 95% confidence level, LSC is 0.026675 g/cm2

Femoral Neck (Left) Statistically significant increase from previous scan.

05/10/2016	72	0.583	-2.4	-0.038(-6.0%)*	0.035(6.4%)*
08/25/2014	71	0.548	-2.7	-0.073(-11.7%)*	-0.060(-9.8%)*
08/21/2013	70	0.608	-2.2	-0.013(-2.1%)	-0.014(-2.2%)
08/15/2012	69	0.621	-2.1	0.000(0.1%)	-0.001(-0.2%)
08/08/2011	68	0.623	-2.0	0.002(0.3%)	0.014(2.2%)
07/28/2010	67	0.609	-2.2	-0.012(-1.9%)	-0.003(-0.6%)
07/16/2009	66	0.612	-2.1	-0.009(-1.4%)	-0.009(-1.4%)
07/13/2007	64	0.621	-2.1		

*Denotes significance at 95% confidence level, LSC is 0.028808 g/cm2

Fig. 7.1 Sample bone density exam results

essential microminerals including boron, silicon, zinc, and copper. Same formula contained 350 µg of vitamin K2 in menaquinone-7 (MK7) form. Additionally, we have added 45 mg of menaquinone-4 (MK4) form of vitamin K2. Mary was already very active, but we still recommended she adds Tai Chi to her routine to improve balance to decrease risk of falls. Nearly 2 years later, we saw Mary for follow-up consultation after she obtained repeat DEXA scan that showed that her hip density remained stable and her spine improved significantly. (See Fig. 7.1.) Needless to say, Mary was very happy; she also reported that her horse riding has improved with practicing Tai Chi and unexpected "side effect" of adding this low-impact but powerful form of traditional Chinese medicine practice.

References

1. Akishita M, Ishii S, Kojima T, Kozaki K, Kuzuya M, Arai H, et al. Priorities of health care outcomes for the elderly. J Am Med Dir Assoc. 2013;14(7):479–84.
2. Franco OH, de Laet C, Peeters A, Jonker J, Mackenbach J, Nusselder W. Effects of physical activity on life expectancy with cardiovascular disease. Arch Intern Med. 2005;165(20):2355–60.
3. Kogan M, Weil A. Common rheumatic diseases in the elderly. Integrative geriatric medicine. Oxford Online; 2018. p. 463.
4. Pizzorno JE, Murray MT. Textbook of natural medicine. 4th ed. St. Louis: Churchill Livingstone; 2012.
5. Zhang Y, Neogi T, Chen C, Chaisson C, Hunter DJ, Choi HK. Cherry consumption and decreased risk of recurrent gout attacks. Arthritis Rheum. 2012;64(12):4004–11.
6. Huang H-Y, Appel LJ, Choi MJ, Gelber AC, Charleston J, Norkus EP, et al. The effects of vitamin C supplementation on serum concentrations of uric acid: results of a randomized controlled trial. Arthritis Rheum. 2005;52(6):1843–7.
7. Daily JW, Yang M, Park S. Efficacy of turmeric extracts and curcumin for alleviating the symptoms of joint arthritis: a systematic review and meta-analysis of randomized clinical trials. J Med Food. 2016;19(8):717–29.
8. Ogata T, Ideno Y, Akai M, Seichi A, Hagino H, Iwaya T, et al. Effects of glucosamine in patients with osteoarthritis of the knee: a systematic review and meta-analysis. Clin Rheumatol. 2018;37(9):2479–87.
9. Henrotin Y, Mathy M, Sanchez C, Lambert C. Chondroitin sulfate in the treatment of osteoarthritis: from in vitro studies to clinical recommendations. Ther Adv Musculoskelet Dis. 2010;2(6):335–48.
10. Najm WI, Reinsch S, Hoehler F, Tobis JS, Harvey PW. S-adenosyl methionine (SAMe) versus celecoxib for the treatment of osteoarthritis symptoms: a double-blind cross-over trial. [ISRCTN36233495]. BMC Musculoskelet Disord. 2004;5:6.
11. Galizia I, Oldani L, Macritchie K, Amari E, Dougall D, Jones TN, et al. S-adenosyl methionine (SAMe) for depression in adults. Cochrane Database Syst Rev. 2016;10:CD011286.
12. Leong DJ, Choudhury M, Hanstein R, Hirsh DM, Kim SJ, Majeska RJ, et al. Green tea polyphenol treatment is chondroprotective, anti-inflammatory and palliative in a mouse post-traumatic osteoarthritis model. Arthritis Res Ther. 2014;16(6):508.
13. Ahmed S. Green tea polyphenol epigallocatechin 3-gallate in arthritis: progress and promise. Arthritis Res Ther. 2010;12(2):208.
14. Senftleber NK, Nielsen SM, Andersen JR, Bliddal H, Tarp S, Lauritzen L, et al. Marine oil supplements for arthritis pain: a systematic review and meta-analysis of randomized trials. Nutrients. 2017;9(1):42.

15. NIH. Omega-3 Fatty Acids [Internet]. NIH Office of Dietary Supplements. 2020 [cited 2021 Mar 4]. Available from: https://ods.od.nih.gov/factsheets/Omega3FattyAcids-HealthProfessional/.
16. Marouf BH, Hussain SA, Ali ZS, Ahmmad RS. Resveratrol supplementation reduces pain and inflammation in knee osteoarthritis patients treated with meloxicam: a randomized placebo-controlled study. J Med Food. 2018; https://doi.org/10.1089/jmf.2017.4176.
17. Chachay VS, Kirkpatrick CMJ, Hickman IJ, Ferguson M, Prins JB, Martin JH. Resveratrol--pills to replace a healthy diet? Br J Clin Pharmacol. 2011;72(1):27–38.
18. Christiansen BA, Bhatti S, Goudarzi R, Emami S. Management of osteoarthritis with avocado/soybean unsaponifiables. Cartilage. 2015;6(1):30–44.
19. Bruni N, Della Pepa C, Oliaro-Bosso S, Pessione E, Gastaldi D, Dosio F. Cannabinoid delivery systems for pain and inflammation treatment. Molecules. 2018;23(10):2478.
20. Kim LS, Axelrod LJ, Howard P, Buratovich N, Waters RF. Efficacy of methylsulfonyl-methane (MSM) in osteoarthritis pain of the knee: a pilot clinical trial. Osteoarthr Cartil. 2006;14(3):286–94.
21. Chai SC, Davis K, Zhang Z, Zha L, Kirschner KF. Effects of tart cherry juice on biomarkers of inflammation and oxidative stress in older adults. Nutrients. 2019;11(2):228.
22. Valério DA, Georgetti SR, Magro DA, Casagrande R, Cunha TM, Vicentini FTMC, et al. Quercetin reduces inflammatory pain: inhibition of oxidative stress and cytokine production. J Nat Prod. 2009;72(11):1975–9.
23. Mlcek J, Jurikova T, Skrovankova S, Sochor J. Quercetin and its anti-allergic immune response. Molecules. 2016;12:21(5).
24. Brien S, Lewith G, Walker A, Hicks SM, Middleton D. Bromelain as a treatment for osteoar-thritis: a review of clinical studies. Evid Based Complement Alternat Med. 2004;1(3):251–7.
25. Zhang M, Han W, Hu S, Xu H. Methylcobalamin: a potential vitamin of pain killer. Neural Plast. 2013;2013:424651.
26. Vitamin B12 [Internet]. NIH National Institutes of Health Office of Dietary Supplements. 2020 [cited 2021 Jan 2]. Available from: https://ods.od.nih.gov/factsheets/VitaminB12-HealthProfessional/.
27. Litchford MD. Counteracting the trajectory of frailty and sarcopenia in older adults. Nutr Clin Pract. 2014;29(4):428–34.
28. Iwamoto J. Vitamin K2 therapy for postmenopausal osteoporosis. Nutrients. 2014;6(5):1971–80.
29. Mangano KM, Sahni S, Kerstetter JE. Dietary protein is beneficial to bone health under condi-tions of adequate calcium intake: an update on clinical research. Curr Opin Clin Nutr Metab Care. 2014;17(1):69–74.
30. Sandhaus S. Osteoporosis [Internet]. Life Extension. 2021 [cited 2021 Mar 4]. Available from: https://www.lifeextension.com/protocols/metabolic-health/osteoporosis.
31. Body JJ, Bergmann P, Boonen S, Boutsen Y, Bruyere O, Devogelaer JP, et al. Non-pharmacological management of osteoporosis: a consensus of the Belgian bone Club. Osteoporos Int. 2011;22(11):2769–88.
32. Bischoff-Ferrari HA, Dawson-Hughes B, Staehelin HB, Orav JE, Stuck AE, Theiler R, et al. Fall prevention with supplemental and active forms of vitamin D: a meta-analysis of ran-domised controlled trials. BMJ. 2009;339:b3692.
33. Ersoy FF. Osteoporosis in the elderly with chronic kidney disease. Int Urol Nephrol. 2007;39(1):321–31.
34. Munson JC, Wahl PM, Daniel G, Kimmel SE, Hennessy S. Factors associated with the ini-tiation of proton pump inhibitors in corticosteroid users. Pharmacoepidemiol Drug Saf. 2012;21(4):366–74.
35. Clarke BL, Khosla S. Physiology of bone loss. Radiol Clin N Am. 2010;48(3):483–95.
36. Epsley S, Tadros S, Farid A, Kargilis D, Mehta S, Rajapakse CS. The effect of inflammation on bone. Front Physiol. 2020;11:511799.
37. Kogan M, Weil A. Common rheumatic diseases in the elderly. In: Integrative geriatric medi-cine. New York: Oxford University Press; 2018. p. 273.

38. Bolland MJ, Grey A, Reid IR. Calcium supplements and cardiovascular risk: 5 years on. Ther Adv Drug Saf. 2013;4(5):199–210.
39. NIH. Vitamin D [Internet]. NIH National Institutes of Health Office of Dietary Suppolements. 2020 [cited 2020 Dec 31]. Available from: https://ods.od.nih.gov/factsheets/VitaminD-HealthProfessional/
40. Schwalfenberg GK. Vitamins K1 and K2: the emerging group of vitamins required for human health. J Nutr Metab. 2017;2017:6254836.
41. Shen C-L, Yeh JK, Cao JJ, Wang J-S. Green tea and bone metabolism. Nutr Res. 2009;29(7):437–56.
42. Wuttke W, Gorkow C, Seidlová-Wuttke D. Effects of black cohosh (Cimicifuga racemosa) on bone turnover, vaginal mucosa, and various blood parameters in postmenopausal women: a double-blind, placebo-controlled, and conjugated estrogens-controlled study. Menopause. 2006;13(2):185–96.
43. Song J, Lee SH, Lee D, Kim H. Astragalus extract mixture HT042 improves bone growth, mass, and microarchitecture in prepubertal female rats: a microcomputed tomographic study. Evid Based Complement Alternat Med. 2017;2017:5219418.
44. Khanizadeh F, Rahmani A, Asadollahi K, Ahmadi MRH. Combination therapy of curcumin and alendronate modulates bone turnover markers and enhances bone mineral density in post-menopausal women with osteoporosis. Arch Endocrinol Metab. 2018;62(4):438–45.
45. Riva A, Togni S, Giacomelli L, Franceschi F, Eggenhoffner R, Feragalli B, et al. Effects of a curcumin-based supplementation in asymptomatic subjects with low bone density: a prelimi-nary 24-week supplement study. Eur Rev Med Pharmacol Sci. 2017;21(7):1684–9.
46. Castiglioni S, Cazzaniga A, Albisetti W, Maier JAM. Magnesium and osteoporosis: current state of knowledge and future research directions. Nutrients. 2013;5(8):3022–33.
47. Maggio M, Artoni A, Lauretani F, Borghi L, Nouvenne A, Valenti G, et al. The impact of omega-3 fatty acids on osteoporosis. Curr Pharm Des. 2009;15(36):4157–64.
48. Elam ML, Johnson SA, Hooshmand S, Feresin RG, Payton ME, Gu J, et al. A calcium-collagen chelate dietary supplement attenuates bone loss in postmenopausal women with osteopenia: a randomized controlled trial. J Med Food. 2015;18(3):324–31.
49. NIH. Calcium [Internet]. NIH Office of Dietary Supplements. 2021 [cited 2021 Apr 1]. Available from: https://ods.od.nih.gov/factsheets/Calcium-HealthProfessional/.
50. Kogan M. Integrative geriatrics: evidence based modalities to advance older adult health. Geriatrics and integrative medicine; New York: Oxford University Press; 2019.
51. Haring B, Crandall CJ, Wu C, LeBlanc ES, Shikany JM, Carbone L, et al. Dietary patterns and fractures in postmenopausal women: results from the women's health initiative. JAMA Intern Med. 2016;176(5):645–52.
52. Nettleton JA. Omega-3 fatty acids: comparison of plant and seafood sources in human nutri-tion. J Am Diet Assoc. 1991;91(3):331–7.
53. Vannucci L, Fossi C, Quattrini S, Guasti L, Pampaloni B, Gronchi G, et al. Calcium intake in bone health: a focus on calcium-rich mineral waters. Nutrients. 2018;10(12):1930.
54. Price CT, Langford JR, Liporace FA. Essential nutrients for bone health and a review of their availability in the average north American diet. Open Orthop J. 2012;6:143–9.
55. NIH. Magnesium [Internet]. National Institutes of Health Office of Dietary Supplements. 2020 [cited 2020 Dec 30]. Available from: https://ods.od.nih.gov/factsheets/Magnesium-HealthProfessional/#:~:text=Magnesium%20is%20widely%20distributed%20in,cereals%20and%20other%20fortified%20foods.
56. Laird E, Ward M, McSorley E, Strain JJ, Wallace J. Vitamin D and bone health: potential mechanisms. Nutrients. 2010;2(7):693–724.
57. Spedding S. Vitamin D and depression: a systematic review and meta-analysis comparing studies with and without biological flaws. Nutrients. 2014;6(4):1501–18.
58. NIH. Vitamin K [Internet]. NIH Office of Dietary Supplements. 2021 [cited 2021 Apr 1]. Available from: https://ods.od.nih.gov/factsheets/VitaminK-HealthProfessional/.

59. NIH. Boron [Internet]. NIH Office of Dietary Supplements. 2021 [cited 2021 Apr 1]. Available from: https://ods.od.nih.gov/factsheets/Boron-HealthProfessional/#:~:text=The%20main%20 sources%20of%20boron,cheese%20%5B6%2C20%5D.
60. Jugdaohsingh R. Silicon and bone health. J Nutr Health Aging. 2007;11(2):99–110.
61. Genuis SJ, Bouchard TP. Combination of micronutrients for bone (COMB) study: bone density after micronutrient intervention. J Environ Public Health. 2012;2012:354151.
62. NIH. Vitamin C [Internet]. National Institutes of Health Office of Dietary Supplements. 2020 [cited 2020 Dec 30]. Available from: https://ods.od.nih.gov/factsheets/ VitaminC-HealthProfessional/.
63. Too much vitamin C: is it harmful? – Mayo Clinic [Internet]. [cited 2021 Apr 1]. Available from: https://www.mayoclinic.org/healthy-lifestyle/nutrition-and-healthy-eating/expert-answers/vitamin-c/faq-20058030#:~:text=Advertisement&text=For%20adults%2C%20 the%20recommended%20daily,Diarrhea.
64. Pepa GD, Brandi ML. Microelements for bone boost: the last but not the least. Clin Cases Miner Bone Metab. 2016;13(3):181–5.
65. Evans GR, Masullo LN. Manganese toxicity. StatPearls. Treasure Island (FL): StatPearls Publishing.
66. Zheng D, Cui C, Yu M, Li X, Wang L, Chen X, et al. Coenzyme Q10 promotes osteoblast proliferation and differentiation and protects against ovariectomy-induced osteoporosis. Mol Med Rep. 2018;17(1):400–7.
67. Hidaka T, Fujii K, Funahashi I, Fukutomi N, Hosoe K. Safety assessment of coenzyme Q10 (CoQ10). Biofactors. 2008;32(1–4):199–208.
68. Candow DG, Forbes SC, Chilibeck PD, Cornish SM, Antonio J, Kreider RB. Effectiveness of creatine supplementation on aging muscle and bone: focus on falls prevention and inflammation. J Clin Med. 2019;8(4):488.
69. Lonnie M, Hooker E, Brunstrom JM, Corfe BM, Green MA, Watson AW, et al. Protein for life: review of optimal protein intake, sustainable dietary sources and the effect on appetite in ageing adults. Nutrients. 2018;10(3):360.
70. Wallace TC. Optimizing dietary protein for lifelong bone health. Nutr Today. 2019;54(3):107–15.
71. Dai Z, Koh W-P. B-vitamins and bone health–a review of the current evidence. Nutrients. 2015;7(5):3322–46.

Chapter 8
Psychological and Sleep

Contents

8.1 Depression

"Until we solve nutritional problems, no amount of medication and psychotherapy is going to stem the tide of mental issues in our society." Dr. Uma Naidoo, Nutritional Psychiatrist, Harvard Medical School.

Like so many other pathologies discussed in this book, new research points to the intimate connection between the gut and mental health. This is largely due to the diverse role the gut plays, as an influential player in metabolic, endocrine, and immune systems [1]. The quality of diet and the health of the microbiome are equally influential. A recent systemic review and meta-analysis observed that a healthy diet is significantly associated with a reduced odds for depression [2]. Moreover, depressive symptoms prompt the increased consumption of high-fat, sugary foods, contributing to a damaging positive-feedback loop [1]. The composition of the microbiota, influenced by probiotics and antibiotics, can influence depression-like behaviors [1]. This is very likely due to the bidirectional nature of the gut-brain axis. The microbiota recruits the axis to exert effects on the CNS. In return, the CNS moderates gut motility and secretion. This relationship is likely driven by both humoral and neural mechanisms, with particular emphasis on the vagus nerve [1]. The vagus nerve sends signals "down" from the brain to the gut through efferent nerve fibers (accounting for 10–20% of all fibers) and sends signals "up" from the gut to the brain (accounting for 80–90% of all fibers) [3].

Prior medical understanding of the etiology of depression as a serotonin receptor deficiency has been replaced by the recognition of the role inflammation plays as the primary driver of depressive symptoms. For example, research abounds with reports of similar or better symptom relief from regular exercise than the standard medication for depression, SSRIs [4]. Although the mechanism for symptomatic relief has not yet been clearly elucidated, a wide range of explanations exist, including reducing inflammation, increasing endorphin and monoamine levels, reduction in the stress hormone cortisol, altered neurotransmitter function, and hippocampus growth [5]. Of note, the impact of therapeutic lifestyle interventions such as exercise is multifaceted showing benefits across multiple body systems. Further, our standard medical approach to treating depression lacks efficacy, yet we continue to rely heavily on this approach. Just 40–60% of patients receive some relief from psychopharmacy approaches, and only 30–45% of patients see symptom resolution [6]. Around 95% of serotonin is produced in the gut, providing further evidence of the interconnectedness between the brain and the gut [7, 8]. Serotonin is produced by the enterochromaffin cells lining the digestive tract [9]. These cells are under direct influence of the gut microbiota. Therefore, ensuring a healthy microbiota is at the center of supporting a healthy brain-gut connection and, ultimately, supports mental health [3]. Thus, our focus for nutritional approaches to address depression revolves around controlling neuroinflammation, healing the gut, and supporting other lifestyle habits proven effective in easing depression – exercise, meditation, and sleep [10]. This starts with balanced nutrition, as outlined in Table 8.1.

Depression-Isolation-Malnutrition Triad in the Elderly
The complex interplay between depression and nutritional deficiencies in the elderly is exacerbated by isolation. Often, depression is missed in its early stages for older adults because they are less likely to initially present with a depressed mood but rather as functional decline, change in nutrient intake, self-isolation, and frequently resurgence of alcohol abuse as a form of self-medication. This sets the patient up for a negative spiral between worsened general nutritional status (caloric, protein, and micronutrient deficiencies), worsened depressive symptoms, and increased isolation. Recovery can be difficult due to lack of resilience and often delayed diagnosis. Regular screening, such as asking about diet history and social health, can help prompt a conversation about depression.

Table 8.1 Nutrition for Depression

	Dose	Mechanism of action	Food sources	Clinical observations/side effects
Probiotics	*Lactobacillus acidophilus*, *Lactobacillus casei*, *B. bifidum*, *Lactobacillus helveticus*, and *B. longum* 20 billion CFU [11]	Not fully elucidated, but mood-altering properties due to bidirectional brain-gut axis [11]	Fermented foods (kimchi, sauerkraut, kombucha), yogurt, kefir, and natto	Sepsis, fungemia, and GI ischemia (generally critically ill patients in intensive care units) [12]
Omega-3	2 g/day with EPA/DHA ratio of 3.5/1 to 7/1	Low levels of omega-3 FA seen in patients diagnosed with both anxiety and depression [13]	Fatty fish (salmon, mackerel, anchovies, herring, sardines). Consult NRDC.org for low-toxin options	Rare allergy, fishy taste, and mercury and dioxins in larger fish (shark or swordfish) [14]
Fiber	25 g for women and 35 g for men	Thought to be related to anti-inflammatory and probiotic effects [15]	Resistant starch (10 g/day), grains, fruits, and vegetables	Flatus, belching, fullness, and bloating [16]
B vitamins	Methylated B complex, EnLyte	Collective effects are prevalent to numerous aspects of brain function, including energy production, DNA/RNA synthesis/repair, genomic and non-genomic methylation, and synthesis of neurochemicals and signaling molecules [17]	Leafy greens however patients with MTHFR variants may need methylated vitamins as enzyme conversion is inhibited	Some patients may react to overmethylation and display symptoms of anxiety, insomnia, hyperactivity, and jitteriness [18]

(continued)

Table 8.1 (continued)

	Dose	Mechanism of action	Food sources	Clinical observations/side effects
Methylfolate	15 mg 1–5 mg	Enhances response to antidepressant. Cofactor in production of serotonin, dopamine, and norepinephrine [19]	Beer liver, spinach, black-eyed pea, asparagus, Brussels sprouts, and fortified breakfast cereal [20]	15 mg was used in the Deplin study [19], as part of a comprehensive approach Our recommendation is to use 1–5 mg
SAMe	800–1600 mg/day	Uncertain. May enhance monoamine systems (5-HT and norepinephrine), may increase fluidity in cell membranes that is linked to an increase in B-adrenoreceptor and muscarinic receptor density, and may influence expression of key genes in the brain affecting behavior, memory, learning, and cognition [21]	Poultry, red meat, bread, milk, and cheese [22]	*Bipolar warning*: may trigger manic episodes Often lower doses may work; start with 200 mg/day [23]
Dehydroepiandrosterone (DHEA)	5–25 mg/day for women and 10–50 mg/day for men	Partially metabolized to testosterone and estrogen (both of which may have mood effects of their own), may modulate bioavailability of testosterone, antagonize certain effects of cortisol, stimulate or antagonize GABA receptors, alter NMDA neurotransmission, and increase serotonin levels [24]	Soy and wild yam	Mild hirsutism and acne [25]

Table 8.1 (continued)

	Dose	Mechanism of action	Food sources	Clinical observations/side effects
Rhodiola	340–1360 mg daily	May enhance central neurotransmission and reduce or modulate excessive HPA axis activity (Mao, 2014). When it is combined with tricyclic antidepressants, *Rhodiola* use has been associated with reduction of side effects, particularly sedation, fatigue, and sexual dysfunction, as well as an improvement in depressive symptoms [26]	Arctic root, golden root, and roseroot	Is generally uncommon and mild and may include allergy, irritability, insomnia, increased blood pressure, and chest pain [26]
Saffron	15 mg	May be due to inhibition of dopamine, norepinephrine, and serotonin reuptake [27]	Colorant and flavoring agent [27]	Mild (anxiety, decreased appetite, sedation, nausea, headache, constipation) [28]
Turmeric	500–1000 mg/day	Anti-inflammatory and antioxidant	Curcumin	Diarrhea, headache, rash, and yellow stool [29]
St. John's wort	0.3% hypericin and 1–4% hyperforin, 900–1800 mg per day [30]	Inhibits monoamine oxidase A and B activity and also inhibits uptake of serotonin, dopamine, and norepinephrine. May also have affinity for adenosine, GABA, and glutamate receptors [31]	*Hypericum perforatum*	Not recommended due to interactions with many different medications

8.2 Anxiety

The conventional approach to anxiety, benzodiazepines, has serious side effects in the elderly. Benzodiazepines are not only overprescribed in the elderly but are included in the Beers Criteria. The Beers Criteria for Potentially Inappropriate Medication Use in Older Adults is used by the American Geriatrics Society to provide guidance regarding medications that should be avoided in the elderly [32]. As such, alternative interventions are imperative to treat anxiety in the older adult.

Some of our more common expressions such as "butterflies in my stomach" or having to go to the bathroom when we are nervous illustrate the more accepted connection between anxious thoughts and our gut. This very direct connection is felt by most people at one time or another in their life and is driven by the exchange of neurotransmitters and peptides that travel on the vagus nerve between the gut and the brain. Research has shown that individuals that suffer anxiety have a different composition of microbes in the gut that produce less anti-inflammatory short-chain fatty acids and more pathogenic microbes [33]. Both an excess and deficiency in fat and sugar can prompt high anxiety states [34]. The frequency and regularity of eating can also affect hormones and impact behavior due to effects on the circadian rhythms of the regulatory feeding and reward systems [34]. Weight on its own can be an anxiety-inducing state; in one study, an overall U-shaped association was observed between anxiety and BMI [35]. Additionally, a common side effect of food sensitivities is anxiety [36]. Thus our approach to treating anxiety nutritionally focuses on avoiding triggering foods, incorporating gut-healing and microbe-friendly foods, normalizing weight, and using supplements to heal the gut, diversify the microbiome, and fight systemic inflammation.

The standard American diet (SAD) is characterized by meals high in fat and refined carbohydrate that lack substantial amounts of fruits and vegetables. This diet is lacking in the fiber that produces a healthy gut microbiome as well as the anti-inflammatory phytonutrients that come from colorful fruits and vegetables. Additionally, the SAD contributes to weight gain which has been shown to contribute to neuroinflammation [37].

Foods to avoid are as follows [34]:

- Stimulants such as caffeine, energy drinks, chocolate, ginseng, guarana, taurine, and gotu kola.
- Food sensitivities: particularly gluten but any food that is creating inflammation via immune reactivity can trigger anxiety. Consider food sensitivity testing or an elimination diet to identify.
- Chemicals from preservatives, artificial flavor, and color.
- Alcohol.
- High-glycemic foods that spike blood sugar can trigger anxiety via the resultant spike in cortisol that comes from the blood sugar drop. For detailed list, see https://www.health.harvard.edu/diseases-and-conditions/glycemic-index-and-glycemic-load-for-100-foods.

Foods that can be helpful due to their nutrient content are as follows:

- Fatty fish and other sources of omega-3 fats eaten 2–3 times per week [38].
- High-fiber foods (beans, raspberries, avocados, winter squash, whole grains). Complex carbohydrates that provide various fiber sources to feed microbes that produce vitamins, minerals, and SCFA [39].
- Fermented foods such as sauerkraut, kimchi, kombucha, kefir, yogurt, and other raw, live culture foods (cannot be canned or contain vinegar which inhibits beneficial bacteria growth).
- High-tryptophan foods (poultry, red meat, soy, salmon) [40].
- Foods high in magnesium (nuts and seeds, greens, whole grains) [41].
- Herbal teas (lavender, passionflower, chamomile, kava, hops, lemon balm).
- Please see Table 8.2 for a summary of recommended nutritional support for anxiety.

8.3 Insomnia

A close relative of anxiety, insomnia occurs in 30–40% of older adults, creating an underlying cuase for many systemic imbalances affecting mood and cognition [63]. Among older adults with insomnia, up to 50% also suffer from chronic pain [64]. Many other cases related to insomnia are due to iatrogenic causes, such as inappropriate medication management, or frequent disturbances in a hospital or healthcare setting. Managing insomnia in the elderly is critical as severe insomnia leads to increased morbidity and mortality [65]. Moreover, insomnia, like pain, can be all consuming and contribute to deficiencies in a number of other systems. The high risk of hypnotics in treating insomnia in the elderly cannot be overstated [66]. Hypnotics cause unwanted effects on daytime mood and behavior, rebound effects associated with withdrawal, and dependency with continued use. The elderly are more vulnerable to these problems for two reasons. First, age-related changes in pharmacodynamic and pharmacokinetic processes heighten the behavioral impact of hypnotics. Second, the structure and quality of sleep changes associated with aging increase the perceived need for hypnotics [67]. Working to resolve insomnia requires a multipronged approach that looks deeper than the melatonin-cortisol balance which is often not the driving issue as it is with other life stages into sources of chronic pain, medications, frequent nighttime urination, and foods and supplements that can promote or hinder sleep.

The natural shifts in the sleep-wake cycle of the older adult explain a part of the frequency with which older adults experience insomnia (see Table 8.3 for expected changes). Older adults experience a decrease in both sleep length and quality. Primary drivers include changing circadian rhythms, lowered melatonin levels, and higher rates of comorbidities [68]. In a study of 6800 adults over 65 years, 93% had

Table 8.2 Nutritional support for anxiety

	MOA	Daily dose	Food sources	Clinical observations/side effects
B vitamins	Cofactors in synthesis and regulation of dopaminergic and serotonergic neurotransmitters [42]	Thiamine, 1 mg Riboflavin, 1.6 mg Niacin, 30 mg Vitamin B6, 3 mg Folate, 1000 µg Vitamin B12, 263 µg Biotin, 334 µg Pantothenic acid, 3.3 mg [43]	Salmon, leafy greens, liver and other organ meats, eggs, milk, beef, oysters, and legumes	Some patients will be sensitive to active forms of B12 (methylcobalamin) and should be given adeno- or hydroxycobalamin to avoid overmethylation
L-theanine	Structure resembles L-glutamic acid; MOA may be mediated through glutamate receptors. Has been associated with an increase in expression of BDNF in the hippocampus [44]	200–400 BID or TID depending on the severity	Green tea or matcha powder	Caffeine may not be well tolerated; one can get L-theanine from decaf green tea
GABA	Major inhibitory neurotransmitter in the CNS [45]	100 mg/kg [46]	Whole grains, fava beans, soy, lentils, nuts, fish, citrus, tomatoes, berries, spinach, broccoli, potatoes, and cocoa	May lower blood pressure in hypertensive patients [47]
Inositol	Can affect response to serotonergic, muscarinic, and noradrenergic stimulation [48]	12 g divided into three doses	Cantaloupe, citrus, fruit, beans, brown rice, corn, and wheat bran	Lowers blood glucose and with concomitant use with antidiabetic patients may cause hypoglycemia [49]
Botanicals				
Lavender	Inhibition of voltage-gated calcium channels, reduction of 5-HT1A receptor activity, and increased parasympathetic tone [50]	80–160 mg [50]	Oral capsules and aromatherapy effective	

Table 8.2 (continued)

	MOA	Daily dose	Food sources	Clinical observations/side effects
Passionflower	Affinity to GABA (A) and GABA (B) receptors and effects on GABA uptake [51]	45 drops (800 mg) [52]	Can cause dizziness, confusion, sedation, hypersensitivity, and ataxia in some patients [52]	
Chamomile	Anti-inflammatory and antiphlogistic. Sedative effects may be due to the flavonoid, apigenin that binds to benzodiazepine receptors [53]	500–1500 mg (extract) [54]	German chamomile, taken for 8 weeks. Also good for digestion due to its MOA [55]	
CBD/medical cannabis	Serotonin 5-HT1A receptor partial agonist. Allosteric modulator of the μ- and δ-opioid receptors [56]	CBD 15–50 mg BID if low-dose THC is used, keep CBD/THC ratio at 10:1 or more. Often adding low-dose THC can boost CBD effect	At the time of this writing, availability of CBD and cannabis varies from state to state best guidance is to start small and slowly increase to determine therapeutic dose	
Kava	Block voltage-gated sodium-ion channels, enhance ligand binding to GABA (A) receptors, diminish excitatory neurotransmitter release due to calcium ion channel blockade, and reduce neuronal reuptake of noradrenaline [57]	300 mg [58]	Contraindication with CNS depressants, alcohol, barbiturates, and benzodiazepines Use extracts standardized to 70% kavalactone [59]	
Melissa	Rosmarinic acid and triterpenoids oleanolic acid and ursolic acid inhibit GABA transaminase activity, resulting in increased GABA levels [60]	600 mg [61]	Taken in combination with 13 other herbs, 0.23 mL/kg body weight three times daily for 8 weeks [62]	

Table 8.3 Expected sleep architecture changes in older adults [70]

Total sleep time decreases	Increased stage 1 and 2 sleep
Sleep onset or latency becomes delayed	Decreased stage 3 and 4 sleep or slow-wave sleep (SWS)
Increased daytime napping	Circadian phase advanced (i.e., early to bed and early to rise)
Increase in awakenings and arousals	Decreased rapid-eye movement (REM) sleep
Decreased sleep efficiency	Fewer sleep cycles through per night

one or more comorbid conditions, including depression, chronic pain, cancer, chronic obstructive pulmonary disease, cardiovascular disease, and polypharmacy [63]. These drivers manifest as a number of experienced changes; see below table for details.

Sleep problems, especially in the elderly, are multifaceted and can be treated with a variety of non-pharmacological therapies such as exercise, bright-light exposure, nighttime continence care, cognitive behavioral interventions, and treating the primary comorbidity. However, the most common treatment is pharmacological, with benzodiazepines [68].

Although benzodiazepines are associated with small improvements in sleep latency and longer sleep duration, they also reduce deep sleep, which compromises sleep's restorative effects. Benzodiazepines also carry with them a long list of adverse effects, including daytime drowsiness, lethargy, fatigue, agitation, memory loss, impaired coordination, and falls [68].The adverse effects of benzodiazepines far outweigh the benefits, especially in the elderly. Older people have increased sensitivity to adverse effects, despite a growing tolerance to the sedative effects [68].

Despite the known risks of benzodiazepine use in the elderly, only one third of prescriptions are considered appropriate [69]. It is imperative to consider and implement alternative strategies to treat insomnia in older adults. Table 8.4 summarizes recommended nutritional and botanical support for insomnia.

8.3.1 Light Therapy

The foundation of light as therapy for insomnia is based on modeling circadian rhythms. Circadian rhythms influence sleep-wake cycles, melatonin secretion, cortisol, and core body temperature. Circadian rhythm problems are common with advancing age [71]. Over two-dozen studies have evaluated the efficacy of light therapy in treating insomnia (and/or depression) in older persons. Findings are mixed but overall suggest a favorable effect in older adults. These favorable effects include reduction in nighttime awakening and daytime sleeping, improved sleep efficiency, and greater increase in sleep time [71].

Table 8.4 Nutritional and botanical support for insomnia

	MOA	Dose	Food sources	Side effects and prescriber notes
			Source	
CBD/medical cannabis	Cannabis may act centrally as a zeitgeber, facilitating circadian rhythms, [78] and decreases cortisol [79]	1–10 mg of THC equivalent at bedtime. Often lower doses work well CBD alone at doses of 15–50 mg could occasionally work		Need medical cannabis recommendation and use sublingual or oral forms. Sublingual cannabis has a quicker onset but does not last as long
Melatonin	Acts on melatonin 1 and 2 receptors in the suprachiasmatic nucleus of the hypothalamus, reducing sleep onset time and increasing sleep duration [80]	3–5 mg sublingual or time-released formula	Goji berries, almonds, tart cherries, dairy, orange bell pepper, walnuts, and flax	Early morning light therapy helps shift circadian rhythm better than melatonin when there is not a deficiency in melatonin production
Magnesium	Is a muscle relaxant; improves sleep efficiency, sleep time and sleep onset latency, and early morning awakening; increases serum renin and melatonin; and decreases serum cortisol [81]	400–600 mg taken at bedtime, glycinate form preferred	Dark leafy greens: Cooking increases mineral bioavailability (spinach, kale, mustard greens, Collards, arugula) ~70 mg/cup Black beans, 120 mg/cup kidney beans, 70 mg/cup Brown rice, 94/cup Lentils, 72 mg/cup Oatmeal, 61 mg/cup Quinoa, 118 mg/0.5 cup Pumpkin seeds, 151 mg/oz. Brazil nuts, 107 mg/oz. Almonds, 78 mg/oz. Peanuts, 63 mg/oz	Preferred form of magnesium for insomnia is glycinate. Avoid citrate or hydroxide version as it is not well absorbed and causes loose stools

(continued)

Table 8.4 (continued)

	MOA	Dose	Food sources	Side effects and prescriber notes
GABA	Major inhibitory neurotransmitter in the CNS [45]	100 mg/kg [82]	Whole grains, fava beans, soy, lentils, nuts, fish, citrus, tomatoes, berries, spinach, broccoli, potatoes, and cocoa	Mild/moderate: Abdominal discomfort, headache, and drowsiness [83]
5-HTP	Plays major roles in circadian rhythmicity, thermoregulation, emotion, cognition, and nociception [84]	200 mg [85]	Sources of tryptophan (seeds, milk, eggs, cheese, pork, potato, sweet potato, whey)	Most concerning for serotonin syndrome; characterized by mental status changes, autonomic dysfunction, and dystonias [86]
Tryptophan/LNAAA (tryptophan/large neutral amino acids)	Precursor to serotonin	1 g [87]	Seeds, milk, eggs, cheese, pork, potato, sweet potato, and whey	LNAA (large neutral amino acids) help transport tryptophan across the BBB to work as precursor to serotonin
L-theanine	Structure resembles L-glutamic acid; MOA may be mediated through glutamate receptors. Has been associated with an increase in expression of BDNF in the hippocampus [44]	250 mg and 400 mg	Green tea (decaf)	Best for those that can't fall asleep or wake up because of a racing mind. In such patients, treatment is geared toward antianxiety vs. anti-insomnia

Herbs

	Mechanism	Dose		Adverse effects
Chamomile	Anti-inflammatory and antiphlogistic. Sedative effects may be due to the flavonoid, apigenin that binds to benzodiazepine receptors [53]	Chamomile: 500–1500 mg	Best used as nighttime tea infusions	Anaphlaxis, contact dermatitis, eye irritation, hypersensitivity, and vomiting (when taken in large amounts) [88]
Lemon balm	Rosmarinic acid and triterpenoids oleanolic acid and ursolic acid inhibit GABA transaminase activity, resulting in increased GABA levels [60]	600 mg		Headache, dysuria, pyuria, nausea, vomiting, stomach pain, dizziness, and wheezing [89]
Kava	Block voltage-gated sodium-ion channels, enhance ligand binding to GABA (A) receptors, diminish excitatory neurotransmitter release due to calcium ion channel blockade, and reduce neuronal reuptake of noradrenaline [57]	300 mg		Allergic skin reactions, dizziness, drowsiness, enlarged pupils, GI upset, headache, liver damage, visual changes, and motor reflex impairment [90]
Passionflower	Affinity to GABA (A) and GABA (B) receptors and effects on GABA uptake [51]	45 drops (800 mg)		Confusion, dizziness, drowsiness, nausea/vomiting, pancreas toxicity, prolonged QT interval, vasculitis, and tachycardia [91]
Valerian	Inhibits sympathetic nervous system neurons by modifying the transport and liberation of GABA [92]	225–1215 mg [93]		Can cause dizziness, confusion, sedation, hypersensitivity, and ataxia in some patients [52]
Hops	Modulates GABA activity by modulation GABA receptors [94]	2 mg [94]		Drowsiness, dizziness, and hypersensitivity reactions [95]
Whey protein	Increases tryptophan (precursor of serotonin and melatonin) [96]	24 g [97]	Dairy products	May cause liver and kidney dysfunction [98] *No casein, isolate (no inflammatory additives)

8.3.2 *Vitamin D Deficiency*

Vitamin D deficiency has been associated with an 8–14% increase in depression and a 50% increase in suicide [72]. However, causality and efficacy of supplementation remain controversial. As a hormone, vitamin D regulates a variety of nutritional pathways and is involved in the circadian rhythm [72]. It is very difficult to get enough vitamin D synthesized or ingested from food. For most patients, supplementation to replete and then maintain normal levels is required. Despite confirmatory evidence that vitamin D treats depression, we recommend supplementation with vitamin D (D3) combining with vitamin K2 in supplemental form due to the synergistic contribution each makes to immune, cardiovascular, and bone health [73]. Prophylactic supplementation with vitamin D may also serve to prevent late-life depression [74]. Supplementing may also support concomitant insomnia [75] or anxiety [76].

8.3.3 *Scheduling Meals*

The timing of meals can influence nighttime waking and should be considered when a pattern surfaces of easy transition to sleep with waking between 1:00 AM and 3:00 AM that has cortisol-related symptoms: wide awake, rapid heart rate, racing mind, and inability to settle back into rest. For someone with reactive hypoglycemia, it is recommended for them to consume a high-quality and well-balanced snack before bed to help sustain a normal blood sugar throughout the night. Examples include plain Greek yogurt with walnuts and blueberries or whole-grain toast with unsweetened peanut butter. These patients would also be well served to eat within 30 min of waking and every 3–4 h in between. Better daytime blood sugar management will dictate the quality of blood sugar management at night.

CBT-I (CBT for insomnia) is the gold standard for treating insomnia in the elderly and should be covered by Medicare. Unfortunately, the overlap between providers trained in CBT-I and those that accept Medicare is marginal, making this approach inaccessible and unaffordable for most older adults. Group CBT-I and group mind-body approaches can also be very effective and more affordable and can be delivered via telemedicine with equal benefits [77].

8.3.4 *Therapeutic Diets*

8.3.4.1 Mediterranean Diet

The Mediterranean diet has substantial evidence showing its effectiveness in reducing depression. A meta-analysis of 22 studies exploring the protective effects of a Mediterranean diet concluded that higher adherence to the diet was associated with both a reduced risk for depression and a cognitive decline [99]. The SMILES study, a 12-week, parallel-group, single-blind, randomized controlled trial of adjunctive personalized dietary intervention to treat moderate to severe depression, revealed that dietary improvement may provide not only an effective but widely accessible treatment for depression [100]. Mental health scores were improved with the Mediterranean diet plus fish oil supplement [101]. Nuts had a beneficial effect on the depressive risk of diabetes mellitus [101]. This is in contrast to a Western diet, which is considered an aggravator for depression [101]. The saturated fats and refined carbohydrates typical of a Western diet may induce inflammation and oxidative stress, disrupt the gut microbiome and brain-gut axis, cause hippocampal degeneration, and lead to nutrient inadequacies, which are all risk factors for depression [101]. See appendix for detailed description of the Mediterranean diet.

8.3.4.2 Elimination Diet

The most common foods that cause reactions that can impact mental health are gluten, dairy, corn, soy, and peanuts [102]. Often, the extent of the elimination diet needs to be established based on the overall context for the patient. Taking a depressed patient who lacks motivation and asking them to eliminate all convenience and comfort foods will likely not go well. Thus, starting with the removal of gluten and/or dairy to see if enough improvement happens that will help motivate additional changes is effective. More details for the elimination diet can be found in the appendix.

8.3.4.3 Intermittent Fasting

It is well established that calorie restriction in the right settings can result in favorable physiologic changes, such as fat distribution, body temperature, fasting insulin, T3 and T4, and ghrelin levels. Furthermore, calorie restriction can reduce the risk of cardiovascular disease, improve insulin sensitivity in diabetes, alleviate oxidative stress, and enhance cognitive function. Intermittent fasting has been shown to increase global quality of sleep, daytime concentration, vigor, and emotional balance. Clinicians have found that fasting relieves negative moods like tension, anger, and confusion and enhanced a sense of euphoria [103]. Sustained calorie reduction by 24% for 6 months reduced depressive symptoms while producing no obvious negative effects on mood [104]. In a prospective uncontrolled trial of severe calorie restriction in patients with chronic pain, more than 80% of the subjects showed an effective improvement in depressive mood [105], thought be due to increased availability of serotonin and endogenous opioids [106].

Intermittent fasting has multiple possible implementation methods, and the correct choice is the one that the patient can implement. Well-studied methods include the 5:2 fast where 5 days of regular eating is interspersed with 2 days of restricted 500–600 calorie intake, each week. Alternatively, a nightly fast of 12–16 h is effective and requires fasting between dinner and the first meal of the next day is 12–16 h. Intake of non-calorie fluids is allowed. And lastly, the fasting-mimicking diet (FMD) is a monthly 5-day fast with prepackaged meals. FMD benefits from extensive research due to its easily replicated approach.

8.3.4.4   Blood Sugar Balancing Diet

An important trigger for anxiety can be a drop in blood sugar. Food choices exert a large influence on the course our blood sugar takes over the course of a day and thus establish a well-balanced diet that manages blood sugar may reduce symptoms. Patients should be advised to eat within 30 min of waking a breakfast that contains high levels of protein (20–30 g) with healthy fats. Throughout the day, foods should be combined such that complex carbohydrates are always consumed with protein and fat at each meal. For patients that display insomnia with night waking that has a cortisol-spike quality (heart racing, mind unable to settle), a pre-bed snack of protein and fat can help set blood sugar for the night and prevent the drop that causes the nighttime waking.

Table 8.5 summarizes recommended micronutrients to support psychological health.

8.4   Case Studies

8.4.1   Case 1: Depression

Alex, a 72-year-old engineer, has struggled with depression since his wife passed away 3 years ago. They have been married for 37 years and she died suddenly in a car accident. He has done extensive grief and depression counseling and several different antidepressants, but neither helped much. During more detailed history, he explained that even before her passing, he had struggled with low mood and energy for a long time. But he always felt that his wife who was very engaged in life was one who kept them both going. Alex's other medical problems included high blood pressure controlled with lisinopril, constipation which he managed with extra fiber and prune juice, and chronic osteoarthritis in both knees which at times required Tylenol with codeine, but most of the time, regular Tylenol was enough. Alex always kept up with all needed screenings and rarely drank alcohol and never smoked, but he was overweight with BMI of 28. He was taking 1000 units of daily vitamin D and a multivitamin. His laboratory results were significant for borderline low B12 level of 310 ng/ml. Additional functional tests revealed DHEA at 27 µg/dL and C-reactive protein at 3.5. We also decided to obtain MTHFR genetic tests that revealed that Alex had two copies of A1298C making him more difficult to convert folic acid to biologically active, methylated form.

Table 8.5 Micronutrients of primary concern for psychological support

	MOA	Food sources	RDA for 55+	Side effects/comments for providers
Omega-3	As highly unsaturated fatty acids, they are important components of neuronal cell membranes, modulating mechanisms of brain signaling, including the dopaminergic and serotonergic pathways [107]	Flaxseed (oil), chia seeds, walnuts, salmon, canola oil, and sardines [108]	1.6 g M and 1.1 g F [108]	Preferred source is fatty fish since conversion to EPA/DHA is only 5–8% effective from vegetarian sources
Magnesium	Cofactor for enzymes that breakdown neurotransmitters	Pumpkin seeds, chia seeds, almonds, spinach, cashews, and peanuts [41]	420 mg M and 320 mg F [41]	Best forms for absorption are glycinate and L-threonate
B vitamins	Cofactors in methionine and folate cycles, in synthesis, and in regulation of dopaminergic and serotonergic neurotransmitters [42]	Salmon, leafy greens, liver and other organ meats, eggs, milk, beef, oysters, and legumes	Thiamine, 1 mg Riboflavin, 1.6 mg Niacin, 30 mg Vitamin B6, 3 mg Folate, 400 μg Vitamin B12, 263 μg Biotin, 334 μg Pantothenic acid. 3.3 mg [43]	Methylated or active forms of B vitamins preferred for efficacy
Vitamin A	Retinoid acid, bioactive metabolite of vitamin A, is a potent signaling molecule that modulates neurogenesis, neuronal survival, and synaptic plasticity [109]	Beef liver, sweet potato, spinach, pumpkin pie, and carrots [110]	900 μg M and 700 μg F [110]	Associated with chronic vitamin A toxicity, including vision disturbances, joint and bone pain, poor appetite, nausea/vomiting, hair loss, headache, sunlight sensitivity, and dry skin [111]
Ashwagandha	Anti-inflammatory, antioxidant, and adaptogen, with the ability to regulate physiological processes and stabilize the body's response to stress [112]	Ashwagandha	125–600 mg [112]	As an adaptogenic herb, beneficial effects take 2–3 weeks to notice

Alex's diet became much worse since his wife passed; he started eating more premade dinners and cooked a lot less, even though he loved to cook with his wife and food has always been a big part of his life. While he was not interested in psychotherapy, he was open to joining our mind-body medical shared support group for patients with depression, anxiety, and insomnia. Instead of counseling Alex about his meals given lack of energy and motivation, we decided to recommend that he purchases much better-quality premade meals. Additionally, we asked Alex to stop his poor-quality multivitamin and instead started him on magnesium citrate 400 mg at bedtime, high-potency B complex with 1000 mcg of methyl B12 and 1000 mcg of methylfolate, as well as 100 mg of thiamine, riboflavin, niacin, vitamin B6, biotin, and vitamin B5 (pantothenic acid).

Given that Alex suffered from low energy, osteoarthritis, and depression, we recommended to start SAMe at 200 mg once daily, slowly titrating up to 400 mg twice daily. Due to borderline DHEA deficiency, we also started DHEA 25 mg once daily. Since he did not like the taste of turmeric, we started him on a highly concentrated form of curcumin at 1000 mg/day of clinically studied form called Meriva™.

Over the course of the next 3 months, Alex felt more energy which allowed him to get more active and ride his bike which he always enjoyed. His constipation nearly completely resolved because of magnesium citrate addition. He also felt that his knees felt a lot less achy and he now needed to take regular Tylenol occasionally. At the repeat blood work, his vitamin B12 was over 1000 ng/ml, DHEA 120 μg/dL, and C-reactive protein 1.2. At the next follow-up in 12 months, Alex came with his new much younger girlfriend. He was doing very well, his mood was good, and he stayed very active and enjoyed a new circle of friends through his girlfriend.

8.4.2 Case 2: Anxiety

Susan, a 71-year-old teacher, suffered from severe chronic anxiety for decades. Her other problems included restless leg syndrome and neuropathic leg pain on both sides that felt like stinging and burning and only added to worsening Susan's sleep and anxiety. Susan was followed by a primary care doctor and neurologist and has been tried on many different medications. She found that combination of Lyrica 75 mg and lorazepam 0.5 mg twice daily made her conditions livable. However, over time, medications became less effective, and she found her way to see us in the clinic. During nutritional history, she disclosed eating dessert with each meal and strong cravings for sweets, especially after dinner. She routinely ate one cup of ice cream every night claiming that it "calmed her and helped her to fall asleep." Her primary care doctor recommended a trial of acupuncture, massage, and gentle Yoga. She felt that these were very helpful, especially acupuncture to help her leg pain and anxiety. Unfortunately she could not afford regular acupuncture and had to do it only monthly.

Our recommendations were to start microdosing of medical cannabis with 10:1 CBD/THC ratio in the PM with additional 15–30 mg of CBD in the AM. We also initiated magnesium citrate 300 mg taken at bedtime and as needed sublingual liposomal form of L-theanine at 300 mg 2–3 times daily. Additionally, Susan has joined our weekly mind-body telemedicine group to participate in regular meditative practices and to get additional group support. 3 months later, Susan reported that a combination of mind-body class, cannabinoids, magnesium, and occasional massage and acupuncture hit the sweet spot and her anxiety has been completely controlled. Several years later, Susan continued to participate in group classes and reported much better quality of life due to controlled anxiety. She also reported that her chronic neuropathic pain has gotten gradually better and she has been doing more exercises and living a more active lifestyle.

8.4.3   Case 3: Insomnia

John is a 68-year-old obese man with long-standing history of depression, insomnia, hypertension, and coronary artery disease with history of multiple stents on complex cardiac regimen with hydrochlorothiazide, lisinopril, clopidogrel, Cymbalta, and high-dose atorvastatin. In the prior 12 months before presenting to our clinic, John's overuse of zolpidem became very problematic after he had several arguments with his internist who was refusing to provide refills ahead of schedule. But the last point that led John's wife Sara to bring him in was the fall during the night. Unable to navigate stairs, John fell on his way to the bathroom and ended up with broken ribs. Lucky he did not have any other complications and recovered quickly. During the intake process, we learned that John liked to combine zolpidem with whisky shot at night for "better efficacy." He also often had either a strong cup of tea or coffee with dinner around 7 PM. John relished his nightcap and getting him to stop it was clearly not possible, so we agreed that he will take his whisky drink with dinner and stop all caffeine containing beverages with lunch around 1 PM.

To make something resembling his nightcap, we added a teaspoon of alcohol-based valerian tincture in combination with 30 mg of CBD oil and 450 mg of magnesium citrate. This allowed us to cut his zolpidem dose in half from 10 mg to 5 mg. On follow-up visit in 8 weeks, John felt that sleep was about the same but he felt more energy, likely an improvement in overall sleep architecture now that the dose of zolpidem was much lower. Interestingly at the same time, John's blood pressure improved significantly, and instead of his usual 140–150 mmHg systolic, it has now been mostly under 120 mmHg. With this change and the fact that John often had to go to the bathroom at night, we have stopped hydrochlorothiazide. At the next follow-up in 3 months, John was a different person. He was much happier and more energetic. He had a big smile with a big thank you and a strong hug. Cutting down diuretic stopped his nocturia almost completely, and with that, he felt his sleep got a lot better which led to even more improvement in the energy and the mood. And despite cutting down diuretic, his blood pressure stayed steadily under 130 mmHg systolic.

References

1. Dash S, Clarke G, Berk M, Jacka FN. The gut microbiome and diet in psychiatry: focus on depression. Curr Opin Psychiatry. 2015;28(1):1–6.
2. Lai JS, Hiles S, Bisquera A, Hure AJ, McEvoy M, Attia J. A systematic review and meta-analysis of dietary patterns and depression in community-dwelling adults. Am J Clin Nutr. 2014;99(1):181–97.
3. Breit S, Kupferberg A, Rogler G, Hasler G. Vagus nerve as modulator of the brain-gut axis in psychiatric and inflammatory disorders. Front Psych. 2018;9:44.
4. Craft LL, Perna FM. The benefits of exercise for the clinically depressed. Prim Care Companion J Clin Psychiatry. 2004;6(3):104–11.
5. Blake H. Physical activity and exercise in the treatment of depression. Front Psych. 2012;3:106.
6. Carvalho AF, Cavalcante JL, Castelo MS, Lima MCO. Augmentation strategies for treatment-resistant depression: a literature review. J Clin Pharm Ther. 2007;32(5):415–28.
7. Terry N, Margolis KG. Serotonergic mechanisms regulating the GI tract: experimental evidence and therapeutic relevance. Handb Exp Pharmacol. 2016;239:319.
8. Berger M, Gray JA, Roth BL. The expanded biology of serotonin. Annu Rev Med. 2009;60:355–66.
9. Mawe GM, Hoffman JM. Serotonin signalling in the gut–functions, dysfunctions and therapeutic targets. Nat Rev Gastroenterol Hepatol. 2013;10(8):473–86.
10. Sarris J, O'Neil A, Coulson CE, Schweitzer I, Berk M. Lifestyle medicine for depression. BMC Psychiatry. 2014;14(1):107.
11. Nikolova V, Zaidi SY, Young AH, Cleare AJ, Stone JM. Gut feeling: randomized controlled trials of probiotics for the treatment of clinical depression: systematic review and meta-analysis. Ther Adv Psychopharmacol. 2019;9:2045125319859963.
12. Didari T, Solki S, Mozaffari S, Nikfar S, Abdollahi M. A systematic review of the safety of probiotics. Expert Opin Drug Saf. 2014;13(2):227–39.
13. Larrieu T, Layé S. Food for mood: relevance of nutritional omega-3 fatty acids for depression and anxiety. Front Physiol. 2018;9:1047.
14. Schwalfenberg G. Omega-3 fatty acids: their beneficial role in cardiovascular health. Can Fam Physician. 2006;52:734–40.
15. Swann OG, Kilpatrick M, Breslin M, Oddy WH. Dietary fiber and its associations with depression and inflammation. Nutr Rev. 2020;78(5):394–411.
16. Bliss DZ, Savik K, Jung H-JG, Whitebird R, Lowry A. Symptoms associated with dietary fiber supplementation over time in individuals with fecal incontinence. Nurs Res. 2011;60(3 Suppl):S58–67.
17. Kennedy DO. B vitamins and the brain: mechanisms, dose and efficacy–a review. Nutrients. 2016;8(2):68.
18. Miller AL. The methylation, neurotransmitter, and antioxidant connections between folate and depression. Altern Med Rev. 2008;13(3):216–26.
19. Shelton RC, Sloan Manning J, Barrentine LW, Tipa EV. Assessing effects of l-methylfolate in depression management: results of a real-world patient experience trial. Prim Care Companion CNS Disord. 2013;15(4):PCC.13m01520.
20. NIH. Folate [Internet]. National Institutes of Health Office of Dietary Supplements. 2020 [cited 2020 Dec 30]. Available from: https://ods.od.nih.gov/factsheets/Folate-HealthProfessional/.
21. Galizia I, Oldani L, Macritchie K, Amari E, Dougall D, Jones TN, et al. S-adenosyl methionine (SAMe) for depression in adults. Cochrane Database Syst Rev. 2016;10:CD011286.
22. Górska-Warsewicz H, Laskowski W, Kulykovets O, Kudlińska-Chylak A, Czeczotko M, Rejman K. Food products as sources of protein and amino acids-the case of Poland. Nutrients. 2018;10(12):1977.
23. Berigan TR. A case report of a manic episode triggered by S-Adenosylmethionine (SAMe). Prim Care Companion J Clin Psychiatry. 2002;4(4):159.

24. Wolkowitz OM, Reus VI, Keebler A, Nelson N, Friedland M, Brizendine L, et al. Double-blind treatment of major depression with dehydroepiandrosterone. Am J Psychiatry. 1999;156(4):646–9.

25. Bentley C, Hazeldine J, Greig C, Lord J, Foster M. Dehydroepiandrosterone: a potential therapeutic agent in the treatment and rehabilitation of the traumatically injured patient. Burns Trauma. 2019;7:26.

26. Mental Health America. Rhodiola Rosea [Internet]. Mental Health America. 2020 [cited 2021 Mar 3]. Available from: https://www.mhanational.org/rhodiola-rosea

27. Siddiqui MJ, Saleh MSM, Basharuddin SNBB, Zamri SHB, Mohd Najib MHB, Che Ibrahim MZB, et al. Saffron (Crocus sativus L.): as an antidepressant. J Pharm Bioallied Sci. 2018;10(4):173–80.

28. Bostan HB, Mehri S, Hosseinzadeh H. Toxicology effects of saffron and its constituents: a review. Iran J Basic Med Sci. 2017;20(2):110–21.

29. Hewlings SJ, Kalman DS. Curcumin: a review of its effects on human health. Foods. 2017;6(10):92.

30. Gaster B, Holroyd J. St John's wort for depression: a systematic review. Arch Intern Med. 2000;160(2):152–6.

31. Butterweck V. Mechanism of action of St John's wort in depression: what is known? CNS Drugs. 2003;17(8):539–62.

32. Croke LM. Beers criteria for inappropriate medication use in older patients: an update from the AGS. Am Fam Physician. 2020;101(1):56–7.

33. Jiang H-Y, Zhang X, Yu Z-H, Zhang Z, Deng M, Zhao J-H, et al. Altered gut microbiota profile in patients with generalized anxiety disorder. J Psychiatr Res. 2018;104:130–6.

34. Murphy M, Mercer JG. Diet-regulated anxiety. Int J Endocrinol. 2013;2013:701967.

35. DeJesus RS, Breitkopf CR, Ebbert JO, Rutten LJF, Jacobson RM, Jacobson DJ, et al. Associations between anxiety disorder diagnoses and body mass index differ by age, sex and race: a population based study. Clin Pract Epidemiol Ment Health. 2016;12:67–74.

36. Teufel M, Biedermann T, Rapps N, Hausteiner C, Henningsen P, Enck P, et al. Psychological burden of food allergy. World J Gastroenterol. 2007;13(25):3456–65.

37. Fonseka TM, Müller DJ, Kennedy SH. Inflammatory cytokines and antipsychotic-induced weight gain: review and clinical implications. Mol Neuropsychiatry. 2016;2(1):1–14.

38. Naidoo U. This is your brain on food (an Indispensible guide to the surprising foods that fight depression, anxiety, PTSD, OCD, ADHD, and more). 1st ed. Brown Spark: Little; 2020.

39. Whitbread D. Top 10 Foods Highest in Fiber [Internet]. My Food Data. 2020 [cited 2021 Mar 3]. Available from: https://www.myfooddata.com/articles/foods-high-in-dietary-fiber.php.

40. Friedman M. Analysis, nutrition, and health benefits of tryptophan. Int J Tryptophan Res. 2018;11:1178646918802282.

41. NIH. Magnesium [Internet]. National Institutes of Health Office of Dietary Supplements. 2020 [cited 2020 Dec 30]. Available from: https://ods.od.nih.gov/factsheets/Magnesium-HealthProfessional/#:~:text=Magnesium%20is%20widely%20distributed%20in,cereals%20 and%20other%20fortified%20foods.

42. Young LM, Pipingas A, White DJ, Gauci S, Scholey A. A systematic review and meta-analysis of B vitamin supplementation on depressive symptoms, anxiety, and stress: effects on healthy and "at-risk" individuals. Nutrients. 2019;11(9):2232.

43. Lewis JE, Tiozzo E, Melillo AB, Leonard S, Chen L, Mendez A, et al. The effect of methylated vitamin B complex on depressive and anxiety symptoms and quality of life in adults with depression. ISRN Psychiatry. 2013;2013:621453.

44. Hidese S, Ogawa S, Ota M, Ishida I, Yasukawa Z, Ozeki M, et al. Effects of L-theanine administration on stress-related symptoms and cognitive functions in healthy adults: a randomized controlled trial. Nutrients. 2019;11(10):2362.

45. Nuss P. Anxiety disorders and GABA neurotransmission: a disturbance of modulation. Neuropsychiatr Dis Treat. 2015;11:165–75.

46. Ngo D-H, Vo TS. An updated review on pharmaceutical properties of gamma-aminobutyric acid. Molecules. 2019;24(15):2678.

47. Shimada M, Hasegawa T, Nishimura C, Kan H, Kanno T, Nakamura T, et al. Anti-hypertensive effect of gamma-aminobutyric acid (GABA)-rich Chlorella on high-normal blood pressure and borderline hypertension in placebo-controlled double blind study. Clin Exp Hypertens. 2009;31(4):342–54.
48. Kofman O, Einat H, Cohen H, Tenne H, Shoshana C. The anxiolytic effect of chronic inositol depends on the baseline level of anxiety. J Neural Transm. 2000;107(2):241–53.
49. Zheng X, Liu Z, Zhang Y, Lin Y, Song J, Zheng L, et al. Relationship between Myo-inositol supplementary and gestational diabetes mellitus: a meta-analysis. Medicine (Baltimore). 2015;94(42):e1604.
50. Malcolm BJ, Tallian K. Essential oil of lavender in anxiety disorders: ready for prime time? Ment Health Clin. 2017;7(4):147–55.
51. Appel K, Rose T, Fiebich B, Kammler T, Hoffmann C, Weiss G. Modulation of the γ-aminobutyric acid (GABA) system by Passiflora incarnata L. Phytother Res. 2011;25(6):838–43.
52. Akhondzadeh S, Naghavi HR, Vazirian M, Shayeganpour A, Rashidi H, Khani M. Passionflower in the treatment of generalized anxiety: a pilot double-blind randomized controlled trial with oxazepam. J Clin Pharm Ther. 2001;26(5):363–7.
53. Srivastava JK, Shankar E, Gupta S. Chamomile: a herbal medicine of the past with bright future. Mol Med Report. 2010;3(6):895–901.
54. Mao JJ, Li QS, Soeller I, Rockwell K, Xie SX, Amsterdam JD. Long-term chamomile therapy of generalized anxiety disorder: a study protocol for a randomized, double-blind, placebo- controlled trial. J Clin Trials. 2014;4(5):188.
55. Mao JJ, Li QS, Soeller I, Xie SX, Amsterdam JD. Rhodiola rosea therapy for major depressive disorder: a study protocol for a randomized, double-blind, placebo- controlled trial. J Clin Trials. 2014;4:170.
56. Meissner H, Cascella M. Cannabidiol (CBD) [Internet]. PubMed. 2021 [cited 2021 Mar 3]. Available from: https://www.ncbi.nlm.nih.gov/books/NBK556048/.
57. Singh YN, Singh NN. Therapeutic potential of kava in the treatment of anxiety disorders. CNS Drugs. 2002;16(11):731–43.
58. Geier FP, Konstantinowicz T. Kava treatment in patients with anxiety. Phytother Res. 2004;18(4):297–300.
59. Pittler MH, Ernst E. Efficacy of kava extract for treating anxiety: systematic review and meta-analysis. J Clin Psychopharmacol. 2000;20(1):84–9.
60. Ibarra A, Feuillere N, Roller M, Lesburgere E, Beracochea D. Effects of chronic administration of Melissa officinalis L. extract on anxiety-like reactivity and on circadian and exploratory activities in mice. Phytomedicine. 2010;17(6):397–403.
61. Cases J, Ibarra A, Feuillère N, Roller M, Sukkar SG. Pilot trial of Melissa officinalis L. leaf extract in the treatment of volunteers suffering from mild-to-moderate anxiety disorders and sleep disturbances. Med J Nutr Metab. 2011;4(3):211–8.
62. Büchner KH, Hellings H, Huber M, Peukert E, Späth L, Deininger R. Double blind study as evidence of the therapeutic effect of Melissengeist on psycho-vegetative syndromes (author's transl). Med Klin. 1974;69(23):1032–6.
63. Patel D, Steinberg J, Patel P. Insomnia in the elderly: a review. J Clin Sleep Med. 2018;14(6):1017–24.
64. Curtis AF, Williams JM, McCoy KJM, McCrae CS. Chronic pain, sleep, and cognition in older adults with insomnia: a daily multilevel analysis. J Clin Sleep Med. 2018;14(10):1765–72.
65. Miner B, Kryger MH. Sleep in the aging population. Sleep Med Clin. 2017;12(1):31–8.
66. Rumble R, Morgan K. Hypnotics, sleep, and mortality in elderly people. J Am Geriatr Soc. 1992;40(8):787–91.
67. Morgan K. Hypnotics in the elderly. What cause for concern? Drugs. 1990;40(5):688–96.
68. Chen L, Bell JS, Visvanathan R, Hilmer SN, Emery T, Robson L, et al. The association between benzodiazepine use and sleep quality in residential aged care facilities: a cross-sectional study. BMC Geriatr. 2016;16(1):196.

69. Airagnes G, Pelissolo A, Lavallée M, Flament M, Limosin F. Benzodiazepine misuse in the elderly: risk factors, consequences, and management. Curr Psychiatry Rep. 2016;18(10):89.

70. Edwards BA, O'Driscoll DM, Ali A, Jordan AS, Trinder J, Malhotra A. Aging and sleep: physiology and pathophysiology. Semin Respir Crit Care Med. 2010;31(5):618–33.

71. Sloane PD, Figueiro M, Cohen L. Light as therapy for sleep disorders and depression in older adults. Clin Geriatr. 2008;16(3):25–31.

72. Spedding S. Vitamin D and depression: a systematic review and meta-analysis comparing studies with and without biological flaws. Nutrients. 2014;6(4):1501–18.

73. van Ballegooijen AJ, Cepelis A, Visser M, Brouwer IA, van Schoor NM, Beulens JW. Joint association of low vitamin D and vitamin K status with blood pressure and hypertension. Hypertension. 2017;69(6):1165–72.

74. Okereke OI, Singh A. The role of vitamin D in the prevention of late-life depression. J Affect Disord. 2016;198:1–14.

75. Gao Q, Kou T, Zhuang B, Ren Y, Dong X, Wang Q. The association between vitamin D deficiency and sleep disorders: a systematic review and meta-analysis. Nutrients. 2018;10(10):1395.

76. Bičíková M, Dušková M, Vítků J, Kalvachová B, Řípová D, Mohr P, et al. Vitamin D in anxiety and affective disorders. Physiol Res. 2015;64(Suppl 2):S101–3.

77. Gehrman P, Shah MT, Miles A, Kuna S, Godleski L. Feasibility of group cognitive-behavioral treatment of insomnia delivered by clinical video telehealth. Telemed J E Health. 2016;22(12):1041–6.

78. Whitehurst LN, Fogler K, Hall K, Hartmann M, Dyche J. The effects of chronic marijuana use on circadian entrainment. Chronobiol Int. 2015;32(4):561–7.

79. Shannon S, Lewis N, Lee H, Hughes S. Cannabidiol in anxiety and sleep: a large case series. Perm J. 2019;23:18–041.

80. Srinivasan V, Pandi-Perumal SR, Trahkt I, Spence DW, Poeggeler B, Hardeland R, et al. Melatonin and melatonergic drugs on sleep: possible mechanisms of action. Int J Neurosci. 2009;119(6):821–46.

81. Djokic G, Vojvodić P, Korcok D, Agic A, Rankovic A, Djordjevic V, et al. The effects of magnesium – melatonin – Vit B complex supplementation in treatment of insomnia. Open Access Maced J Med Sci. 2019;7(18):3101–5.

82. Kim S, Jo K, Hong K-B, Han SH, Suh HJ. GABA and l-theanine mixture decreases sleep latency and improves NREM sleep. Pharm Biol. 2019;57(1):65–73.

83. Byun JI, Shin YY, Chung SE, Shin WC. Safety and efficacy of gamma-aminobutyric acid from fermented rice germ in patients with insomnia symptoms: a randomized, Double-Blind Trial. J Clin Neurol. 2018;14(3):291–5.

84. Rancillac A. Serotonin and sleep-promoting neurons. Oncotarget. 2016;7(48):78222–3.

85. Hinz M, Stein A, Uncini T. 5-HTP efficacy and contraindications. Neuropsychiatr Dis Treat. 2012;8:323–8.

86. Ferguson JM. SSRI antidepressant medications: adverse effects and tolerability. Prim Care Companion J Clin Psychiatry. 2001;3(1):22–7.

87. Schneider-Helmert D, Spinweber CL. Evaluation of L-tryptophan for treatment of insomnia: a review. Psychopharmacology. 1986;89(1):1–7.

88. Cunha JP. Chamomile [Internet]. RxList. 2021 [cited 2021 Mar 3]. Available from: https://www.rxlist.com/consumer_chamomile/drugs-condition.htm.

89. Healthline. 10 Benefits of Lemon Balm and How to Use It [Internet]. Healthline. 2017 [cited 2021 Mar 4]. Available from: https://www.healthline.com/health/lemon-balm-uses.

90. Cunha JP. Kava [Internet]. RxList. 2017 [cited 2021 Mar 4]. Available from: https://www.rxlist.com/consumer_kava/drugs-condition.htm.

91. Cunha JP. Passion Flower [Internet]. RxList. 2021 [cited 2021 Mar 3]. Available from: https://www.rxlist.com/consumer_passion_flower/drugs-condition.htm.

92. Fernández-San-Martín MI, Masa-Font R, Palacios-Soler L, Sancho-Gómez P, Calbó-Caldentey C, Flores-Mateo G. Effectiveness of valerian on insomnia: a meta-analysis of randomized placebo-controlled trials. Sleep Med. 2010;11(6):505–11.
93. Bent S, Padula A, Moore D, Patterson M, Mehling W. Valerian for sleep: a systematic review and meta-analysis. Am J Med. 2006;119(12):1005–12.
94. Franco L, Sánchez C, Bravo R, Rodriguez A, Barriga C, Juánez JC. The sedative effects of hops (Humulus lupulus), a component of beer, on the activity/rest rhythm. Acta Physiol Hung. 2012;99(2):133–9.
95. Hops. LiverTox: clinical and research information on drug-induced liver injury. Bethesda: National Institute of Diabetes and Digestive and Kidney Diseases; 2012.
96. Doherty R, Madigan S, Warrington G, Ellis J. Sleep and nutrition interactions: implications for athletes. Nutrients. 2019;11(4):822.
97. Madzima TA, Melanson JT, Black JR, Nepocatych S. Pre-sleep consumption of casein and whey protein: effects on morning metabolism and resistance exercise performance in active women. Nutrients. 2018;10(9):1273.
98. Vasconcelos QDJS, Bachur TPR, Aragão GF. Whey protein supplementation and its potentially adverse effects on health: a systematic review. Appl Physiol Nutr Metab. 2021;46(1):27–33.
99. Psaltopoulou T, Sergentanis TN, Panagiotakos DB, Sergentanis IN, Kosti R, Scarmeas N. Mediterranean diet, stroke, cognitive impairment, and depression: a meta-analysis. Ann Neurol. 2013;74(4):580–91.
100. Jacka FN, O'Neil A, Opie R, Itsiopoulos C, Cotton S, Mohebbi M, et al. A randomised controlled trial of dietary improvement for adults with major depression (the "SMILES" trial). BMC Med. 2017;15(1):23.
101. Huang Q, Liu H, Suzuki K, Ma S, Liu C. Linking what we eat to our mood: a review of diet, dietary antioxidants, and depression. Antioxidants (Basel). 2019;8(9):376.
102. Bressan P, Kramer P. Bread and other edible agents of mental disease. Front Hum Neurosci. 2016;10:130.
103. Hussin NM, Shahar S, Teng NIMF, Ngah WZW, Das SK. Efficacy of fasting and calorie restriction (FCR) on mood and depression among ageing men. J Nutr Health Aging. 2013;17(8):674–80.
104. Redman LM, Martin CK, Williamson DA, Ravussin E. Effect of caloric restriction in non-obese humans on physiological, psychological and behavioral outcomes. Physiol Behav. 2008;94(5):643–8.
105. Michalsen A, Weidenhammer W, Melchart D, Langhorst J, Saha J, Dobos G. Short-term therapeutic fasting in the treatment of chronic pain and fatigue syndromes–well-being and side effects with and without mineral supplements. Forsch Komplementarmed Klass Naturheilkd. 2002;9(4):221–7.
106. Zhang Y, Liu C, Zhao Y, Zhang X, Li B, Cui R. The effects of calorie restriction in depression and potential mechanisms. Curr Neuropharmacol. 2015;13(4):536–42.
107. Bozzatello P, Brignolo E, De Grandi E, Bellino S. Supplementation with omega-3 fatty acids in psychiatric disorders: a review of literature data. J Clin Med. 2016;5(8):67.
108. NIH. Omega-3 Fatty Acids [Internet]. NIH Office of Dietary Supplements. 2020 [cited 2021 Mar 4]. Available from: https://ods.od.nih.gov/factsheets/Omega3FattyAcids-HealthProfessional/.
109. Olson CR, Mello CV. Significance of vitamin a to brain function, behavior and learning. Mol Nutr Food Res. 2010;54(4):489–95.
110. NIH. Vitamin A [Internet]. Vitamin A. 2020 [cited 2021 Jan 30]. Available from: https://ods.od.nih.gov/factsheets/VitaminA-HealthProfessional/.
111. Kubala J. Vitamin A: benefits, deficiency, toxicity and more [Internet]. Healthline. 2018 [cited 2021 Mar 4]. Available from: https://www.healthline.com/nutrition/vitamin-a.
112. Pratte MA, Nanavati KB, Young V, Morley CP. An alternative treatment for anxiety: a systematic review of human trial results reported for the Ayurvedic herb ashwagandha (Withania somnifera). J Altern Complement Med. 2014;20(12):901–8.

Chapter 9
Neurodegenerative

Contents

Integrative nutrition addresses neurodegenerative disease though the system-based approach that begins in the gut and encompasses diet and nutraceutical support as the primary interventions, in concert with fine-tuning all areas of lifestyle medicine. We address Parkinson's disease, Alzheimer's disease, and multiple sclerosis in turn, highlighting the most clinically relevant aspects of nutrition care.

9.1   Parkinson's Disease

According to a 2018 NIH study by Dorsey et al., Parkinson's disease(PD) is the fastest-growing neurological disease in the world and is expected to double by 2040 to 12 to 17 million cases worldwide [1]. Key elements of the pathogenesis that are modifiable through diet and lifestyle change include oxidative stress, impaired autophagy, inflammation, mitochondrial dysfunction, and impaired detoxification pathways [2]. Thus, the complex pathophysiology of PD provides two targets for nutritional intervention: the gut and mitochondria [3]. A well-established connection between gut and brain health via the vagus nerve encourages the inspection of gut health wherever concerns exist in the brain. Assessment using a comprehensive stool test that analyzes using PCR, culture, and microscopic methods provides detailed information regarding microbiome balance, digestive sufficiency, inflammation status, and pathogen load. Table 9.1 describes nutritional interventions indicated for various imbalances highlighted in comprehensive stool testing. Table 9.2 discusses key supplements recommended to support Parkinson's disease.

The mitochondria are particularly susceptible to the negative effects of toxin exposure. The link between exposure to toxins such as heavy metals, pesticides, solvents, and other pollutants and PD has been shown in the research literature for

Table 9.1 Comprehensive stool testing [4, 5]

Concern	Symptom	Intervention
Pancreatic insufficiency	Maldigestion Pain Undigested food in stool	Smaller meals, more frequently. Add comprehensive digestive enzyme with each meal. Add Swedish bitters before meals to stimulate digestive process. Reduce alcohol intake. Smoking cessation.
Elevated fecal fat	Frequent greasy, foul-smelling, loose stools Indigestion Gas Cramps Unintentional weight loss [6]	Consider SIBO breath testing. Assess for/reduce the use of acid-blocking medications.
Elevated products of protein breakdown	Protein maldigestion and absorption	Assess for the use of acid-blocking medications. Consider addition of betaine HCl. Support with PERT.
High secretory IgA	Immune upregulation in the gut	Investigate infectious causes. Consider food antibody testing.
High eosinophil protein X	Increased intestinal permeability and GI inflammation	Consider IgE food antibody panel and elimination diet.
Positive fecal occult blood test	Anemia, overt bleeding, non-bloody diarrhea, iron deficiency, and dyspepsia [7]	Assess causes of bleeding (ulcers, polyps, diverticulitis, IBD, colorectal cancer).
Microbiome imbalances	Abdominal pain and alternating bowel habits	Increase dietary SCFAs to include prebiotic food sources (FOS, inulin, psyllium, oat bran, xylooligosaccharide, beta-glucan, arabinogalactan). Increase intake of fiber and whole complex carbohydrate and resistant starch. Add multi-strain probiotic. Increase fermented foods (kefir, yogurt, kim chee). Elevated beta-glucuronidase: add calcium-d-glucarate.

Table 9.2 Top ten nutritional supplements to support Parkinson's disease

Supplement	Daily dose
B12	0.5–5 mg
Methylfolate	0.45–5 mg
Melatonin	5–10 mg
Omega-3	1000–3000 mg/day of EPA/DHA. Avoid over 4 gm
CoQ10	100–200 mg
Vitamin E	200–400 IU
N-acetyl cysteine	600–1200 mg
Resveratrol	400–1000 mg
Turmeric	500–1500 mg of concentrated highly absorbable form
Green tea	Food or capsules 500–1000 mg of EGCG
M. pruriens[a]	15,000–30,000 mg [56]

[a]*M. pruriens and Sinemet:* The amount of levodopa in any supply of *M. pruriens* is unreliable and inconsistent. *M. pruriens* should not be combined with other levodopa-containing medications. Data remains limited to support widespread *M. pruriens* in treatment of Parkinson's

decades [2]. Targeting this driver requires not only a reduction in exposure to toxins by choosing organic food and using natural cleaning and personal care products (see www.ewg.org for more details) but also specific support of detoxification pathways using nutritional supplements, diet, and lifestyle habits such as regular use of infrared sauna. Table 9.3 identifies specific nutritional supplements and foods that support liver detoxification and mitochondrial health [8, 9].

9.1.1 Case 1

Frank came to see Dr. Kogan at the age of 71 after being diagnosed with early PD. His symptoms were mild but progressing. He had right-sided tremor for several years prior to diagnosis, but shuffling gait and several falls triggered evaluation. When he first presented to the clinic, his other PD-related problems were constipation, difficulty sleeping, and frequent leg cramps. Frank, now retired from his office job, lived with his wife who recently committed to cooking healthy meals for both of them. Frank's diet was not very healthy but had increased the amount of vegetables per his neurologist's recommendation. Additional nutrition changes were optimized including his vitamin D level. Melatonin 3 mg was added to help with sleep.

Upon comprehensive intake, it became clear that Frank consumed an excess of simple carbohydrates especially with dinner, taking 1–2 glasses of wine and a large bowl of ice cream. While he was getting an adequate amount of protein, he consumed very little beneficial fats. He often ate very late at night.

Frank's therapeutic diet consisted of cutting out alcohol, which likely interfered with sleep, as well as most simple carbohydrates. Dr. Kogan advised substituting them with high-quality oils such as olive, avocado, and nuts and seeds and complex carbohydrates from grains, vegetables, and some fruits, especially fresh or frozen

Table 9.3 Nutritional supplements and foods to support detoxification and mitochondrial health

Name	Function	Dosing	Nutritional supplement alternative	Comments
Antioxidants [8, 10] lutein, quercetin, and resveratrol found in fruits and vegetables	Stimulate hormetic response to oxidants providing antioxidant effect	8–10 servings/ day (4–6 cups)	Vitamins C and E, selenium, and carotenoids, such as beta-carotene, lycopene, lutein, and zeaxanthin [11]	Food sources are preferred since trials of single antioxidants have never shown benefits
Protein and amino acids (fish, soy, legumes, nuts/ seeds)	Provide key amino acids and antioxidants	0.83 g/kg [12]	High-quality, organic plant and animal protein supplemental powders (1–1.3 g/kg/d) [13]	High-quality, organic plant and animal sources reduce the body burden of toxins and supports. See www. nrdc.org for list of low-toxin fish
Brassicas (broccoli, Brussels sprouts, cabbage, cauliflower, collard greens, kale, and turnips)	Provide sulfur compounds to support liver detox and fiber for gut health	1–2 cups/ day	Methylsulfonylmethane (MSM) typical dose is 1–2 gm/day [14]	Patients sensitive to sulfur need to be careful with supplemental forms and start with 500 mg or less daily
Leafy greens (kale, spinach, romaine, chard, collards, mustard, arugula)	Bitters that support digestion and reduce oxidative stress	Two cups/day	Nitrate (1.2–3.0 mg/d), lutein (10 mg), and phylloquinone (limited studies) [15, 16]	Cephalic vagal responses and/or local response to reduce dyspepsia [17]
Allium (onion, garlic, leek, shallot)	Sulfur-containing foods that support liver detoxification and provide fermentable fibers for gut microbiome health	Daily use in cooking	Methylsulfonylmethane (MSM) typical dose is 1–2 gm/day	Supports key biological compounds such as glutathione Supports sulfation, a necessary step in liver detoxification Enhances immune function
Liver/kidney support (asparagus, artichoke, beets, celery, sprouts)	Enhances urine flow and alkalization	½ cup/ day	2–50 mg/kg/d retinoic acid suspension in corn oil and 500 mg/d quercetin [18]	

Table 9.3 (continued)

Name	Function	Dosing	Nutritional supplement alternative	Comments
Herbal tea (green, dandelion)	High content of polyphenols	2–3c/day [19]	Chamomile, gentian, or dandelion root [20]	The total polyphenol content of green and black teas is similar, but with different types of flavonoids present due to the degree of oxidation during processing [21]
Herbs (curry, dill, rosemary, cilantro, turmeric)	Anti-inflammatory support and specific compounds that absorb toxins	Varies by herb	Coenzyme Q10, krill oil, lipoic acid, resveratrol, grape-seed oil, α-tocopherol, and selenium	Antioxidative, anti-amyloidogenic, and antiapoptotic [22]

berries. Additionally, we prescribed magnesium citrate 300 mg at bedtime (targeting his constipation and insomnia) and increased his melatonin to 10 mg. We also asked him to stop eating at 7 PM and have a first-day meal at 10–11 AM, making sure he gets close to 16 h of intermittent fasting every night.

While Frank's PD tremor stayed the same, his constipation and cramps resolved and his sleep improved. Additionally Frank felt more energy and took on PD boxing and Tai Chi. His lifestyle modifications improved his quality of life significantly.

9.2   Alzheimer's Disease (AD)

The projections for AD and other dementias reveal a healthcare crisis that is as costly financially as it is to the quality of life for our elders. As a slowly progressing disease whose pathology begins decades prior to the onset of symptoms that would bring a patient in for medical care, the work of a geriatric practitioner becomes less preventative and more mitigative. And yet, there are much research and clinical exploration in the field of integrative medicine to address the cognitive changes associated with aging. All attempts at a pharmacological intervention have failed. Thus, more than simply tracking the cognitive changes in an assessment such as the MoCA or Mini-Cog, diving into the common drivers of cognitive decline can help stop and often reverse its progression. Of note, once a patient has entered into advanced decline, there is little integrative medicine that has been able to do to address it. Early and aggressive intervention is critical. Recognizing the immense social stigma around cognitive decline, practitioners will serve their patients best by normalizing the concern and actively seeking to assess cognitive function in all patients. Instead of brushing it off as a normal part of aging, understanding that this is a symptom of imbalance just like a fever lets us know of the presence of a virus.

One of the new systems that categorizes AD according to key drivers, separates it in number of types [23].

Drivers of AD are as follows:

1. Type 1 – inflammatory, "hot" – inflammatory markers (hs-CRP), infection (Lyme, fungal, dental), leaky gut, and poor diet.
2. Type 1.5 – glycotoxic, "sweet" – inflammatory and atrophic features, high glucose, and insulin.
3. Type 2 – atrophic "cold" (hormonal deficiencies) – sex hormones, vitamin D, insulin, and neurotrophins.
4. Type 3 – toxic or "vile" – begins with problems with numbers, speech, organizing, and depression.
5. Vascular – leaky brain, high homocysteine, and vascular amyloid.
6. Traumatic – amyloid produced as a result of brain trauma can be cleared over time.

How does epigenetics contribute? The primary genetic single-nucleotide polymorphism (SNP) that drives risk of AD is APOE4. As such, knowing the APOE4 status of patients is central to supporting their medical management so as to optimize health span. As decades of monotherapy is replaced by a robust multifactorial disease model, APOE4 plays this central role, driving varied system dysfunction including inflammatory, cardiovascular, and neurodegenerative [24]. Other SNPs associated with AD include ADNP, APP, HLA-DR/DQs, MTHFR, and *Presenilin* [25, 26] [27].

Dr. Dale Bredesen has extensively researched lifestyle modifications to support neurocognition. Figure 9.1 summarizes his findings.

Treating and preventing neurocognitive decline come in many forms. Table 9.4 summarizes these interventions and their intended effects. Table 9.5 reviews key nutrients to support Alzheimer's.

Fig. 9.1 Lifestyle modifications to support cognition [28]

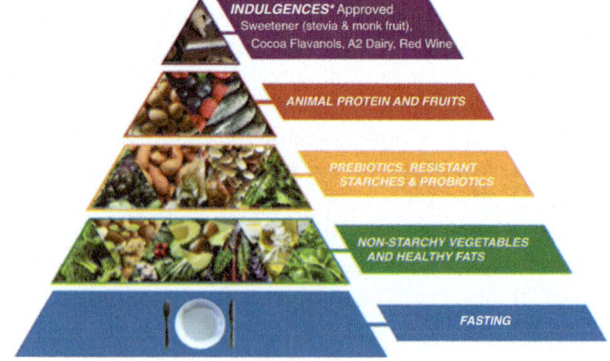

Table 9.4 Integrative interventions to combat Alzheimer's

Intervention	Details	Targeted effect
Intermittent fasting	Fasting: 3 h before bed and minimum of 12 h, APOE4 = 16+ For non-APOE4, 5:2 fasting may be considered (2 days with 500–600 calories, rest of the week normal intake)	Allows prolonged decrease in insulin resulting in anti-inflammatory affect, BDNF stimulation, and amyloid breakdown [29, 30]. Increases autophagy [31]
Cognitive games	BrainHQ and Lumosity, 10–20 min per day Sudoku, card games, and learning a new language or instrument	Helps exercise memory, cognition, and emotional control [32]
Smoking cessation	Single most important factor in reducing all chronic diseases	Reduces cerebral oxidative stress associated with AD [33, 34]
Physical activity	30–60 min of exercise, 5–6 days per week Reduced sedentary time and the use of standing desks and active recreation like dancing rather than watching TV	Improves mitochondrial respiratory activity, reduces apoptotic signaling and neuronal death, and stimulates plasticity of brain network [35]
Social connection	Screening for social isolation and loneliness and encouraging socialization	Feeling of loneliness and isolation triggers inflammation and increases risk of AD and dementia [36]
Mindfulness and meditation	Regular practice of tai chi, transcendental meditation, and yoga	Dose-dependent relationship between tai chi attendance and some cognitive measures [37]
Hearing support	Regular testing and assessment of hearing with follow-up treatment as needed	Hearing loss is associated with an increased risk of AD [38]
Mood stabilization	Regular anxiety and depression screening with follow-up treatment as needed	Depression is associated with an increased risk of AD onset [39]

Table 9.5 Top ten nutritional supplements to support Alzheimer's disease

Supplement	Daily dose
B12	0.5–5 mg
Methylfolate	0.4–5 mg
Zinc	15–30 mg
Vitamin E	200–400 IU
Alpha lipoic acid	300–1200 mg. Not every day, in pulses
Omega-3 fatty acid	1000–3000 mg/day of EPA/DHA. Avoid over 4 gm
Coenzyme Q10	100–200 mg
Acetyl-L-carnitine	1500–3000 mg
N-acetyl cysteine	600–1200 mg
Alpha-glycerylphosphorylcholine, (alpha-GPC) and cytidine 5′-diphosphocholine (CDP-choline)	600–1200 mg
Turmeric	500–1500 mg of concentrated highly absorbable form
B. monnieri	300–1000 mg

9.2.1 Case 2: Francis

Francis, previously healthy except for episodic GI issues that were diagnosed as irritable bowel syndrome decades earlier in her late 50s, started noticing cognitive fatigue, problems with running multiple cognitive tasks and remembering small details on which her work often depended. As a highly energetic leadership executive in charge of a large firm, she felt that she could no longer sustain her "game." Subtle at first, Francis attributed these changes to an increased workload and stressors in the last year or two, but after she took an extended vacation and did in-depth mind-body training, she got more concerned that the cognitive concerns were slowly progressing. She went to her PCP who completed a Mini-Cog screening and basic blood work; both were normal. Francis insisted that something was wrong, and her PCP referred her for a neuropsychiatric evaluation that showed essentially normal performance on all scales for her age. Despite the normal results, Francis was convinced that something was wrong and on her own pursued a substantial amount of reading. She found the work of Dr. Dale Bredesen most convincing after reading *The End of Alzheimer's: The First Program to Prevent and Reverse Cognitive Decline*. Before coming to see us in the clinic, she checked her APOE4 status which turned out negative (no APOE4 alleles) and started on a ketogenic diet with nightly 14-h intermittent fasting. She felt significantly better within 3 months, and although her symptoms did not resolve completely, she felt very encouraged. After beginning to work with her, we decided to maintain her on a ketogenic diet given subjective improvement. We carefully monitored her blood lipids and reduced her intake of animal fat (high in saturated fats) while increasing beneficial plant-based oils, mostly olive, and increasing nighttime fasting to 16 h. We also addressed several other issues including borderline low vitamin B12 level, elevated homocysteine, slightly off thyroid levels, and identification of mild SIBO that we thought was likely the cause of Francis' long-lasting IBS. While the ketogenic diet likely improved SIBO, we added a course of antimicrobial herbs, see Chap. 4, which resolved all IBS symptoms. After 12 months, Francis stated that her symptoms improved nearly 90% and she was maintaining her ketogenic diet in combination with several supplements and low dose of thyroid hormone. Several years later, Francis continues to work and be fully engaged in life without any signs of progressive decline.

9.3 Multiple Sclerosis (MS) [40]

The typical geriatric patient that has survived into their golden years with MS is very likely to have it well controlled, leaving the practitioner less likely to diagnose the disease than they are to work with it as a comorbidity. To the extent that a patient seeks to optimize their lifestyle to alleviate additional stressors, there are several approaches that have been gaining traction in the integrative community as research supports clinical understanding of the disease drivers. Two rather extreme diet interventions have come to the forefront of clinical care of MS: the vegan diet and the Wahls protocol. While protein sources differ between the two, a consistent theme is that of a large amount of high-quality vegetables. The vegan diet's focus should remain on organic, whole foods rather than incorporating vegan convenience foods. Great care should be taken with supplementation of key nutrients commonly deficient in a vegan diet – EPA/DHA omega-3 fats, iron, B12, calcium, vitamin D, and iodine [41]. Alternatively, the Wahls protocol focuses on 6–9 cups of non-starchy vegetables and 4 ounces of fish, twice weekly [40]. The use of cannabis as part of MS treatment is an emerging field that shows great promise. Cannabis has been shown to reduce patient-reported spasticity, mobility, and pain [42].

9.3.1 Case 3

In her mid 30s, Kate, who was previously a perfectly healthy project manager at the International Monetary Fund (IMF), came down with sudden onset of vision disturbances and one-sided weakness. Kate was quickly diagnosed with Multiple Sclerosis (MS) and was started on an aggressive course of IV steroids. Throughout her life, Kate had a healthy lifestyle with a good exercise routine and balanced diet that she characterized as mostly organic, high in vegetables and omnivore type. After Kate rapidly improved with the course of steroids she spent weeks researching MS and as part of her plan decided to proceed with a consultation at the integrative medicine center. In addition to correcting her significant vitamin D deficiency, we changed Kate to a plant-based organic diet and added a number of anti-inflammatory supplements including curcumin, fish oil, and later CBD oil. Kate chose to avoid all MS medications but she never needed them, now over 10 years later Kate is symptoms free and has stayed in continuous remission giving the most of the benefit to a combination of vitamin D deficiency correction and plant-based diet. For a list of recommended nutrients to support Kate and other's with MS, please see Table 9.6

Table 9.6 Top ten nutritional supplements to support multiple sclerosis [57]

Supplement	Daily dose
Omega-3 fatty acids	1000–3000 mg/day of EPA/DHA. Avoid over 4 gm/day
CoQ10	500 mg CoQ10/day
Vitamin B7	100–300 mg/day
Vitamin D	50,000 IU weekly OR 5000 IU daily. Should be combined with vitamin K2
Vitamin A	25,000 IU
Acetyl L-carnitine	1500–3000 mg
SOD	500 mg [58]
Methylated vitamin B12	1–5 mg orally or sublingual
Melatonin	5–10 mg

9.4   Therapeutic Neurodegenerative Diets

9.4.1   Ketogenic Diet

The goal of a ketogenic diet is to shift the patient's primary metabolism from glucose dominant to ketone dominant by reducing dietary carbohydrate to 10–15%, protein to 10–15%, and fat to 70% of total intake. The metabolic effect of this shift allows fasting glucose and insulin to decrease, insulin sensitivity to be re-established, weight optimized, and markers of inflammation reduced [43]. The ketogenic diet is an effective tool for cognition in patients that have diabetes, insulin resistance, and obesity as comorbidities. As this therapeutic diet is highly specific and requires detailed guidance and support for most patients, referral to a nutrition professional specialized in it is strongly recommended. See appendix for more details.

9.4.2   Anti-inflammatory Mediterranean Diet

The Mediterranean diet centers on antioxidant-rich fruits and vegetables, whole grains, lean protein, and high intake of extra-virgin olive oil which addresses one of the key drivers of cognitive decline – oxidative stress. For patients that are on a standard American diet with minimal fruits and vegetables, fried foods, and abundant added sugars, the Mediterranean diet is an appropriate first step toward improving cognition by reducing inflammatory foods. See appendix for more details [44].

9.4.3   Detox Diet

Toxins are a primary driver in many cases of cognitive decline with known cases of reversal of diagnosed AD being resolved through detoxification protocol [45]. A detox diet uses high doses of specific foods to support the body's detoxification pathway while also prioritizing the avoidance of toxins in conventionally raised food [46]. Often, toxin buildup is linked to specific genetic SNPs that alter the efficacy of the detoxification enzymes and allow toxins to accumulate. For more details, see appendix.

Table 9.7 summarizes key micronutrients to support neurologic health.

L-carnitine vs. Acetyl-L-carnitine: What's the Difference?
L-carnitine is an amino acid that can be found in foods like beef, chicken, fish, dairy, and other natural sources. Acetyl-L-carnitine is a different version of L-carnitine, with a few noticeable distinctions. Acetyl L-carnitine is more easily absorbed by the gut and more readily and effectively crosses the

blood-brain barrier. As such, acetyl-L-carnitine is more commonly utilized to support brain health [59]. This difference comes at a price; acetyl-L-carnitine is more expensive. On the other hand, L-carnitine does not cross the BBB but is helpful for building muscle and treating cachexia. The lower price point of L-carnitine makes the necessary higher doses required for muscle wasting more cost-effective.

*Alzheimer's – data conflicting. Doses: 0.5–3 g orally daily [60].

Table 9.7 Micronutrients of primary concern for neurologic health

Micronutrient	Function	Dietary sources	Symptoms of deficiency	RDA* male (>70 years)	RDA female (>70 years)
B12 [47]	Required for proper RBC formation, neurological function, and DNA synthesis [47]	Clams, liver, beef, salmon, trout, tuna, and nutritional yeast [47]	Fatigue, weakness, weight loss, numbness and tingling in hands and feet, balance problems, depression, confusion, dementia, and memory problems [47]	2.4 µg [47]	2.4 µg [47]
Folate [48]	Coenzyme in DNA and RNA synthesis and metabolism of amino acids [48]	Beef liver, spinach, black-eyed peas, breakfast cereals (fortified), rice, asparagus, and Brussels sprouts [48]	Weakness, difficulty concentrating, irritability, and headache [48]	400 µg DFE [48]	400 µg DFE [48]
CoQ10 [49]	Cofactor in electron transport chain (ETC), significant lipid antioxidant [49]	Salmon, tuna, liver, and whole grains [49]	Dysfunction in respiratory chain, cerebellar ataxia, seizures, intellectual disability, hypotonia, dystonia, spasticity, nystagmus, sensorineural hearing loss, and vision loss [50]	30–90 mg/d [49]	30–90 mg/d [49]

(continued)

Table 9.7 (continued)

Micronutrient	Function	Dietary sources	Symptoms of deficiency	RDA* male (>70 years)	RDA female (>70 years)
Omega-3 fatty acid (EPA/DHA) [51]	Components of the phospholipids that form structures of cell membranes and provide energy [51]	Salmon, sardines, trout, oysters, and sea bass [51]	Rough, scaly skin and dermatitis [51]	1.6 g^a [51]	1.1 g^a [51]
Alpha linolenic acid [51]		Flaxseed (oil), chia seeds, English walnuts, canola oil, salmon, and soybean oil [51]		1.6 g^a [51]	1.1 g^a [51]
Vitamin D [52, 53]	Promotes Ca absorption in the gut and maintains serum Ca and Phos concentrations to enable normal bone mineralization and growth. Reduces inflammation and modulates cell growth, neuromuscular and immune function, and glucose metabolism [53]	Cod liver oil, trout, salmon (sockeye), mushrooms, milk, and fortified cereal [52]	Osteomalacia [52]	20 µg (800 IU) [52]	20 µg (800 IU) [52]
Carnitine [54]	Critical role in energy production. Transports toxic compounds out of cellular organelles to prevent accumulation and shuttles fatty acids across the mitochondrial membrane to drive ATP production [54]	Beef steak, ground beef, milk (whole), and codfish [54]	Hypotonia, fatigue, irritability, muscle weakness, shortness of breath, and edema [54]	No RDA established. RDA of protein: 0.8 g/kg/d [55]	No RDA established. RDA of protein: 0.8 g/kg/d [55]

^{a}Adequate intake, data not sufficient to claim RDA*

Acknowledgement *Chapter created with research from Dr. Dale Bredesen's work, author of The End of Alzheimer's and Chief Science Officer of Apollo Health.*

References

1. Dorsey ER, Sherer T, Okun MS, Bloem BR. The emerging evidence of the Parkinson pandemic. J Parkinsons Dis. 2018;8(s1):S3–8.
2. Goldman SM. Environmental toxins and Parkinson's disease. Annu Rev Pharmacol Toxicol. 2014;54:141–64.
3. Felice VD, Quigley EM, Sullivan AM, O'Keeffe GW, O'Mahony SM. Microbiota-gut-brain signalling in Parkinson's disease: implications for non-motor symptoms. Parkinsonism Relat Disord. 2016;27:1–8.
4. Struyvenberg MR, Martin CR, Freedman SD. Practical guide to exocrine pancreatic insufficiency – breaking the myths. BMC Med. 2017;15(1):29.
5. GI Effects: Comprehensive Profile – Stool [Internet]. Genova Diagnostics. 2020 [cited 2021 Mar 5]. Available from: https://www.gdx.net/product/gi-effects-comprehensive-stool-test.
6. Ruiz, Jr AR. Overview of Malabsorption [Internet]. Merck Manual Professional Version. 2019 [cited 2021 Mar 5]. Available from: https://www.merckmanuals.com/professional/gastrointestinal-disorders/malabsorption-syndromes/overview-of-malabsorption.
7. Narula N, Ulic D, Al-Dabbagh R, Ibrahim A, Mansour M, Balion C, et al. Fecal occult blood testing as a diagnostic test in symptomatic patients is not useful: a retrospective chart review. Can J Gastroenterol Hepatol. 2014;28(8):421–6.
8. Calabrese V, Cornelius C, Trovato A, Cavallaro M, Mancuso C, Di Rienzo L, et al. The hormetic role of dietary antioxidants in free radical-related diseases. Curr Pharm Des. 2010;16(7):877–83.
9. Licznerska B, Szaefer H, Matuszak I, Murias M, Baer-Dubowska W. Modulating potential of L-sulforaphane in the expression of cytochrome p450 to identify potential targets for breast cancer chemoprevention and therapy using breast cell lines. Phytother Res. 2015;29(1):93–9.
10. Kalyanaraman B. Teaching the basics of redox biology to medical and graduate students: oxidants, antioxidants and disease mechanisms. Redox Biol. 2013;1:244–57.
11. Antioxidants: In Dept [Internet]. National Center for Integrative and Complementary Health. 2013 [cited 2021 Mar 5]. Available from: https://www.nccih.nih.gov/health/antioxidants-in-depth.
12. Klein AV, Kiat H. Detox diets for toxin elimination and weight management: a critical review of the evidence. J Hum Nutr Diet. 2015;28(6):675–86.
13. Nowson C, O'Connell S. Protein requirements and recommendations for older people: a review. Nutrients. 2015;7(8):6874–99.
14. Wong T, Bloomer RJ, Benjamin RL, Buddington RK. Small intestinal absorption of methylsulfonylmethane (MSM) and accumulation of the sulfur moiety in selected tissues of mice. Nutrients. 2017;10(1):19.
15. Morris MC, Wang Y, Barnes LL, Bennett DA, Dawson-Hughes B, Booth SL. Nutrients and bioactives in green leafy vegetables and cognitive decline: prospective study. Neurology. 2018;90(3):e214–22.
16. Ma L, Hu L, Feng X, Wang S. Nitrate and nitrite in health and disease. Aging Dis. 2018;9(5):938–45.
17. McMullen MK, Whitehouse JM, Towell A. Bitters: time for a new paradigm. Evid Based Complement Alternat Med. 2015;2015:670504.
18. Hodges RE, Minich DM. Modulation of metabolic detoxification pathways using foods and food-derived components: a scientific review with clinical application. J Nutr Metab. 2015;2015:760689.

19. Khan N, Mukhtar H. Tea and health: studies in humans. Curr Pharm Des. 2013;19(34):6141–7.
20. Koithan M, Niemeyer K. Using herbal remedies to maintain optimal weight. J Nurse Pract. 2010;6(2):153–4.
21. Stangl V, Lorenz M, Stangl K. The role of tea and tea flavonoids in cardiovascular health. Mol Nutr Food Res. 2006;50(2):218–28.
22. Iriti M, Vitalini S, Fico G, Faoro F. Neuroprotective herbs and foods from different traditional medicines and diets. Molecules. 2010;15(5):3517–55.
23. Shetty P, Youngberg W. Clinical lifestyle medicine strategies for preventing and reversing memory loss in Alzheimer's. Am J Lifestyle Med. 2018;12(5):391–5.
24. Theendakara V, Peters-Libeu CA, Spilman P, Poksay KS, Bredesen DE, Rao RV. Direct transcriptional effects of apolipoprotein E. J Neurosci. 2016;36(3):685–700.
25. Román GC, Mancera-Páez O, Bernal C. Epigenetic factors in late-onset Alzheimer's disease: MTHFR and CTH gene polymorphisms, metabolic transsulfuration and methylation pathways, and B vitamins. Int J Mol Sci. 2019;20(2):319.
26. Giri M, Zhang M, Lü Y. Genes associated with Alzheimer's disease: an overview and current status. Clin Interv Aging. 2016;11:665–81.
27. Malishkevich A, Marshall GA, Schultz AP, Sperling RA, Aharon-Peretz J, Gozes I. Blood-borne activity-dependent neuroprotective protein (ADNP) is correlated with premorbid intelligence, clinical stage, and Alzheimer's disease biomarkers. J Alzheimers Dis. 2016;50(1):249–60.
28. Bresden. KetoFLEX 12/3 [Internet]. Apollo Health. 2021 [cited 2021 Mar 4]. Available from: https://www.apollohealthco.com/ketoflex-12-3/.
29. Zhang J, Zhan Z, Li X, Xing A, Jiang C, Chen Y, et al. Intermittent fasting protects against Alzheimer's disease possible through restoring Aquaporin-4 polarity. Front Mol Neurosci. 2017;10:395.
30. Baik S-H, Rajeev V, Fann DY-W, Jo D-G, Arumugam TV. Intermittent fasting increases adult hippocampal neurogenesis. Brain Behav. 2020;10(1):e01444.
31. Bagheriya M, Butler AE, Barreto GE, Sahebkar A. The effect of fasting or calorie restriction on autophagy induction: a review of the literature. Ageing Res Rev. 2018;47:183–97.
32. Ning H, Li R, Ye X, Zhang Y, Liu L. A review on serious games for dementia care in ageing societies. IEEE J Transl Eng Health Med. 2020;8:1400411.
33. Choi D, Choi S, Park SM. Effect of smoking cessation on the risk of dementia: a longitudinal study. Ann Clin Transl Neurol. 2018;5(10):1192–9.
34. Durazzo TC, Mattsson N, Weiner MW. Alzheimer's Disease Neuroimaging Initiative. Smoking and increased Alzheimer's disease risk: a review of potential mechanisms. Alzheimers Dement. 2014;10(3 Suppl):S122–45.
35. Gronek P, Balko S, Gronek J, Zajac A, Maszczyk A, Celka R, et al. Physical activity and Alzheimer's disease: a narrative review. Aging Dis. 2019;10(6):1282–92.
36. Shankar A, Hamer M, McMunn A, Steptoe A. Social isolation and loneliness: relationships with cognitive function during 4 years of follow-up in the English longitudinal study of ageing. Psychosom Med. 2013;75(2):161–70.
37. Chang JY, Tsai P-F, Beck C, Hagen JL, Huff DC, Anand KJS, et al. The effect of tai chi on cognition in elders with cognitive impairment. Medsurg Nurs. 2011;20(2):63–9; quiz 70
38. Thomson RS, Auduong P, Miller AT, Gurgel RK. Hearing loss as a risk factor for dementia: a systematic review. Laryngoscope Investig Otolaryngol. 2017;2(2):69–79.
39. Sanmugam K. Depression is a risk factor for Alzheimer disease-review. Rese Jour of Pharm and Technol. 2015;8(8):1056.
40. Wahls T, Scott MO, Alshare Z, Rubenstein L, Darling W, Carr L, et al. Dietary approaches to treat MS-related fatigue: comparing the modified Paleolithic (Wahls Elimination) and low saturated fat (Swank) diets on perceived fatigue in persons with relapsing-remitting multiple sclerosis: study protocol for a randomized controlled trial. Trials. 2018;19(1):309.

41. Elorinne A-L, Alfthan G, Erlund I, Kivimäki H, Paju A, Salminen I, et al. Food and nutrient intake and nutritional status of Finnish vegans and non-vegetarians. PLoS One. 2016;11(2):e0148235.
42. Zajicek J, Fox P, Sanders H, Wright D, Vickery J, Nunn A, et al. Cannabinoids for treatment of spasticity and other symptoms related to multiple sclerosis (CAMS study): multicentre randomised placebo-controlled trial. Lancet. 2003;362(9395):1517–26.
43. Broom GM, Shaw IC, Rucklidge JJ. The ketogenic diet as a potential treatment and prevention strategy for Alzheimer's disease. Nutrition. 2019;60:118–21.
44. Valls-Pedret C, Sala-Vila A, Serra-Mir M, Corella D, de la Torre R, Martínez-González MÁ, et al. Mediterranean diet and age-related cognitive decline: a randomized clinical trial. JAMA Intern Med. 2015;175(7):1094–103.
45. Foley MM, Seidel I, Sevier J, Wendt J, Kogan M. One man's swordfish story: the link between Alzheimer's disease and mercury exposure. Complement Ther Med. 2020;52:102499.
46. Jeffery EH. Diet and detoxification enzymes. Altern Ther Health Med. 2007;13(2):S98–9.
47. Vitamin B12 [Internet]. NIH National Institutes of Health Office of Dietary Supplements. 2020 [cited 2021 Jan 2]. Available from: https://ods.od.nih.gov/factsheets/VitaminB12-HealthProfessional/.
48. NIH. Folate [Internet]. National Institutes of Health Office of Dietary Supplements. 2020 [cited 2020 Dec 30]. Available from: https://ods.od.nih.gov/factsheets/Folate-HealthProfessional/.
49. Saini R. Coenzyme Q10: the essential nutrient. J Pharm Bioallied Sci. 2011;3(3):466–7.
50. Primary coenzyme Q10 deficiency [Internet]. Genetics Home Reference. 2020 [cited 2021 Mar 5]. Available from: https://ghr.nlm.nih.gov/condition/primary-coenzyme-q10-deficiency.
51. NIH. Omega-3 Fatty Acids [Internet]. NIH Office of Dietary Supplements. 2020 [cited 2021 Mar 4]. Available from: https://ods.od.nih.gov/factsheets/Omega3FattyAcids-HealthProfessional/.
52. NIH. Vitamin D [Internet]. NIH National Institutes of Health Office of Dietary Suppolements. 2020 [cited 2020 Dec 31]. Available from: https://ods.od.nih.gov/factsheets/VitaminD-HealthProfessional/.
53. Berridge MJ. Vitamin D deficiency accelerates ageing and age-related diseases: a novel hypothesis. J Physiol Lond. 2017;595(22):6825–36.
54. NIH. Carnitine [Internet]. NIH National Institutes of Health Office of Dietary Supplements. 2017 [cited 2021 Jan 2]. Available from: https://ods.od.nih.gov/factsheets/Carnitine-HealthProfessional/.
55. Baum JI, Kim I-Y, Wolfe RR. Protein consumption and the elderly: what is the optimal level of intake? Nutrients. 2016;8(6):359.
56. Katzenschlager R, Evans A, Manson A, Patsalos PN, Ratnaraj N, Watt H, et al. Mucuna pruriens in Parkinson's disease: a double blind clinical and pharmacological study. J Neurol Neurosurg Psychiatry. 2004;75(12):1672–7.
57. Tryfonos C, Mantzorou M, Fotiou D, Vrizas M, Vadikolias K, Pavlidou E, et al. Dietary supplements on controlling multiple sclerosis symptoms and relapses: current clinical evidence and future perspectives. Medicines (Basel). 2019;6(3):95.
58. Skarpanska-Stejnborn A, Pilaczynska-Szczesniak L, Basta P, Deskur-Smielecka E, Woitas-Slubowska D, Adach Z. Effects of oral supplementation with plant superoxide dismutase extract on selected redox parameters and an inflammatory marker in a 2,000-m rowing-ergometer test. Int J Sport Nutr Exerc Metab. 2011;21(2):124–34.
59. Liu J, Head E, Kuratsune H, Cotman CW, Ames BN. Comparison of the effects of L-carnitine and acetyl-L-carnitine on carnitine levels, ambulatory activity, and oxidative stress biomarkers in the brain of old rats. Ann N Y Acad Sci. 2004;1033:117–31.
60. Pennisi M, Lanza G, Cantone M, D'Amico E, Fisicaro F, Puglisi V, et al. Acetyl-L-carnitine in dementia and other cognitive disorders: a critical update. Nutrients. 2020;12(5):1389.

Chapter 10
Oncology

Contents

Integrative nutrition care must support the nutritional status of the patient with cancer with a moderated approach. The phrase "Good, Better, Best" should become the guiding mantra for working with diet and lifestyle in the context of cancer. The recommendations in this book must be used in the context of the patient in order to be effective. If time is restricted, the use of pre-appointment questionnaires to understand the hurdles that patients face will allow the provider to determine the appropriate recommendations. The older adult is more vulnerable to malnutrition and sarcopenia; therefore, nutrition interventions should consider the difficulty in bouncing back from weight loss or nutrient deficiency.

The etiology of cancer requires a nutritional approach that seeks to:

- Limit exposure to toxins from environmental sources as much as possible. See www.ewg.org for up-to-date research on all things environmental toxins:

  - Organic produce when possible.
  - Air and water filters for inside the home.
  - Nonreactive cookware and food storage.
  - Chemical-free home and body care products.

- Support the nutrient needs for optimal gene expression:

  - Ensure adequate diet to meet nutritional needs and identify genetic SNPs that require methylation support with targeted vitamins.
  - High intake of phytonutrients from colorful fruits and vegetables.

© The Author(s), under exclusive license to Springer Nature
Switzerland AG 2021
J. Wendt et al., *Integrative Geriatric Nutrition*,
https://doi.org/10.1007/978-3-030-81758-9_10

- Provide for regular support of apoptosis:

  - Integration of any type of fasting supports the removal of rogue cells before systemic issues present; see the appendix for more details.

10.1   Nutritional Support for Cancer Prevention

Diet and lifestyle play a critical role in the prevention of cancer. Over 70% of cancer cases in the United States are potentially preventable because a majority of risk factors are modifiable such as obesity, excess alcohol consumption, cigarette smoking, and hepatitis B and C viruses [6]. The American Cancer Society (ACS) estimates that 45% of cancer deaths in the United States are preventable with diet and lifestyle modifications [7]. ACS's guidelines for prevention are in direct alignment with the integrative approach to oncology care: diet and lifestyle are the pillars.

Oncogenes may be responsive to specific dietary approaches such as intermittent fasting and antioxidant-rich plant-based diets in the context of normalized body weight. Fasting prior to chemotherapy has been shown to protect healthy, noncancerous cells from treatment toxicity by reducing expression of oncogenes, such as RAS and the AKT signaling pathways [8]. A plant-based diet, full of colorful fruits and vegetables, rich in antioxidants, and balanced with clean proteins and healthy fats, is the goal for optimal health which includes prevention of cancer [9]. Key aspects of a preventative diet are as follows:

- *A rainbow of colors on the plate*: each color imparts specific attributes that support the optimal function of our genome, our gut, and our biochemistry. Ideally, 80% of the plate should contain vegetables and fruits. See Table 10.1 for more detail.
- *Adequate protein based on the specific patient:* protein calculations vary widely, and for older adults, the requirements are higher; therefore, it is important to consider patient activity levels, digestive capacity, and health concerns when establishing protein recommendations. Ideally, if animal protein is included in the diet (and there is no evidence to suggest it should not be), encourage wild caught, pasture-raised animal products which reduce toxin exposure and improve the quality of the nutrients such as increasing the amount of anti-inflammatory omega-3 fats.
- *Fiber-rich foods to feed a healthy microbiome and support digestion function:* fiber-rich foods include fruits, vegetables, as well as whole grains and legumes. Beneficial bacteria consume fiber and produce anti-inflammatory fats called short-chain fatty acids which nourish the gut lining and circulate systemically to resolve inflammation [10]. Further, fiber supports healthy, regular elimination which moves toxins out of the body and prevents recirculation. Anything short of daily bowel movements should be investigated and corrected.

Table 10.1 Why "eating the rainbow" is chemoprotective and anticancer [12]

Color	Phytochemical	Food sources	MOA
Red	Capsaicin	Chili pepper	Chemopreventive, tumor suppressing, radiosensitizing, and anticancer agent
Red	Lycopenes	Tomatoes, watermelons, papaya, pink grapefruit, pink guava, and red carrot	Is an antioxidant and suppresses tumor development by inhibiting tumor neo-angiogenesis
Green	Sulforaphanes [13]	Broccoli and broccoli sprouts	Chemopreventive
Green	Cucurbitacin B	Traditional Chinese medicinal plant	Antiangiogenic and tumor suppressor
Green	Lutein [14]	Kale, spinach, and broccoli	Is anticancer, inhibits cancer cell growth, and induces cell cycle arrest
	Catechins	Green tea	Antioxidant and chemoprotective
Green-white	Indoles [15]	Broccoli, Brussels sprouts, cabbage, and cauliflower	Chemopreventive
Green-white	Benzyl isothiocyanate	Broccoli, watercress, Brussels sprouts, cabbage, cauliflower, and Japanese radish	Chemopreventive activity. Mediate anticarcinogenic activity by suppressing the activation of carcinogens and increasing their detoxification
Green-white	Phenethyl isothiocyanate	Broccoli, watercress, and garden cress	Chemopreventive and immune modulator
Brown	Piperlongumine	Long pepper	Anti-inflammatory, antinociceptive, and antitumor properties. Significant chemotherapeutic and chemopreventive
Yellow-brown	Isoflavones	Soy, lentil, bean, and chickpeas	Chemoprotective, estrogenic or antiestrogenic [16]

- *Healthy fats allow the absorption of fat-soluble vitamins*: dietary fat allows the body to absorb vitamins A, D, E, and K which all play a role in cancer prevention [9]. Additionally, certain fats, like omega-3 s, are the building blocks for cancer-fighting anti-inflammatory compounds.
- *Avoid chemicals from processed food and supplements*: packaged foods that are processed with added flavors, colors, and preservatives increase the toxin load and reduce nutritional value from the diet through substitution of healthy foods. Under current regulatory oversight, care must be made with the selection of nutritional supplements. Over 79% of adults over 55 consume supplements which can be a source of contaminants if they are not coming from a reputable source [11]. The authors strongly encourage practitioners to become educated in the brands that are high quality or refer to a practitioner that can advise on this for patients.

10.2   Nutritional Support for Acute Cancer

Older adults facing cancer treatment can be supported nutritionally to alleviate side effects from treatment and to provide foundational support that allows for the best quality of life during treatment. The question of which dietary approach is the best during treatment is a common question. When it comes to recommendations on diet, the older adult in particular may have some lifestyle considerations that are paramount to defining the best approach. Depending on the level of support, the side effects from treatment, and the habits of the patient around food, the dietary recommendation needs to be adjusted. Please see Table 10.2 for nutritional support recommendations based on common treatment concerns in oncology patients:

1. First and foremost, adequate caloric intake should be well established.
2. If possible, the quality of the food can be enhanced to include a plant-based, nutrient-dense diet such as the Mediterranean diet.
3. Some patients may want to consider eliminating all refined carbohydrates and sweeteners which is ideal as long as this does not cause weight gain.
4. For well-supported, enthusiastic patients, a ketogenic diet with or without fasting may be appropriate. If this type of therapeutic diet is desired, connecting with a licensed nutritionist or dietician who is trained in the ketogenic diet is strongly advised.

Many older patients exhibit nutrition deficiencies which contribute to and perpetuate chronic disease, including cancer. Further, in patients with a health history of cancer treatment, nutritional deficiencies are common. Common causes for nutritional deficiencies in older adults with cancer include the following [47]:

1. Deterioration in taste, smell, and appetite as a consequence of the tumor, therapy, or both.
2. Altered food preferences, food avoidance, and food aversion.
3. Eating problems (teeth, chewing).
4. Dysphagia, odynophagia, or partial or total gastrointestinal obstruction.
5. Early satiety, nausea, and vomiting.
6. Soreness, xerostomia, sticky saliva, painful throat, and trismus.
7. Oral lesions and esophagitis.
8. Radiotherapy- or chemotherapy-induced mucositis and cute or chronic radiation enteritis during and after radiotherapy.
9. Depression and anxiety.
10. Pain.

Understanding these concerns as they relate to older adults will allow the provider to create a nutrition plan that adequately addresses these concomitant concerns that will improve the nutrition status which will, in turn, reduce the risks of remission.

Table 10.2 Nutritional support for common treatment concerns [17]

Concern	Dietary recommendation	Supplemental considerations and daily dose
Diarrhea	BRAT (bananas, rice, applesauce, toast) diet increases clear liquids Consume foods high in sodium and potassium [18]	Glutamine 10 g [19] short course. Long courses can theoretically worsen outcomes Omega-3 fatty acids 1.5 g [20] Prebiotics 450 billion/g [21]
Anemia	Anti-inflammatory diet [22] Increase foods high in heme iron such as red meat and liver	Vitamin A 10,000 IU (data mixed) [23] Folate 1 mg [24] B12 1–2 mg [25] Riboflavin 1.3 mg M and 1.1 mg F [26] Vitamin C 200 mg [27] Vitamin E 600 mg [28] Vitamin B6 125–250 µg [29] Iron: Dose and form individualized (only if deficiency present) Multivitamin [30]
Malabsorption	May benefit from gluten-free diet [31]	Vitamin D 800 IU [32] Folate 400 µg [33] Vitamin B12 250–1000 µg Iron: Dose and form individualized (only if deficiency present) Trace metals [31]
Nausea/ vomiting	Ginger as tea Honey Bone broth	L-glutamine (as mouth rinse) 10–30 g/day divided doses Zinc L-carnosine (as mouth rinse) 15–30 mg with meals
Mucositis	Mouth rinse: ¾ tsp. salt and 1 tsp. baking soda in 4 cups of water Honey	L-glutamine (as mouth rinse) 10–30 g/day divided doses Zinc L-carnosine (as mouth rinse) 15–30 mg with meals
Cancer cachexia	Increase protein and caloric needs. Nutrient-dense shakes: 1 cup of milk, 1 cup of frozen berries, one serving of protein powder, 1 cup of leafy greens, one ripe banana, and 1–2 tsp. nut butter	L-carnitine 2–3 g twice daily (do not use with taxane chemotherapy) Melatonin 20 mg Vitamin E 200–400 mg twice daily Omega-3 1.5–3 g fatty acids Vitamin D 45–65 ng/mL in serum or 2000 IU daily
Fatigue	Increase protein intake Mediterranean and plant-based diets may reduce fatigue [34]	CoQ10 100–200 mg, Reishi/ Cordyceps 500–1000 three times Ginseng 2000 mg twice Melatonin 20 mg Vitamin D 45–65 ng/mL in serum or 2000 IU daily Probiotics 2 billion CFU [35] Ginger 1.2 g [36]

(continued)

Table 10.2 (continued)

Concern	Dietary recommendation	Supplemental considerations and daily dose
Insomnia	Warm-bath immersion to the mid-thorax [37] Phototherapy [38]	Melatonin 20 mg Iron Valerian extract 400–500 mg [39]
Dysgeusia [40]	Add fruits or mint to water and avoid metal utensils Tart foods before meals may improve flavor perception (lemon) [41]	Cinnamon and mint can help mask metallic taste [41]
Inflammation	Low protein consumption can impair tumorigenesis and inflammation Diets rich in fruit, vegetables, legumes, whole grains, fish, low-fat dairy products, and hazelnut reduce oxidative processes and inflammation [42]	CoQ10 100–200 mg Probiotics 2 billion CFU Omega-3 fatty acids 1.1 g F and 1.6 g M [43] Fiber 25 g F and 38 g M Tryptophan 8–12 g [44] SCFAs [42]
Alopecia	Flavonoids contain potential beneficial features [45]	Selenium 200 µg (deficient patients only) *Before therapy*: It is known blood levels of hemoglobin, iron, thyroid hormones, and vitamin D could be associated to hair loss; ensure sufficient blood levels prior to starting therapy *During therapy*: Topical steroids and vasoconstrictors can help prevent massive damage to hair follicle *After therapy*: NAC and calcitriol [46]

10.3 Nutritional Support for Cancer Survivors

Some older patients with a history of cancer may have long-term repercussions from their treatment that impact their concerns, while others are able to return to the same or better quality of life as they had before diagnosis. For the most part, following the recommendations of preventative care is appropriate. Additional considerations are as follows:

- Intermittent fasting as a lifestyle component which is done daily/weekly to allow for continued cell recycling and DNA repair. There are many different eating patterns with seemingly similar approaches but very different indications. Please see Table 10.3 for distinctions.
- Plant-based diets, possible vegan full-time or as part of quarterly cleansing schedule.
- Low-carbohydrate/near-ketogenic dietary approach that balances the need to restrict carbohydrates with the need to have adequate fiber intake for continued gut microbiome health.
- Strict avoidance of simple sugars and refined, processed grains.

Table 10.3 Distinguishing between eating and fasting patterns

Time-restricted feeding	Intermittent fasting	Intermittent fasting + calorie restricted
Eating pattern in which food intake is restricted to a time window of 8–10 h or less every day. No caloric restriction. Distinct from intermittent fasting because it involves timing to optimally align to biological day [48]	Involves 60–100% energy restriction on fast days with ad lib energy intake on fed days. Many intermittent fasting regimens exist, mostly popular being alternate-day fasting and a 5–2 regimen [48]	Calorie cutting plays no role in geriatric population. We do not recommend this practice, specifically in oncology patients that typically need supplemental nutrition

10.4 Therapeutic Diets

Ketogenic Diet The ketogenic diet is explained in detail in the appendix. The use of the ketogenic diet as part of prevention and disease modification in cancer is indicated in some cases based on recent research [49]. In addressing the prevailing understanding that many cancers feed on glucose exclusive to ketones, a ketogenic diet theoretically works as an anticancer agent by starving out the cancer cells while fueling healthy cells via the ketone pathway. For some older patients that are underweight, thought must be given to the pros and cons of this approach since often patients initially lose weight when initiating the ketogenic diet.

Mediterranean Diet For each type of cancer concern, the Mediterranean diet is indicated based on the anti-inflammatory, high antioxidant, and well-balanced nature of this dietary pattern. Foods of the Mediterranean diet, including fresh fruit, legumes, nuts, vegetables, fish, and extra-virgin olive oil, have protective effects in fighting cell degeneration and proliferation of cancer cells [50]. Additionally, research shows the carotenoids, vitamins C and E, folates, and flavonoids present in many of these foods prevent DNA damage [51]. Finally, omega-3, rich in fish and nuts, helps slow cancer cell proliferation, angiogenesis, inflammation, and metastasis [52].

Tube Feed Alternatives Some patients during the course of treatment may have tube-feeding recommended. The composition of traditional tube feeds does not support the anti-inflammatory approach that is ideal for these patients where they eat solid food. Alternatively, there are products on the market that provide for complete enteral nutrition and use high-quality ingredients and bioavailable nutrients and avoid the use of additives. Many of these are also covered by insurance with a doctor's prescription.

A Note on Brands
These are the brands most commonly used in our practice and those we believe to represent good quality. We do not have any financial relationships with these brands but rather hope to share from our experience what works best.
Brands: Kate Farms, Functional Formularies, CWI Medical, Nestle Nutrition, and Ensure Harvest.

Table 10.4 summarizes recommended supplements for oncology patients, and Table 10.5 highlights recommended micronutrients to support this population.

> **IVC**
>
> High-dose IVC or IV ascorbic acid (IVAA) has been proposed as adjunct chemotherapeutic intervention for most solid tumors. IVAA in pharmacologic doses of over 10 grams and often over 50 grams generate blood and intracellular spikes of H2O2 during and for short period after each infusion. While normal cells are well protected against this effect by catalase enzymes, most solid tumors have minimal catalase activity, thus unable to be protected against sudden spike in H2O2 levels. Detailed analysis of 23 controlled trials of IVC as adjunct for treatment of cancers has concluded the following: "The promising results support the need for randomized placebo-controlled trials such as the ongoing placebo-controlled trials of vitamin C and chemotherapy in prostate cancer" (Nauman et al. 2018).

10.5   Case Study

Phil, a 59-year-old computer programmer, presented to the clinic 2 months after diagnosis of stage IV adenocarcinoma of the colon. The patient had primary tumor of 6.5 cm in the cecum with histological grade of moderately differentiated with extension into the serosal surface and at least six positive regional nodes as well as distant metastasis in the omentum. He had initial partial resection of the tumor with idea to debulk it and start adjuvant chemotherapy and radiation. On presentation, his diet included mostly eating out with high amount of processed foods, carbohydrates, and saturated fat. He was on typical Standard American Diet (SAD); he was also a smoker and was ready to quit. In addition to helping him to quit smoking, we started him on Mediterranean rainbow diet with high amount of colored vegetables, berries, and greens and intermittent fasting for at least 24 h before each round of weekly chemotherapy; eventually he could do it for 48 h before each chemo round. In addition, we added and started a number of supplements to support discovered B12 and Vitamin D deficiency, probiotics and high-dose fish oil to attempt to improve his diarrhea that has been continuous since surgery. Additionally, we started on melatonin and slowly increased the dose to 20 mg at bedtime as well as mix of medicinal mushrooms that contained *Agaricus blazei*, *Cordyceps sinensis*, *Grifola frondosa*, *Ganoderma lucidum*, and *Trametes versicolor*. After he quit smoking, he also chose to try high-dose intravenous vitamin C (IVC) 3 times weekly. At 3 months into this regimen, tumors were no longer detectable, and he had Biocept liquid biopsy negative for circulating tumor cells. After chemo was discontinued, he decreased frequency of IVC to once weekly and added a number of strong antioxidant foods including 1 teaspoon twice daily of matcha green tea. He did not like the taste of turmeric and chose to take curcumin extract in capsules

Table 10.4 Nutritional and botanical support for cancer [53]

	MOA	Dose	Food sources	Side effects and prescriber notes	Used for prevention? Y/N. Dose
Protein powder	Improves nutritional status, glutathione levels, immunity, and inflammatory markers [54]	40 g [54]	Whey, collagen, pea, rice, and hemp	Many popular brands, even those made from organic ingredients, were found to contain high levels of lead, cadmium, arsenic, and BPA [55]	N
Vitamin D	Supports adiposity, immunomodulatory, and inflammatory mediators. Risk reduction is most pronounced in individuals with normal weight [56]	45–65 ng/ mL in serum or 2000 IU daily	Cod liver oil, trout, sockeye salmon, mushrooms, and milk [32]	Treats bone strength, fatigue, and arthralgia	Y, cancer specific. Dose varies
Essential fatty acids	Omega-3 fatty acids, EPA and DHA, can exert antineoplastic activity by inducing apoptotic cell death in cancer cells [57]	1.5–3 g EPA + DHA	Fatty fish, flax–/ hemp–/chia seeds, and nuts	Treat cachexia, depression, and fatigue. Have been shown to decrease the risk of skin melanoma, but not other types of cancers	Y, in recommended RDAs
B complex	Essential for biosynthesis of nucleotides, replication of DNA, supply of methyl groups, and growth and repair of cells [58]	One per day, in the morning	Leafy greens however patients with MTHFR variants may need methylated vitamins as enzyme conversion is inhibited	Treats fatigue and depression	N

(continued)

Table 10.4 (continued)

	MOA	Dose	Food sources	Side effects and prescriber notes	Used for prevention? Y/N. Dose
Magnesium	Results are controversial, but most data points to low mg as a contributing factor to tumorigenesis. Mg deficiency increases oxidative stress, inducing DNA damage and impairing DNA repair mechanisms [59]	300 mg	Green leafy vegetables (spinach), legumes, nuts, seeds, and whole grains [60]	Treats muscle cramping, sleep, and fatigue	N
Probiotics	Can both increase and decrease the production of anti-inflammatory cytokines. Can activate phagocytes to eliminate early-stage cancer cells [61]	Varies	Yogurt, cultured buttermilk, cheese, miso, tempeh, sauerkraut, beer, sour dough, bread, chocolate, kimchi, olives, pickles, and kefir [62]	Immune support	Y, possible. Data inconclusive
Melatonin	Is an antioxidant and modulates melatonin receptors MT1 and MT2, stimulation of apoptosis, regulation of pro-survival signaling and tumor metabolism, inhibition of angiogenesis, metastasis, and induction of epigenetic alteration [63]	20 mg [64]	Egg, salmon, chicken, pork, beef, and lamb [65]	Effective against breast, colon, lung, and brain cancers	Y, at high doses [66]

Table 10.4 (continued)

	MOA	Dose	Food sources	Side effects and prescriber notes	Used for prevention? Y/N. Dose
Medicinal mushrooms	Modify cytokines, direct anticancer agents, and interact with chemotherapeutic agents [67]	1.5–3 g [64]	*Agaricus blazei, Cordyceps sinensis, Grifola frondosa, Ganoderma lucidum,* and *Trametes versicolor* [67]	Effective against breast, colon, lung, and brain cancers	Y, highly variable depending on cancer and mushroom specifics
Curcumin	Modulates growth factors, enzymes, transcription factors, kinase, and inflammatory cytokines, upregulates proapoptotic proteins, and downregulates antiapoptotic proteins [68]	1 g liposomal form [64]	Turmeric (2.5–6% curcumin) and curry [69]	Effective against breast, colon, and non-Hodgkin's lymphoma	Y for multiple cancers, dose similar to therapeutic
EGCG	Potent antiproliferative effects. Induces cell cycle arrest in G1 phase and cell apoptosis [70]	500–1000 mg [64]	Green tea	Effective against breast, colon, prostate, and non-Hodgkin's lymphoma	Y for multiple cancers, 2–4 cups daily of green tea
Resveratrol	Can verse multidrug resistance in cancer cells and, when used in combination with other cancer therapies, can sensitize cancer cells to standard chemotherapeutic agents [71]	Unclear	Grapes, wine, peanuts, and soy [72]	Effective against breast, prostate, and pancreas cancer	Inconclusive, dose not clear

Table 10.5 Micronutrients of primary concern [73]

	MOA	Food sources	RDA for 55+	Side effects/comments for providers
Vitamin D	Maintains skeletal health and can be adversely impacted by cancer and cancer treatments [74]	Liver, egg yolk, saltwater fish, and sun	20 μg (800 IU) [32]	Take with calcium Breast, colorectal, pancreatic, and prostate [32]
Vitamin B12	Methylation, synthesis of nucleic acids, and metabolism of fatty acids and amino acids [75]	Fish, meat, poultry, eggs, and milk	2.4 μg	Chemotherapy and radiation-induced diarrhea can damage mucous membranes and adversely affect micronutrient absorption
Vitamin C	Scavenger, antioxidant, immune modulation, induction of apoptosis, and regulation of cell proliferation and differentiation [73]	Fresh fruit (citrus, cantaloupe, mango, berries)	75 mg F and 90 mg M	IV vitamin C used for cancer treatment, selectively cytotoxic to tumor cells See callout box for IVC
Vitamin E	Is an antioxidant and might block formation of carcinogenic nitrosamines and enhance immune function	Vegetable oils, various oil seeds, and wheat germ	15 mg	Effective in bladder, colon, and prostate cancer
Vitamin A	Scavenger, antioxidant, immune modulation, induction of apoptosis, and regulation of cell proliferation and differentiation [73]	Liver, meat, eggs, dairy products, cod liver oil, carrots, pumpkins, mangoes, and papayas	900 μg M and 700 μg F	Nutritional doses at RDA are essential. High doses of vitamin A are highly controversial and may increase risk of lung cancer in smokers
Selenium	Scavenger, antioxidant, immune modulation, induction of apoptosis, and regulation of cell proliferation and differentiation [73]	Brazil nuts, tuna, halibut, sardines, ham, and shrimp	55 μg	Some RCTs have reported a higher incidence of high-grade prostate cancer and type 2 diabetes in patients with selenium supplementation [76]
Zinc	Is proapoptotic and inhibits cell cycle. Inhibits invasion and migration, preventing malignant advancement to metastasis, and alters bioenergetic/metabolic effects [77]	Meat, nuts, beans, wheat germ, oyster, crab, and lobster	11 μg M and 8 μg F	May cause nausea, vomiting, diarrhea, and metallic taste [78]

Table 10.5 (continued)

	MOA	Food sources	RDA for 55+	Side effects/comments for providers
Magnesium	Required in all steps of cell growth (intracellular signaling, transphosphorylation, transcription, protein synthesis) [59]	Almonds, spinach, cashews, and peanuts	420 mg M and 320 mg F	Complex relationship. Also has been shown to have pro-tumor effects such as facilitating tumor implantation at metastatic sites. Magnesium homeostasis is disrupted in many oncology patients [59]
Calcium	Binds to bile acids and fatty acids in the GI tract, forming calcium soaps, reducing ability of acids and their metabolites to damage cells in colon and stimulate proliferation to repair damage [79, 80]	Yogurt, orange juice, cheese, sardines, and milk	1000–1200 mg	Effective in colorectal
L-carnitine	Improves fatigue [81]	Steak, ground beef, and milk [82]	500–2000 mg [83]	Chemotherapy patients often develop L-carnitine deficiency [84]
L-cysteine	Critical for cell survival and growth. Supports protein folding and redox balance	Broccoli, Brussels sprouts, egg yolks, garlic, oats, onions, poultry, red bell peppers, wheat germ, and yeast [85]	500 mg	Toxicity is rare
L-glutathione	Is antioxidant, maintains redox state, and modulates immune response [86]	Cruciferous vegetables, garlic, shallots, and onions [87]	250 mg [88]	Some data shows elevated levels of glutathione in tumor cells are able to protect against therapies [86]
Omega-3 fatty acids	Induce cell cycle arrest an apoptosis by activating protein phosphatases, leading to dephosphorylation of pRB [89]	Fatty fish, flax-/hemp-/chia seeds, and nuts	1.6 g M and 1.1 g F	Adverse effects are rare

(continued)

Table 10.5 (continued)

	MOA	Food sources	RDA for 55+	Side effects/comments for providers
Vitamin B1	Of importance due to chronic malnutrition in many cancer patients [90]	Yeast, meat, and legumes	1.2 g M and 1.1 g F [91]	Interactions with furosemide and fluorouracil [91]
Vitamin K2	Supports cell cycle arrest, cell differentiation, apoptosis, autophagy, and invasion [92]	Natto, collards, turnip, spinach, kale, and broccoli	120 μg M and 90 μg F	Anemia and jaundice [93]

at dose of 1 gm twice daily. While it is hard to say if our support helped this patient to achieve his goal of long-term remission, his oncologist did tell us that he does not usually see this type of improvement in most of his patients.

References

1. Ravasco P. Nutrition in cancer patients. J Clin Med. 2019;8(8):1211.
2. Cancer.net Editorial Board. Aging and Cancer [Internet]. Cancer.net. 2019 [cited 2021 Feb 17]. Available from: https://www.cancer.net/navigating-cancer-care/older-adults/aging-and-cancer#:~:text=Age%20is%20the%20greatest%20risk,are%2060%25%20of%20cancer%20survivors.
3. Berger NA, Savvides P, Koroukian SM, Kahana EF, Deimling GT, Rose JH, et al. Cancer in the elderly. Trans Am Clin Climatol Assoc. 2006;117:147–55; discussion 155.
4. Blevins Primeau A. Cancer Recurrence Statistics [Internet]. Cancer Therapy Advisor. 2018 [cited 2021 Feb 19]. Available from: https://www.cancertherapyadvisor.com/home/tools/fact-sheets/cancer-recurrence-statistics/.
5. NIH. Cancer Types [Internet]. NIH National Cancer institute. 2020 [cited 2021 Feb 17]. Available from: https://www.cancer.gov/types.
6. Siegel RL, Miller KD, Jemal A. Cancer statistics, 2019. CA Cancer J Clin. 2019;69(1):7–34.
7. ACS. More than 4 in 10 Cancers and Cancer Deaths Linked to Modifiable Risk Factors [Internet]. American Cancer Society. 2017 [cited 2021 Feb 21]. Available from: https://www.cancer.org/latest-news/more-than-4-in-10-cancers-and-cancer-deaths-linked-to-modifiable-risk-factors.html.
8. Caccialanza R, Cereda E, De Lorenzo F, Farina G, Pedrazzoli P, AIOM-SINPE-FAVO Working Group. To fast, or not to fast before chemotherapy, that is the question. BMC Cancer. 2018;18(1):337.
9. Saha SK, Lee SB, Won J, Choi HY, Kim K, Yang G-M, et al. Correlation between oxidative stress, nutrition, and cancer initiation. Int J Mol Sci. 2017;18(7):1544.
10. Ríos-Covián D, Ruas-Madiedo P, Margolles A, Gueimonde M, de Los Reyes-Gavilán CG, Salazar N. Intestinal short chain fatty acids and their link with diet and human health. Front Microbiol. 2016;7:185.
11. CRN. 2019 CRN Consumer Survey on Dietary Supplements: Consumer Intelligence to Enhance Business Outcomes [Internet]. CRN The Science Behind the Supplements. 2019 [cited 2021 Feb 21]. Available from: https://www.crnusa.org/resources/2019-crn-consumer-survey-dietary-supplements-consumer-intelligence-enhance-business.

12. Ranjan A, Ramachandran S, Gupta N, Kaushik I, Wright S, Srivastava S, et al. Role of phyto-chemicals in cancer prevention. Int J Mol Sci. 2019;20(21):4981.
13. Tortorella SM, Royce SG, Licciardi PV, Karagiannis TC. Dietary sulforaphane in cancer che-moprevention: the role of epigenetic regulation and HDAC inhibition. Antioxid Redox Signal. 2015;22(16):1382–424.
14. Gong X, Smith JR, Swanson HM, Rubin LP. Carotenoid lutein selectively inhibits breast can-cer cell growth and potentiates the effect of chemotherapeutic agents through ROS-mediated mechanisms. Molecules. 2018;23(4):905.
15. Higdon JV, Delage B, Williams DE, Dashwood RH. Cruciferous vegetables and human cancer risk: epidemiologic evidence and mechanistic basis. Pharmacol Res. 2007;55(3):224–36.
16. Křížová L, Dadáková K, Kašparovská J, Kašparovský T. Isoflavones. Mol. 2019;24(6)
17. Kogan M, Weil A. Integrative oncology. Integrative geriatric medicine. New York: Oxford University Press; 2018. p. 436.
18. PDQ Supportive and Palliative Care Editorial Board. Nutrition in cancer care (PDQ®): health professional version. PDQ cancer information summaries. Bethesda (MD): National Cancer Institute (US); 2002.
19. Lopez-Vaquero D, Gutierrez-Bayard L, Rodriguez-Ruiz J-A, Saldaña-Valderas M, Infante-Cossio P. Double-blind randomized study of oral glutamine on the management of radio/chemotherapy-induced mucositis and dermatitis in head and neck cancer. Mol Clin Oncol. 2017;6(6):931–6.
20. Colomer R, Moreno-Nogueira JM, García-Luna PP, García-Peris P, García-de-Lorenzo A, Zarazaga A, et al. N-3 fatty acids, cancer and cachexia: a systematic review of the literature. Br J Nutr. 2007;97(5):823–31.
21. Delia P, Sansotta G, Donato V, Frosina P, Messina G, De Renzis C, et al. Use of probiotics for prevention of radiation-induced diarrhea. World J Gastroenterol. 2007;13(6):912–5.
22. Bianchi VE. Role of nutrition on anemia in elderly. Clin Nutr ESPEN. 2016;11:e1–11.
23. Pereira RC, Ferreira LOC, Diniz A, da Silva Diniz A, Batista Filho M, Figueirôa JN. Efficacy of iron supplementation with or without vitamin A for anemia control. Cad Saude Publica. 2007;23(6):1415–21.
24. Drugs.com. Folic Acid Dosage [Internet]. Drugs.com. 2020 [cited 2021 Mar 18]. Available from: https://www.drugs.com/dosage/folic-acid.html.
25. Langan RC, Goodbred AJ. Vitamin B12 deficiency: recognition and management. Am Fam Physician. 2017;96(6):384–9.
26. NIH. Riboflavin [Internet]. NIH Office of Dietary Supplements. 2021 [cited 2021 Mar 18]. Available from: https://ods.od.nih.gov/factsheets/Riboflavin-HealthProfessional/.
27. Li N, Zhao G, Wu W, Zhang M, Liu W, Chen Q, et al. The efficacy and safety of vitamin C for iron supplementation in adult patients with iron deficiency anemia: a randomized clinical trial. JAMA Netw Open. 2020;3(11):e2023644.
28. Ono K. Effects of large dose vitamin E supplementation on anemia in hemodialysis patients. Nephron. 1985;40(4):440–5.
29. Mikkelsen K, Prakash MD, Kuol N, Nurgali K, Stojanovska L, Apostolopoulos V. Anti-tumor effects of Vitamin B2, B6 and B9 in promonocytic lymphoma cells. Int J Mol Sci. 2019;1:20(15).
30. Fishman SM, Christian P, West KP. The role of vitamins in the prevention and control of anae-mia. Public Health Nutr. 2000;3(2):125–50.
31. Holt PR. Intestinal malabsorption in the elderly. Dig Dis. 2007;25(2):144–50.
32. NIH. Vitamin D [Internet]. NIH National Institutes of Health Office of Dietary Suppolements. 2020 [cited 2020 Dec 31]. Available from: https://ods.od.nih.gov/factsheets/VitaminD-HealthProfessional/
33. NIH. Folate [Internet]. National Institutes of Health Office of Dietary Supplements. 2020 [cited 2020 Dec 30]. Available from: https://ods.od.n ih.gov/factsheets/Folate-HealthProfessional/.
34. Inglis JE, Lin P-J, Kerns SL, Kleckner IR, Kleckner AS, Castillo DA, et al. Nutritional interven-tions for treating cancer-related fatigue: a qualitative review. Nutr Cancer. 2019;71(1):21–40.

35. Lee J-Y, Chu S-H, Jeon JY, Lee M-K, Park J-H, Lee D-C, et al. Effects of 12 weeks of probiotic supplementation on quality of life in colorectal cancer survivors: a double-blind, randomized, placebo-controlled trial. Dig Liver Dis. 2014 Dec;46(12):1126–32.
36. Marx W, McCarthy AL, Ried K, McKavanagh D, Vitetta L, Sali A, et al. The effect of a standardized ginger extract on chemotherapy-induced nausea-related quality of life in patients undergoing moderately or highly emetogenic chemotherapy: a double blind, randomized. Placebo Controlled Trial Nutrients. 2017;9:867.
37. Liao W-C. Effects of passive body heating on body temperature and sleep regulation in the elderly: a systematic review. Int J Nurs Stud. 2002;39(8):803–10.
38. PCRM. Insomnia [Internet]. PCRM's Nutrition Guide for Clinicians. 2021 [cited 2021 Mar 7]. Available from: https://nutritionguide.pcrm.org/nutritionguide/view/Nutrition_Guide_for_Clinicians/1342071/all/Insomnia.
39. Culpepper L, Wingertzahn MA. Over-the-counter agents for the treatment of occasional disturbed sleep or transient insomnia: a systematic review of efficacy and safety. Prim Care Companion CNS Disord. 2015;17(6)
40. Kalaskar AR. Management of chemotherapy induced dysgeusia: an important step towards nutritional rehabilitation. Int J Phys Med Rehabil. 2014;02(03).
41. BCA Cancer Agency. Nutritional guidelines for symptom management: taste changes [Internet]. BC Cancer Agency Care and Research. 2005 [cited 2021 Mar 7]. Available from: http://www.bccancer.bc.ca/nutrition-site/Documents/Symptom%20management%20guidelines/TasteChanges.pdf.
42. Soldati L, Di Renzo L, Jirillo E, Ascierto PA, Marincola FM, De Lorenzo A. The influence of diet on anti-cancer immune responsiveness. J Transl Med. 2018;16(1):75.
43. NIH. Omega-3 Fatty Acids [Internet]. NIH Office of Dietary Supplements. 2020 [cited 2021 Mar 4]. Available from: https://ods.od.nih.gov/factsheets/Omega3FattyAcids-HealthProfessional/.
44. IBM Watson Health. Tryptophan [Internet]. Mayo Clinic. 2021 [cited 2021 Mar 20]. Available from: https://www.mayoclinic.org/drugs-supplements/tryptophan-oral-route/proper-use/drg-20064453.
45. Bassino E, Gasparri F, Munaron L. Protective role of nutritional plants containing flavonoids in hair follicle disruption: a review. Int J Mol Sci. 2020;21(2):523.
46. Rossi A, Fortuna MC, Caro G, Pranteda G, Garelli V, Pompili U, et al. Chemotherapy-induced alopecia management: clinical experience and practical advice. J Cosmet Dermatol. 2017;16(4):537–41.
47. Ravasco P. Nutritional approaches in cancer: relevance of individualized counseling and supplementation. Nutrition. 2015;31(4):603–4.
48. Rynders CA, Thomas EA, Zaman A, Pan Z, Catenacci VA, Melanson EL. Effectiveness of intermittent fasting and time-restricted feeding compared to continuous energy restriction for weight loss. Nutrients. 2019;11(10):2442.
49. Tan-Shalaby J. Ketogenic diets and cancer: emerging evidence. Fed Pract. 2017 Feb;34(Suppl 1):37S–42S.
50. Mentella MC, Scaldaferri F, Ricci C, Gasbarrini A, Miggiano GAD. Cancer and mediterranean diet: a review. Nutrients. 2019;2:11(9).
51. Pitsavos C, Panagiotakos DB, Tzima N, Chrysohoou C, Economou M, Zampelas A, et al. Adherence to the Mediterranean diet is associated with total antioxidant capacity in healthy adults: the ATTICA study. Am J Clin Nutr. 2005;82(3):694–9.
52. Castelló A, Boldo E, Pérez-Gómez B, Lope V, Altzibar JM, Martín V, et al. Adherence to the Western, prudent and Mediterranean dietary patterns and breast cancer risk: MCC-Spain study. Maturitas. 2017;103:8–15.
53. Kogan M, Weil A. Integrative Oncology. Integrative Geriatric Medicine. New York: Oxford University Press; 2018. p. 231.
54. Bumrungpert A, Pavadhgul P, Nunthanawanich P, Sirikanchanarod A, Adulbhan A. Whey protein supplementation improves nutritional status, glutathione levels, and immune function in cancer patients: a randomized. Double-Blind Controlled Trial J Med Food. 2018;21(6):612–6.

55. Corleone J. Recommended protein powder supplements for cancer patients [Internet]. Livestrong. 2019 [cited 2021 Mar 5]. Available from: https://www.livestrong.com/article/544436-recommended-protein-powder-supplements-for-cancer-patients/.

56. Chandler PD, Chen WY, Ajala ON, Hazra A, Cook N, Bubes V, et al. Effect of vitamin D3 supplements on development of advanced cancer: a secondary analysis of the VITAL randomized clinical trial. JAMA Netw Open. 2020;3(11):e2025850.

57. D'Eliseo D, Velotti F. Omega-3 fatty acids and cancer cell cytotoxicity: implications for multi-targeted cancer therapy. J Clin Med. 2016;26:5(2).

58. Zhang S-L, Chen T-S, Ma C-Y, Meng Y-B, Zhang Y-F, Chen Y-W, et al. Effect of vitamin B supplementation on cancer incidence, death due to cancer, and total mortality: a PRISMA-compliant cumulative meta-analysis of randomized controlled trials. Medicine (Baltimore). 2016;95(31):e3485.

59. Leidi M, Wolf F, Maier JAM. Magnesium and cancer: more questions than answers. In: Vink R, Nechifor M, editors. Magnesium in the central nervous system. Adelaide: University of Adelaide Press; 2011.

60. NIH. Magnesium [Internet]. National Institutes of Health Office of Dietary Supplements. 2020 [cited 2020 Dec 30]. Available from: https://ods.od.nih.gov/factsheets/Magnesium-HealthProfessional/#:~:text=Magnesium%20is%20widely%20distributed%20in,cereals%20and%20other%20fortified%20foods.

61. Górska A, Przystupski D, Niemczura MJ, Kulbacka J. Probiotic bacteria: a promising tool in cancer prevention and therapy. Curr Microbiol. 2019;76(8):939–49.

62. Syngai GG, Gopi R, Bharali R, Dey S, Lakshmanan GMA, Ahmed G. Probiotics – the versatile functional food ingredients. J Food Sci Technol. 2016;53(2):921–33.

63. Li Y, Li S, Zhou Y, Meng X, Zhang J-J, Xu D-P, et al. Melatonin for the prevention and treatment of cancer. Oncotarget. 2017;8(24):39896–921.

64. Kogan M, Weil A. Integrative Oncology. Integrative Geriatric Medicine. New York: Oxford University Press; 2018. p. 433.

65. Meng X, Li Y, Li S, Zhou Y, Gan R-Y, Xu D-P, et al. Dietary sources and bioactivities of melatonin. Nutrients. 2017;9(4):367.

66. Kubatka P, Zubor P, Busselberg D, Kwon TK, Adamek M, Petrovic D, et al. Melatonin and breast cancer: evidences from preclinical and human studies. Crit Rev Oncol Hematol. 2018;122:133–43.

67. Guggenheim AG, Wright KM, Zwickey HL. Immune modulation from five major mushrooms: application to integrative oncology. Integr Med (Encinitas). 2014;13(1):32–44.

68. Giordano A, Tommonaro G. Curcumin and cancer. Nutrients. 2019;11(10):2376.

69. Lee W-H, Loo C-Y, Bebawy M, Luk F, Mason RS, Rohanizadeh R. Curcumin and its derivatives: their application in neuropharmacology and neuroscience in the 21st century. Curr Neuropharmacol. 2013;11(4):338–78.

70. Du G-J, Zhang Z, Wen X-D, Yu C, Calway T, Yuan C-S, et al. Epigallocatechin Gallate (EGCG) is the most effective cancer chemopreventive polyphenol in green tea. Nutrients. 2012;4(11):1679–91.

71. Ko J-H, Sethi G, Um J-Y, Shanmugam MK, Arfuso F, Kumar AP, et al. The role of resveratrol in cancer therapy. Int J Mol Sci. 2017;18(12):2589.

72. Chachay VS, Kirkpatrick CMJ, Hickman IJ, Ferguson M, Prins JB, Martin JH. Resveratrol--pills to replace a healthy diet? Br J Clin Pharmacol. 2011;72(1):27–38.

73. Gröber U. Antioxidants and other micronutrients in complementary oncology. Breast Care (Basel). 2009;4(1):13–20.

74. Kennel KA, Drake MT. Vitamin D in the cancer patient. Curr Opin Support Palliat Care. 2013;7(3):272–7.

75. MSKCC. Vitamin B12 [Internet]. Memorial Sloan Kettering Cancer Cener. 2019 [cited 2021 Mar 15]. Available from: https://www.mskcc.org/cancer-care/integrative-medicine/herbs/vitamin-b12#msk_professional.

76. Vinceti M, Filippini T, Del Giovane C, Dennert G, Zwahlen M, Brinkman M, et al. Selenium for preventing cancer. Cochrane Database Syst Rev. 2018;1:CD005195.
77. Costello LC, Franklin RB. Cytotoxic/tumor suppressor role of zinc for the treatment of cancer: an enigma and an opportunity. Expert Rev Anticancer Ther. 2012;12(1):121–8.
78. NIH. Zinc [Internet]. NIH Office of Dietary Supplements. 2020 [cited 2021 Feb 5]. Available from: https://ods.od.nih.gov/factsheets/Zinc-HealthProfessional/.
79. Milner JA, McDonald SS, Anderson DE, Greenwald P. Molecular targets for nutrients involved with cancer prevention. Nutr Cancer. 2001;41(1–2):1–16.
80. Lamprecht SA, Lipkin M. Cellular mechanisms of calcium and vitamin D in the inhibition of colorectal carcinogenesis. Ann N Y Acad Sci. 2001;952:73–87.
81. Cruciani RA, Dvorkin E, Homel P, Culliney B, Malamud S, Lapin J, et al. L-carnitine supplementation in patients with advanced cancer and carnitine deficiency: a double-blind, placebo-controlled study. J Pain Symptom Manag. 2009;37(4):622–31.
82. NIH. Carnitine [Internet]. NIH National Institutes of Health Office of Dietary Supplements. 2017 [cited 2021 Jan 2]. Available from: https://ods.od.nih.gov/factsheets/Carnitine-HealthProfessional/.
83. Mawer R. L-carnitine: benefits, side effects, sources and dosage [Internet]. Healthline. 2018 [cited 2021 Mar 7]. Available from: https://www.healthline.com/nutrition/l-carnitine.
84. Matsui H, Einama T, Shichi S, Kanazawa R, Shibuya K, Suzuki T, et al. L-carnitine supplementation reduces the general fatigue of cancer patients during chemotherapy. Mol Clin Oncol. 2018;8(3):413–6.
85. Restorative Medicine. Cysteine [Internet]. Restorative Medicine. 2020 [cited 2021 Mar 9]. Available from: https://restorativemedicine.org/library/monographs/cysteine/.
86. Balendiran GK, Dabur R, Fraser D. The role of glutathione in cancer. Cell Biochem Funct. 2004;22(6):343–52.
87. Berkheiser K. 10 Natural ways to increase your glutathione levels [Internet]. Healthline. 2018 [cited 2021 Mar 15]. Available from: https://www.healthline.com/nutrition/how-to-increase-glutathione.
88. Weschawalit S, Thongthip S, Phutrakool P, Asawanonda P. Glutathione and its antiaging and antimelanogenic effects. Clin Cosmet Investig Dermatol. 2017;10:147–53.
89. Siddiqui RA, Shaikh SR, Sech LA, Yount HR, Stillwell W, Zaloga GP. Omega 3-fatty acids: health benefits and cellular mechanisms of action. Mini Rev Med Chem. 2004;4(8):859–71.
90. Kuo S-H, Debnam JM, Fuller GN, de Groot J. Wernicke's encephalopathy: an underrecognized and reversible cause of confusional state in cancer patients. Oncology. 2009;76(1):10–8.
91. NIH. Thiamin [Internet]. National Institues of Health Office of Dietary Supplements. 2020 [cited 2021 Jan 16]. Available from: https://ods.od.nih.gov/factsheets/Thiamin-HealthProfessional/#:~:text=Food%20sources%20of%20thiamin%20include,major%20source%20of%20the%20vitamin.
92. Xv F, Chen J, Duan L, Li S. Research progress on the anticancer effects of vitamin K2. Oncol Lett. 2018;15(6):8926–34.
93. Johnson LE. Vitamin K excess [Internet]. Merck Manual. 2020 [cited 2021 Mar 15]. Available from: https://www.merckmanuals.com/home/disorders-of-nutrition/vitamins/vitamin-k-excess.

Appendix A: Therapeutic Diets

Food is a powerful source of information for our body. The food choices that we make on a daily basis dominant the epigenetic expression of our genome which dictates which genes are expressed, the cofactors available to support biochemical reactions, and the composition of our gut microbiome based on the food sources made available to these synergistic communities. Food choices matter in big and small ways as a foundation for health. Beyond the population-based recommendations for a nutrient-dense diet composed of colorful fruits and vegetables, food choices can be used as the foundation of a therapeutic approach to disease modification. More extreme food plans (ketogenic or elimination diet) should be reserved for those patients that have not responded to basic improvements in the diet such as an anti-inflammatory diet. Please see Table A.1 for a summary of well-studied therapeutic diets.

Mediterranean/Anti-inflammatory

The most-studied diet for health risk reduction, the Mediterranean diet, a type of anti-inflammatory diet, has innumerable benefits, some of which are highlighted below.

Benefits are as follows:

- One study that showed a 30 % lower risk of heart attack, stroke, and death from cardiovascular events [2].
- Several studies point to reduced risk of cognitive decline and Alzheimer's (Morris MC, Tangney CC, Wang Y, et al [3].
- Studies also show a reduction in risk for certain cancers such as the breast, stomach, liver, and prostate [4].

J. Wendt et al., *Integrative Geriatric Nutrition*,
https://doi.org/10.1007/978-3-030-81758-9

Table A.1 Therapeutic diets at a glance

Diet	Target population	Inclusions	Exclusions	Resources
Mediterranean/anti-inflammatory	Hypertension Overweight/obesity Metabolic syndrome Cognitive risk	Whole foods Healthy fats, lean protein sources (plant and/or animal) Organic and non-GMO sources preferred 8+ servings of fruits and vegetables daily Legumes Dairy and alternatives Nuts/seeds and starchy and non-starchy vegetables High-quality dark chocolate 70 %	Processed, refined foods Fried foods	Andrew Weil Center for Integrative Medicine
Low FODMAP	Irritable bowel syndrome Small intestinal bacterial overgrowth	Pure protein foods Pure fats and oils Certain types of carbohydrates that are not fermentable	Foods high in fermentable carbohydrates (e.g., apples, watermelon, beans, milk, wheat, rye, onion, honey, sugar alcohols)	Monash University
Anti-candida	Chronic fatigue Yeast overgrowth Thrush Athlete's foot Nail fungus	Meat, chicken, nuts, non-starchy vegetables, berries, and healthy fats	Refined sugar of any kind, grains, starches, beans/pulses, high-sugar fruit, and fermented foods	www.thecandidadiet.com
Ketogenic	Neuroinflammation Diabetes Obesity PCOS Cancer Epilepsy	High-fat foods such as avocado, full-fat dairy, macadamia nuts, coconut, animal protein, and eggs	Starchy vegetables limited, grains, refined sugar, corn, and beans/lentils	May need to support with additional electrolytes Blood sugar target: 55–65 mg/dL Blood ketone target: 3–5 mM (pathologic is 15–20 mM)

Intermittent fasting*	Neuroinflammation Blood sugar dysregulation Cardiovascular disease Weight loss resistance	Coconut oil, MCT oil, butter-oil coffee, and any pure fat Restricting eating to a shortened window such as 11 AM to 7 PM	All Fluids encouraged	*The Fast Diet*, *The 5:2 Diet Book*, and *The Obesity Code*
Autoimmune paleo (AIP)	Autoimmune diseases	Meat, fish, poultry, vegetables (except nightshades), fruits, bone broth, fermented foods, animal fat, coconut oil, red palm oil, and olive oil	Grains, dairy, legumes/pulses, eggs, nuts/seeds, and nightshades (tomato, potato, pepper, eggplant, paprika)	After the 4-week elimination period and symptoms improve, systematic reintroduction to identify trigger foods. Likely not all categories need to continue to be removed from diet
Detox food plan	Fatigue Metal toxicity	Cruciferous vegetables, nuts/seeds, leafy greens, eggs, beets, berries, animal- and plant-based protein, gluten-free grains, herbs (cilantro, parsley, chives), fluids, and green tea	Dairy, gluten, processed foods, refined sugar, and caffeine	IFM https://www.ifm.org/news-insights/detox-food-plan/
Elimination diet	Mental fog, headache, endocrine disruption, GI disturbance, and autoimmune	Lean meats, rice, soy, nut milks, legumes, vegetables, whole grains, nuts/seeds, and fresh fruits	Absolute: gluten, dairy, eggs, soy, and corn Optional: nightshades, citrus fruits, nuts and seeds, and grains	Gold standard for assessing food sensitivities
Vegan	High blood pressure, obesity, diabetes, and cardiovascular disease [1]	Whole grains, legumes, fruits, vegetables, nuts, and seeds	Animal protein (beef, poultry, fish, dairy, eggs)	www.pcrm.org

Challenges are as follows:

- Increasing prices of some food items of Mediterranean diet [5].
- Not all patients resonate with approach based on their own heritage.

The Mediterranean diet (as shown in Fig. A.1) is also about the Mediterranean lifestyle which encourages non-exercise movement as part of daily living such as walking to the store and gardening as well as focus on family and well-being. Please see Fig. A.2 for a sample Mediterranean diet food plan.

With new information and research come updates to our foundational teaching. At the time of writing this book, Andrew Weil, an integrative medicine practitioner, recommends switching expeller-pressed canola and grape-seed oil with avocado and algae oils.

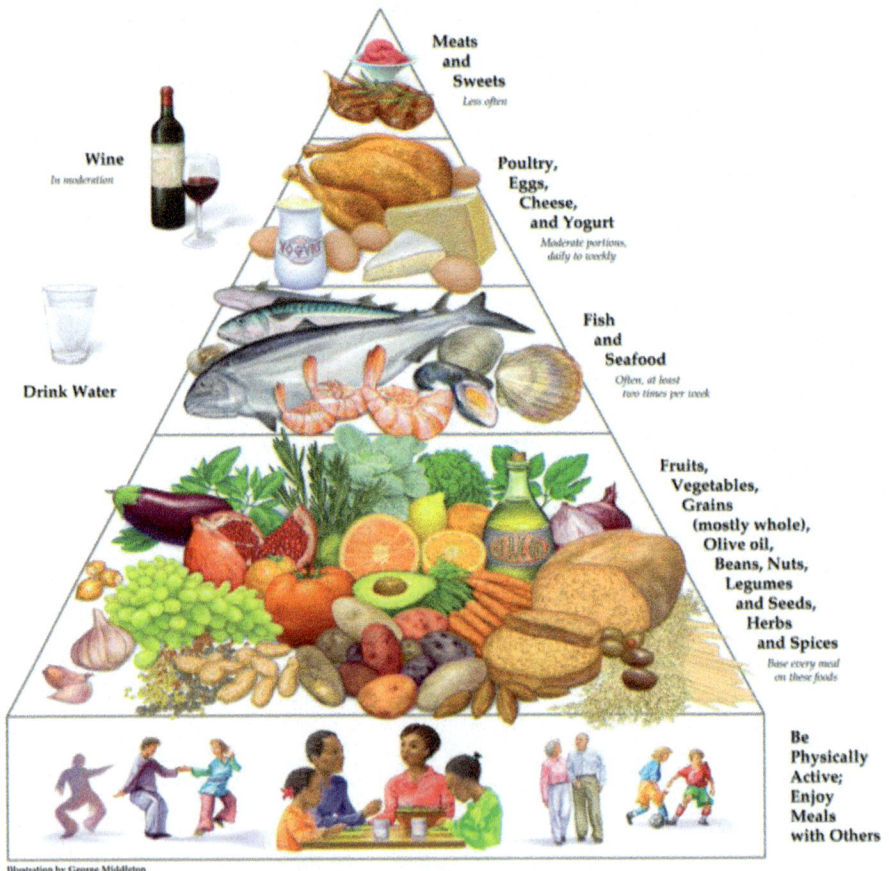

© 2009 Oldways Preservation and Exchange Trust • www.oldwayspt.org

Fig. A.1 Mediterranean diet [6]

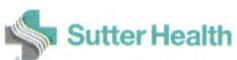

Mediterranean Diet Made Easy

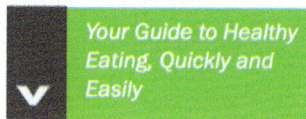

Your Guide to Healthy Eating, Quickly and Easily

Studies show a Mediterranean diet is one of your best defenses against heart disease and other health problems. This easy guide, created by Erika Deshmukh, MS, RD, and Deb Lucus, M.S., R.D., CDE, with Sutter Medical Foundation, gives you simple building blocks for incorporating Mediterranean staples into your everyday life.

A 3-day sample menu plan to fit your busy schedule:

DAY 1

Breakfast:	Oatmeal with fresh berries
Snack:	6 oz Greek yogurt, strawberries and a handful of almonds
Lunch:	Turkey, avocado, tomato, skim-mozzarella and arugula sandwich on whole grain pita
Snack:	Carrots and broccolini with 2 Tbsp hummus
Dinner:	Grilled salmon with fresh herbs, sautéed spinach in light olive oil and tabbouleh salad (bulgur wheat, parsley salad)
Snack:	Watermelon cubes

DAY 2

Breakfast:	Greek yogurt with fresh berries (tsp of sweetener optional)
Snack:	Apple, persimmon or melon cubes
Lunch:	White fish grilled with rosemary and olive oil with quinoa and baked kale
Snack:	Handful cashews and ¼ cup grapes
Dinner:	Chicken kabobs and sautéed spinach with side salad in balsamic vinaigrette
Snack:	Strawberries with light cream and balsamic

DAY 3

Breakfast:	Whole grain toast, 1 oz turkey, ¼ avocado
Snack:	1 medium orange or apple
Lunch:	Pasta with marinara and vegetables with Greek salad
Snack:	1 oz peanuts and string cheese (skim-milk)
Dinner:	Chickpea soup, couscous, grilled asparagus, and arugula salad
Snack:	3 crackers and one glass (5 oz) of red wine

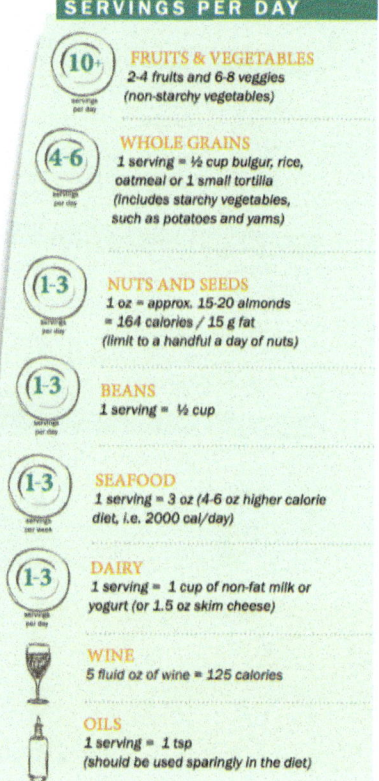

SERVINGS PER DAY

(10+) servings per day
FRUITS & VEGETABLES
2-4 fruits and 6-8 veggies (non-starchy vegetables)

(4-6) servings per day
WHOLE GRAINS
1 serving = ½ cup bulgur, rice, oatmeal or 1 small tortilla (includes starchy vegetables, such as potatoes and yams)

(1-3) servings per day
NUTS AND SEEDS
1 oz = approx. 15-20 almonds = 164 calories / 15 g fat (limit to a handful a day of nuts)

(1-3) servings per day
BEANS
1 serving = ½ cup

(1-3) servings per week
SEAFOOD
1 serving = 3 oz (4-6 oz higher calorie diet, i.e. 2000 cal/day)

(1-3) servings per day
DAIRY
1 serving = 1 cup of non-fat milk or yogurt (or 1.5 oz skim cheese)

WINE
5 fluid oz of wine = 125 calories

OILS
1 serving = 1 tsp (should be used sparingly in the diet)

Fig. A.2 Mediterranean diet food plan [40]

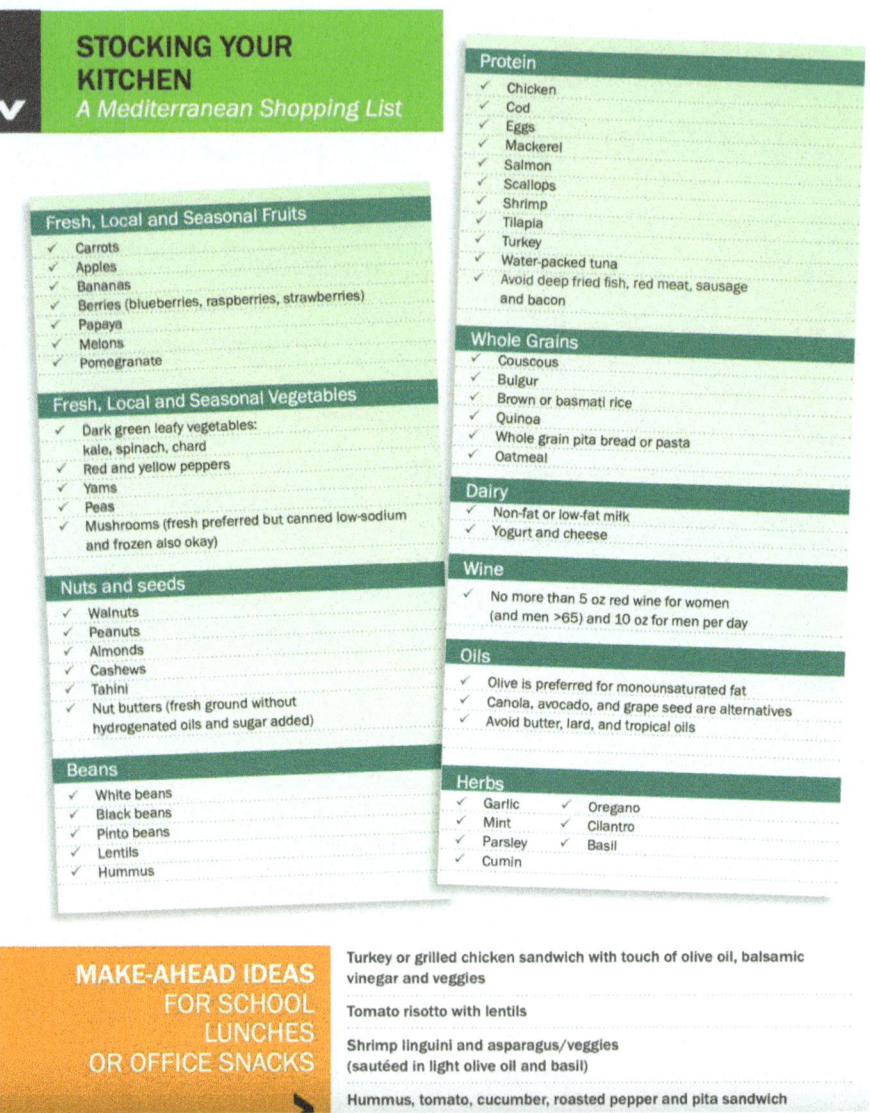

STOCKING YOUR KITCHEN
A Mediterranean Shopping List

Fresh, Local and Seasonal Fruits
- ✓ Carrots
- ✓ Apples
- ✓ Bananas
- ✓ Berries (blueberries, raspberries, strawberries)
- ✓ Papaya
- ✓ Melons
- ✓ Pomegranate

Fresh, Local and Seasonal Vegetables
- ✓ Dark green leafy vegetables: kale, spinach, chard
- ✓ Red and yellow peppers
- ✓ Yams
- ✓ Peas
- ✓ Mushrooms (fresh preferred but canned low-sodium and frozen also okay)

Nuts and seeds
- ✓ Walnuts
- ✓ Peanuts
- ✓ Almonds
- ✓ Cashews
- ✓ Tahini
- ✓ Nut butters (fresh ground without hydrogenated oils and sugar added)

Beans
- ✓ White beans
- ✓ Black beans
- ✓ Pinto beans
- ✓ Lentils
- ✓ Hummus

Protein
- ✓ Chicken
- ✓ Cod
- ✓ Eggs
- ✓ Mackerel
- ✓ Salmon
- ✓ Scallops
- ✓ Shrimp
- ✓ Tilapia
- ✓ Turkey
- ✓ Water-packed tuna
- ✓ Avoid deep fried fish, red meat, sausage and bacon

Whole Grains
- ✓ Couscous
- ✓ Bulgur
- ✓ Brown or basmati rice
- ✓ Quinoa
- ✓ Whole grain pita bread or pasta
- ✓ Oatmeal

Dairy
- ✓ Non-fat or low-fat milk
- ✓ Yogurt and cheese

Wine
- ✓ No more than 5 oz red wine for women (and men >65) and 10 oz for men per day

Oils
- ✓ Olive is preferred for monounsaturated fat
- ✓ Canola, avocado, and grape seed are alternatives
- ✓ Avoid butter, lard, and tropical oils

Herbs
- ✓ Garlic   ✓ Oregano
- ✓ Mint   ✓ Cilantro
- ✓ Parsley   ✓ Basil
- ✓ Cumin

MAKE-AHEAD IDEAS FOR SCHOOL LUNCHES OR OFFICE SNACKS

Turkey or grilled chicken sandwich with touch of olive oil, balsamic vinegar and veggies

Tomato risotto with lentils

Shrimp linguini and asparagus/veggies (sautéed in light olive oil and basil)

Hummus, tomato, cucumber, roasted pepper and pita sandwich

Fig. A.2 (continued)

Low-FODMAP Diet

FODMAPs, or fermentable oligosaccharides, disaccharides, monosaccharides, and polyols, are short-chain carbohydrates that can cause IBS-like symptoms in patients that have bacterial overgrowth in their small intestines (SIBO, small intestinal bacterial overgrowth). Monash University in Australia hosts the lab which tests the

FODMAP content of different foods and is the ultimate source for knowing which foods to avoid when on a low-FODMAP diet.

For comprehensive guidance on food selection and the FODMAP diet, please see www.monashfodmap.com/about-fodmap-and-ibs/high-and-low-fodmap-foods. Please see Fig. A.3 for a sample low-FODMAP plan.

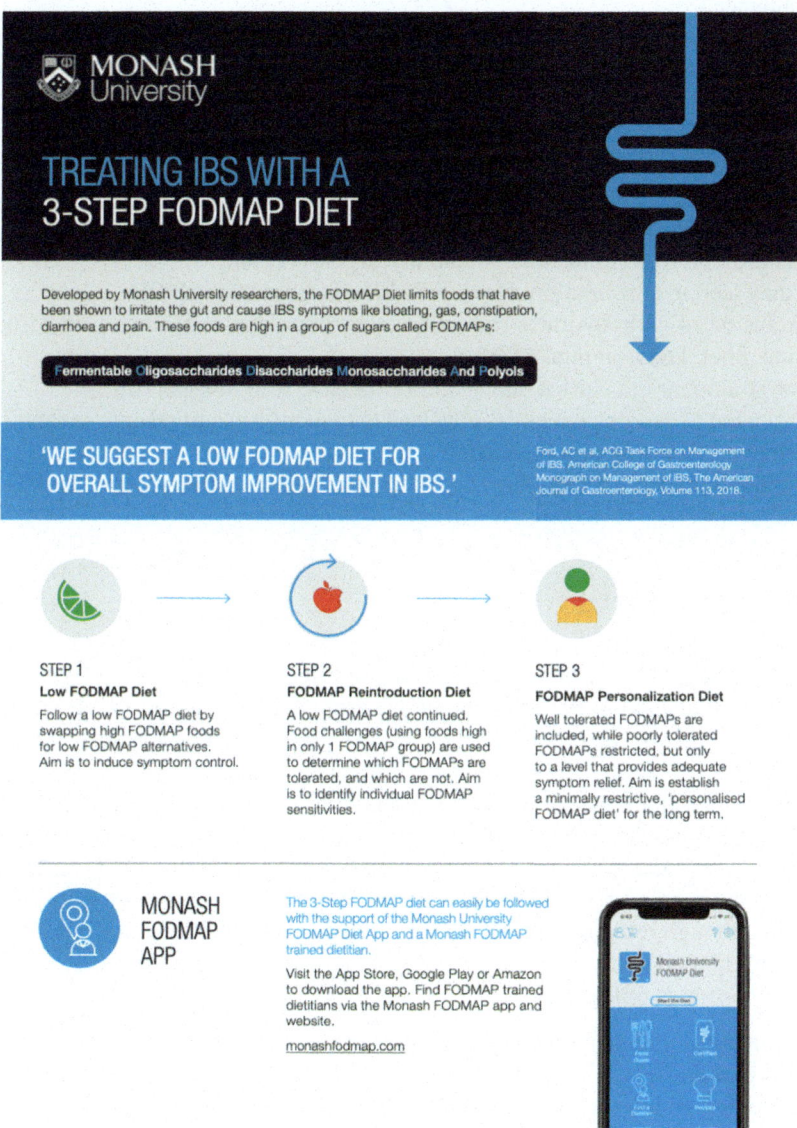

Fig. A.3 Low-FODMAP food plan [41]. (Source: Department of Gastroenterology, Monash University. This patient handout has been reproduced with permission from Monash University (monashfodmap.com). Download the Monash University FODMAP Diet App for a comprehensive food guide containing the FODMAP ratings and serving sizes for hundreds of different foods and beverages. Available on iOS and Android.)

Benefits are as follows:

- Reduces abdominal pain and discomfort, reduces bloating and distension, improves bowel habits, and improves quality of life [7].
- Up to 86 % of patients with IBS have improvement in overall GI symptoms and individual symptoms like abdominal pain, bloating, constipation, diarrhea, and flatulence [8].
- Reduces the osmotic load and gas production in the distal small bowel and proximal colon [8].

Warnings are as follows:

- As a very restrictive diet, it carries risks of disordered eating.
- It may lead to potentially unfavorable gut microbiota [9].
- It is complex and difficult to teach and to learn [10].
- It is difficult to continue and potentially expensive [10].
- It may lead to constipation due to reduction in fiber intake [10].
- Exclusion of carbohydrates rich in fructans may lead to reduction in carbohydrate, fiber, and iron intake [10].
- Lower amount of calories may lead to excessive weight loss [10].
- Exclusion of certain vegetables may lead to reduction in natural antioxidants [10].
- It may result in calcium deficiency [10].
- It is not intended for long-term use (max of 6 months, ideally only 3).

Anti-candida Diet

Candida albicans is the most common human fungal pathogen and is responsible for a variety of infections. Infections arise from *Candida* colonization of the GI tract, where *C. albicans* typically reside [11]. Reducing *C. albicans* overgrowth through dietary intervention can help minimize morbidity and mortality from *C. albicans* systemic infections, reduce infection rate, improve GI symptoms, and improve quality of life. The anti-candida diet has been shown to lower risk of yeast infections and prevent gastrointestinal *Candida* overgrowth [11]. Laboratory research suggests gluten, sugar, and certain dairy products can contribute to yeast growth, although research in humans is still forthcoming. See Fig. A.4 for a sample anti-candida food plan.

Benefits are as follows:

- Eliminating gluten may heal dysbiosis and prevent continued damage to the intestinal lining.
- Removing refined sugars and lactose-rich dairy products may prevent yeast growth by raising pH levels in the digestive tract [12].

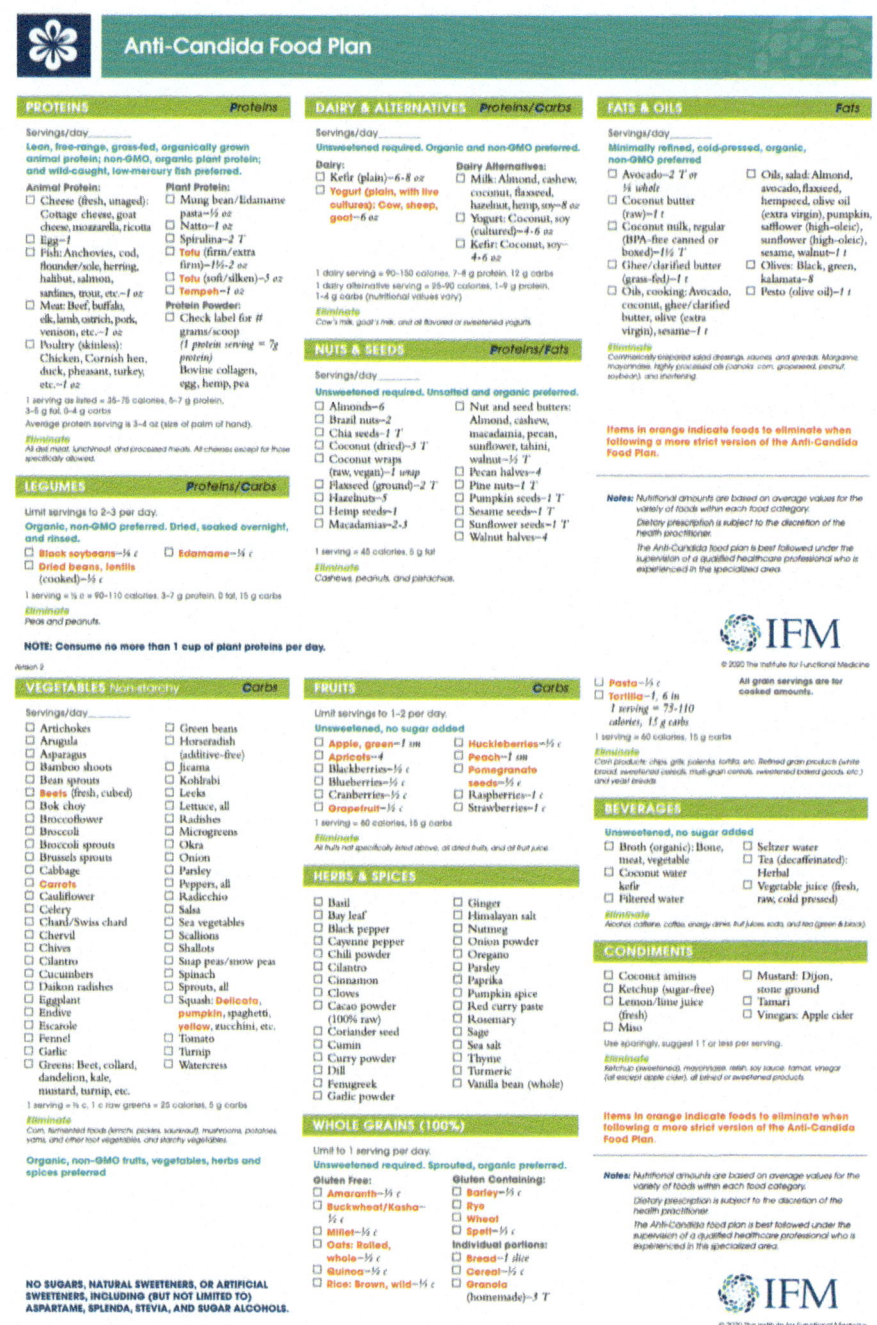

Fig. A.4 Anti-candida food plan [39]. Used with permission from the Institute for Functional Medicine (IFM), a global leader in functional medicine and a collaborator in the transformation of healthcare. IFM is a 501(c)(3) nonprofit organization that believes functional medicine can help every individual reach their full potential for health and well-being. Under no circumstances may the whole or any part of the materials be translated into another language, nor may you create derivative or other works without IFM's prior written permission (for permission, please contact permissions@ifm.org)

- Reducing sugar intake may make it more difficult for yeast to bind to cells inside the mouth [13].

  Warnings are as follows:

- Lacking in human research.
- May be unnecessarily eliminating food groups not proven to promote *C. albicans* growth.
- In the first 2–4 weeks, limit carbohydrates to two servings per day unless vegetarian.
- Limited fat due to maldigestion unless lipase supplementation.

Ketogenic Diet

A ketogenic diet primarily consists of high fats, moderate proteins, and very low carbohydrates. Althought it was originally intended to treat epilepsy, the diet has been used in a number of different patient populations, including diabetes, obesity, PCOS, cancer, and neuroinflammation. See Fig. A.5 for a sample ketogenic food plan.

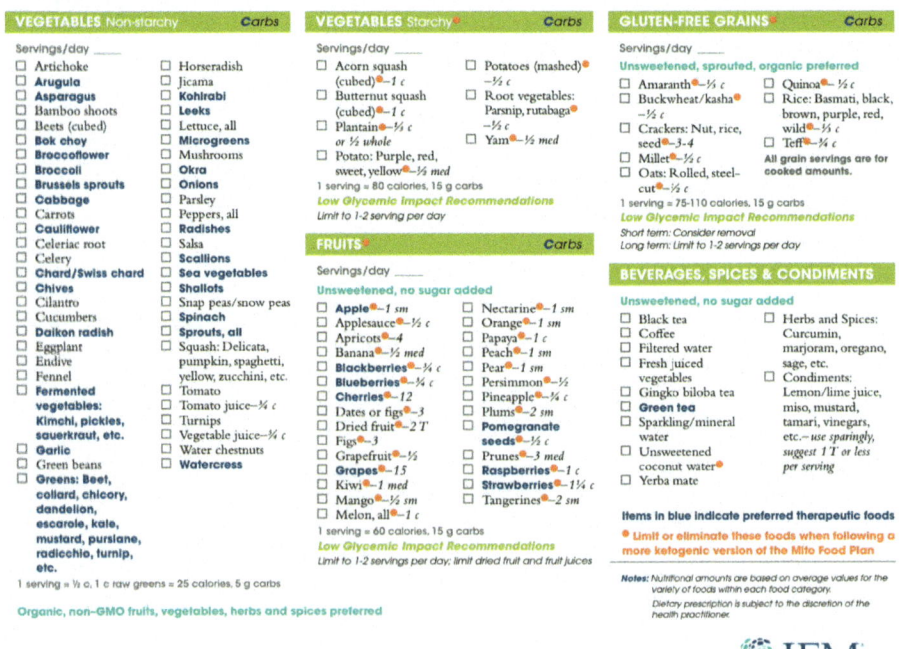

Fig. A.5 Mito food plan [39]. Used with permission from the Institute for Functional Medicine (IFM), a global leader in functional medicine and a collaborator in the transformation of healthcare. IFM is a 501(c)(3) nonprofit organization that believes functional medicine can help every individual reach their full potential for health and well-being. Under no circumstances may the whole or any part of the materials be translated into another language, nor may you create derivative or other works without IFM's prior written permission (for permission, please contact permissions@ifm.org)

Mito Food Plan

PROTEINS — Proteins

Servings/day ____

Free-range, grass-fed, organically grown animal protein; non-GMO, organic plant protein; and wild-caught, low-mercury fish preferred.

Animal Proteins:
- ☐ Cheese (hard)–½ oz
- ☐ Cheese (soft)–1 oz
- ☐ Cottage cheese–¼ c
- ☐ Parmesan cheese–2 T
- ☐ Ricotta cheese–¼ c
- ☐ Egg–1; or 2 egg whites
- ☐ **Fish, Omega-3 rich: Alaskan salmon, cod, halibut, herring, Atlantic mackerel, sardines, shrimp, tuna,** etc.–1 oz
- ☐ **Meat: Beef, buffalo, elk, lamb, venison, other wild game**–1 oz

- ☐ Poultry (skinless): Chicken, Cornish hen, duck, pheasant, turkey, etc.–1 oz

Plant Protein:
- ☐ Spirulina–2 T
- ☐ Tempeh–1 oz
- ☐ Tofu (firm/extra firm)–1½-2 oz
- ☐ Tofu (soft/silken)– 3 oz

Protein Powder:
- ☐ Check label for # grams/scoop (1 protein serving = 7 g protein) Egg, hemp, pea, soy, rice, whey protein

1 serving as listed = 35-75 calories, 5-7 g protein, 3-5 g fat, 0-4 g carbs
Average protein serving is 3-4 oz (size of palm of hand).

LEGUMES — Proteins/Carbs

Servings/day ____

Organic, non-GMO preferred

- ☐ Bean soups●–¾ c
- ☐ Black soybeans (cooked)●–½ c
- ☐ Dried beans, lentils, or peas (cooked)●–⅓ c
- ☐ Edamame (cooked)●– ½ c
- ☐ Flour, legume–¼ c
- ☐ Green peas (cooked)●–½ c

- ☐ Hummus or other bean dips●–⅓ c
- ☐ Refried beans, vegetarian●–½ c

1 serving = 90-110 calories, 3-7 g protein, 0 fat, 15 g carbs

DAIRY & ALTERNATIVES — Proteins/Carb

Servings/day ____

Unsweetened, organic preferred

Dairy:
- ☐ Buttermilk●–8 oz
- ☐ Kefir (plain)●–6-8 oz
- ☐ Milk: Cow, goat●–8 oz
- ☐ Yogurt, Greek (plain)●–6 oz

Dairy Alternatives:
- ☐ Kefir: Coconut, soy (plain)–6-8 oz
- ☐ Milk: Almond, coconut, flaxseed, hazelnut, hemp, oat, soy (plain)–8 oz
- ☐ Yogurt: Coconut, soy (plain, cultured)● –6 oz

1 dairy serving = 90-150 calories, 7-8 g protein, 12 g carbs
1 dairy alternative serving = 12-45 calories, 1-5 g protein, 1-2 g carbs (nutritional values vary)

NUTS & SEEDS — Proteins/Fats

Servings/day ____

Unsweetened, unsalted, organic preferred

- ☐ **Almonds**–6
- ☐ Brazil nuts–2
- ☐ Cashews–6
- ☐ **Chia seeds**–1 T
- ☐ **Coconut (dried)**– 3 T
- ☐ **Flaxseed (ground)**–2 T
- ☐ Hazelnuts–5
- ☐ **Hemp seeds**–1 T
- ☐ Macadamias–2-3
- ☐ Nut and seed butters–½ T

- ☐ Nut cheeses (almond, cashew, etc.)–1 oz
- ☐ **Peanuts**–10
- ☐ Pecan halves–4
- ☐ Pine nuts–1 T
- ☐ Pistachios–16
- ☐ **Pumpkin seeds**–1 T
- ☐ Sesame seeds–1 T
- ☐ Soy nuts–2 T
- ☐ Sunflower seeds–1 T
- ☐ **Walnut halves**–4

1 serving = 45 calories, 5 g fat

FATS & OILS — Fats

Servings/day ____

Minimally refined, cold-pressed, organic, non-GMO preferred

- ☐ **Avocado**–2 T or ¼ whole
- ☐ Butter–1 t; 2 t whipped
- ☐ Chocolate, dark (70% or higher cocoa)–1 oz
- ☐ **Coconut milk, regular (canned)**–1½ T
- ☐ **Coconut milk, light (canned)**–3 T
- ☐ Mayonnaise (unsweetened)–1 t
- ☐ **Oils, cooking: Avocado, coconut, ghee/clarified butter, grapeseed, grass fed butter MCT, olive (extra virgin),** rice bran, sesame–1 t

- ☐ **Oils, salad:** Almond, **Avocado, flaxseed,** grapeseed, hempseed, **MCT, olive (extra virgin),** pumpkin, rice bran, safflower (high-oleic), sesame, sunflower (high-oleic), walnut–1 t
- ☐ **Olives: Black, green, kalamata**–8
- ☐ Pesto (olive oil)–1 T
- ☐ Salad dressing made with the above oils–1 T

1 serving = 45 calories. 5 g fat

Items in blue indicate preferred therapeutic foods

● Limit or eliminate these foods when following a more ketogenic version of the Mito Food Plan

Notes: Nutritional amounts are based on average values for the variety of foods within each food category.

Dietary prescription is subject to the discretion of the health practitioner.

⊛IFM
© 2019 The Institute for Functional Medicine

Version 7

Fig. A.5 (continued)

Benefits are as follows:

- Often provides rapid weight loss [14].
- Improves glucose control, insulin resistance, blood pressure, and triglyceride and HDL levels [14].
- Low-carbohydrate diets have positive effects on body weight, BMI, abdominal circumference, blood pressure, high-density lipoprotein cholesterol, triglycerides, glycemia, hemoglobin A1c, insulin, and CRP. These studies ranged from 3 to 36 months only, so there is insufficient data to support long-term use of the diet [15].
- In PCOS patients, those who followed a strict ketogenic diet showed significantly decreased fasting serum insulin, LH-to-FSH ratio, and free testosterone along with decrease in weight and BMI [15].

Warnings are as follows:

- Contraindicated in patients with pancreatitis, liver failure, disorders of fat metabolism, various enzyme deficiencies, and porphyrias [14].
- May cause nausea, vomiting, headache, fatigue, dizziness, insomnia, exercise intolerance, and constipation [14].

- Long-term adverse effects include hepatic steatosis, hypoproteinemia, kidney stones, osteoporosis, and vitamin and mineral deficiencies [14, 16].
- Can cause dehydration, electrolytes, and hypoglycemia [17].

Autoimmune Paleo Diet

The autoimmune protocol (AIP) diet is an extension of the Paleolithic diet that aims to reduce inflammation in the gut, heal the gastrointestinal tract, and reduce systemic inflammation. The AIP consists of an elimination phase of certain food groups that trigger intestinal inflammation, dysbiosis, and/or symptomatic food intolerance. The elimination phase is followed by the maintenance phase, during which food groups are reintroduced, in a staged approach [15]. Please see Fig. A.6 for a sample autoimmune paleo diet.

Benefits are as follows:

- Can improve symptoms and endoscopic inflammation in patients with IBD [15]
- Lowers systemic inflammation and oxidative stress [18]
- Reduces symptoms of autoimmune disease, including fatigue, muscle and joint pain, bloating, gas, rashes, hair loss, and overall body aches

   Warnings are as follows:

- Restrictive
- Is expensive and can be difficult for vegetarians
- May cause hypoglycemia, sensitivity to certain foods, insomnia, anxiety, and restlessness

Detox Food Plan

The detox food plan supports intestinal and liver function during the metabolic detoxification process. The goal is to eat more foods that support the liver while at the same time reducing exposure to toxic compounds. Unlike other elimination diets, the detox food plan focuses on long-term nutritional support of the major systems involved in detoxification (the gut and the liver). There is a greater focus on eating clean foods for life, reducing plastic or potentially toxic elements, and eating organic whenever possible [19]. See Fig. A.7 for a sample detox food plan.

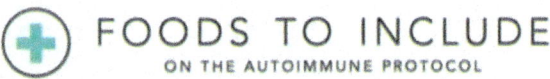

FOODS TO INCLUDE
ON THE AUTOIMMUNE PROTOCOL

VEGETABLES

artichoke	fennel
arugula	green bean
asparagus	kale
bok choi	leek
broccoli	lettuce
brussels sprout	mushroom
cabbage	rhubarb
cauliflower	snap pea
celery	spinach
chard	squash
collard green	watercress
cucumber	

ROOTS

beet	turnip
carrot	radish
celeriac	rutabaga
jicama	shallot
onion	sweet potato
parsnip	yam

FERMENTS

sauerkraut
fermented vegetables
(carrot, beet, etc.)
kombucha
water kefir

FRUIT

apple	lemon
apricot	lime
avocado	mango
banana	marionberry
blackberry	nectarine
blueberry	orange
cantaloupe	papaya
cherry	peach
clementine	pear
coconut	persimmon
date	plum
fig	pineapple
grape	pomegranate
grapefruit	raspberry
guava	strawberry
huckleberry	tangerine
honeydew	watermelon
kiwi	

HERBS

basil	mint
bay leaves	parsley
chamomile	peppermint
chives	rosemary
cilantro	sage
dill	spearmint
lavender	tarragon
lemongrass	thyme
marjoram	

SPICES

cinnamon	saffron
cloves	sea salt
garlic	shallots
ginger	turmeric

MEATS

beef	chicken
bison	turkey
buffalo	duck
lamb	pork
fish	rabbit
shellfish	venison

OFFAL

bone broth	kidney
liver	heart

PANTRY ITEMS

apple-cider vinegar	dates
anchovies	dried fruit
arrowroot powder	olives
coconut flour	salmon
coconut flakes	sardines
coconut vinegar	tuna
coconut aminos	ume plum vinegar

Fig. A.6 Sample autoimmune paleo food plan [43]

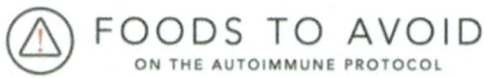

FOODS TO AVOID
ON THE AUTOIMMUNE PROTOCOL

GRAINS	
amaranth	oats
barley	quinoa
buckwheat	rice
bulgur	rye
corn	sorghum
farro	spelt
kamut	teff
millet	wheat

NIGHTSHADES	
cayenne	poblano
chili pepper	potato
eggplant	sweet pepper
goji berry	tobacco
ground cherry	tomato
habañero	tomatillo
jalepeno	wolf berries
paprika	

SPICES	
allspice	cumin
anise	fennel seed
annatto	fennugreek
canola	juniper
caraway	mustard
cardamom	nutmeg
celery seed	pepper
coriander	poppy

BEANS + LEGUMES	
adzuki beans	kidney beans
black beans	lentils
black-eyed peas	lima beans
chickpeas	peanuts
fava beans	soybeans

NUTS + SEEDS	
almond	hemp
brazil	macadamia
cashew	pecan
chestnut	pine
chia	pistachio
coffee	pumpkin
cocoa/chocolate	sesame
flax	sunflower
hazelnut	walnut

DAIRY	
butter	ghee
cheese	milk
cream	yogurt
cream cheese	

EGGS
chicken eggs
duck eggs
goose eggs

ALCOHOL
all alcohol

* Optional Restrictions: fruit, starchy vegetables, gluten cross-reactive foods, FODMAPs

AUTOIMMUNE**PALEO**
Seeking wellness + Building community

Fig. A.6 (continued)

VEGETABLES Non-starchy — Carbs

Servings/day____

Cruciferous
- Arugula
- Bok choy
- Broccoli, broccoli sprouts
- Brussels sprouts
- Cabbage
- Cauliflower
- Collard greens
- Kale
- Kohlrabi
- Mustard greens
- Radishes
- Rutabaga
- Turnips, turnip greens
- Watercress

Leafy Greens
- Chard/Swiss chard
- Endive
- Greens: Beet, spinach, lettuce
- Fresh herbs: cilantro, parsley
- Radicchio

Allium
- Chives
- Garlic
- Leeks
- Onion
- Scallions
- Shallots

Other Non-Starchy Vegetables
- Artichokes
- Asparagus
- Bean sprouts
- Beets
- Carrots
- Celery
- Cucumbers
- Eggplant
- Fennel
- Fermented Vegetables
- Green beans
- Mushrooms
- Nopales
- Peppers, all
- Salsa
- Sea vegetables
- Snap peas/snow peas
- Squash: spaghetti, yellow, zucchini, etc.
- Tomatillo
- Tomato
- Vegetable juice–¾ c

1 serving = ½ c, 1 c raw greens = 25 calories, 5 g carbs

VEGETABLES Starchy — Carbs

Servings/day____
- Acorn squash (cubed)–1 c
- Butternut squash (cubed)–1 c
- Parsnip –½ c
- Plantain–⅓ c or ½ whole
- Potato: Purple, red, sweet, yellow–¼ med

1 serving = 80 calories, 15 g carbs

FRUITS — Carbs

Servings/day____
Unsweetened, no sugar added
- Apple–1 sm
- Applesauce–½ c
- Apricots–4
- Banana, med–½
- Blackberries–¾ c
- Blueberries–¾ c
- Cherries–12
- Dried fruit (no sulfites)–2 T
- Figs–3
- Grapes–15
- Grapefruit–½ med
- Kiwi–1 med
- Mandarins–2 sm
- Mango–½ sm
- Melon, all–1 c
- Nectarine–1 sm
- Orange–1 sm
- Papaya–1 c
- Peach–1 sm
- Pear–1 sm
- Pineapple–¾ c
- Plums–2 sm
- Pomegranate seeds–½ c
- Prunes–3 med
- Raisins–2 T
- Raspberries–1 c
- Rhubarb–½ c
- Strawberries–1¼ c
- Tangerines–2 sm

1 serving = 60 calories, 15 g carbs

Organic, non-GMO fruits, vegetables, herbs and spices

GLUTEN-FREE GRAINS — Carbs

Servings/day____
Unsweetened, sprouted, organic
- Amaranth–¾ c
- Brown rice cakes–2
- Buckwheat/kasha–½ c
- Crackers (nut, seed, rice)–3-4
- Millet–¼ c
- Oats: Rolled or steel-cut–½ c
- Quinoa–½ c
- Rice: Basmati, black, brown, purple, red, jasmine–⅓ c
- Teff–¾ c

1 serving = 75–110 calories, 15 g carbs
All grain servings are for cooked amounts.

BEVERAGES, SPICES & CONDIMENTS

Servings/day____
- Filtered water (with lemon or lime juice)
- Sparkling/mineral water
- Fresh juiced fruits/vegetables
- Coffee
- Kombucha (no added sweeteners)
- Tea: Black, dandelion, **green**, herbal, etc.
- Herbs and spices: curry, dill, ginger, garlic, rosemary, turmeric, etc.
- Condiments: Lemon/lime juice, miso, mustard, tamari, vinegars, etc.– use sparingly, suggest 1 T or less per serving

Items in blue indicate preferred therapeutic foods

Notes: Nutritional amounts are based on average values for the variety of foods within each food category.
Dietary prescription is subject to the discretion of the practitioner.

◈ IFM
© 2021 The Institute for Functional Medicine

◈ **Detox Food Plan**

PROTEINS — Proteins

Servings/day____
Lean, free-range, grass-fed, organically grown animal protein; non-GMO, organic plant protein; and wild-caught, low-mercury fish. Avoid canned meats.

Animal Proteins:
- Egg–1 or 2 egg whites
- Fish: **Anchovy**, halibut, **herring**, sablefish, **salmon**, **sardines**, etc.–1 oz
- Meat: Beef, buffalo, elk, lamb, venison, other wild game–1 oz
- Poultry (skinless): Chicken, duck, pheasant, turkey–1 oz

Plant Protein:
- Tofu (firm/extra firm)–1½-2 oz
- Tofu (soft/silken)–3 oz
- Tempeh–½ c
- Spirulina–2 T

1 serving as listed = 35–75 calories, 5–7 g protein, 3–5 g fat, 0–4 g carbs
Average protein serving is 3–4 oz (size of palm of hand).

LEGUMES — Proteins/Carbs

Servings/day____
Organic, non-GMO
- Bean soups–¾ c
- **Black soybeans** (cooked)–½ c
- Dried peas, beans, or lentils (cooked)–½ c
- Flour, legume–¼ c
- Edamame–½ c
- Green Peas (cooked)–⅓ c
- Hummus or other bean dips–⅓ c
- Refried beans, vegetarian–⅓ c

1 serving = 110 calories, 15 g carbs, 7 g protein

Version 8

DAIRY ALTERNATIVES — Proteins/Carbs

Servings/day____
Unsweetened, organic
- Kefir, coconut or **soy**–4-6 oz
- Yogurt, coconut or **soy** (cultured)–4-6 oz
- Milk (homemade preferred): Almond, coconut, flaxseed, hazelnut, hemp, nut, oat, **soy**–8 oz

1 serving = 50–100 calories, 12 g carbs, 7 g protein

NUTS & SEEDS — Proteins/Fats

Servings/day____
Unsweetened, unsalted organic
- Almonds–6
- Brazil nuts–2
- Cashews–6
- Chia seeds–1 T
- Coconut(dried)–3 T
- **Flaxseed**, ground–2 T
- Hazelnuts–5
- Hemp seeds–1 T
- Macadamias–2-3
- Nut and seed butters–½ T
- Pecan halves–4
- Pine nuts–1 T
- Pistachios–16
- Pumpkin seeds–1 T
- Sunflower seed kernels–1 t
- **Sesame seeds**–1 T
- **Soy nuts**–2 T
- Walnut halves–4

1 serving = 45 calories, 5 g fat

FATS & OILS — Fats

Servings/day____
Minimally refined, cold-pressed, organic, non-GMO
- **Avocado**–2 T or ¼ whole
- Coconut milk, regular (canned)–1½ T
- Coconut milk, light (canned)–3 T
- Ghee/clarified butter–1 t
- Oils, cooking: **Avocado**, coconut, grapeseed, **olive** (extra virgin), **sesame**–1 t
- Oils, salad: Almond, **avocado**, canola, **flaxseed**, grapeseed, **hempseed, olive** (extra virgin), pumpkin seed, rice bran, safflower (high-oleic), **sesame**, sunflower (high-oleic), walnut–1 t
- Olives: Black, green, kalamata–8

1 serving = 45 calories, 5 g fat

Items in blue indicate preferred therapeutic foods

Notes: Nutritional amounts are based on average values for the variety of foods within each food category.
Dietary prescription is subject to the discretion of the health practitioner.

◈ IFM
© 2021 The Institute for Functional Medicine

Fig. A.7 Detox Food Plan [39]. Used with permission from the Institute for Functional Medicine (IFM), a global leader in functional medicine and a collaborator in the transformation of healthcare. IFM is a 501(c)(3) nonprofit organization that believes functional medicine can help every individual reach their full potential for health and well-being. Under no circumstances may the whole or any part of the materials be translated into another language, nor may you create derivative or other works without IFM's prior written permission (for permission, please contact permissions@ifm.org)

Benefits are as follows [19]:

- Increases energy and supports immune system
- Provides nutritional support for facilitating pathways involved in removing toxins
- Improves symptoms such as pain, fatigue levels, cognitive function and moods, more effective and satisfying sleep cycles, and weight loss and increases well-being for most individuals
- Reduces food triggers
- Supports liver function
- Reduces toxic burden and encourages healthy elimination of toxins
- Provides targeted antioxidants
- Supports nutrient-dependent pathways
- Balances hormone metabolism

Warnings are as follows [19]:

- Restrictive
- Often involves more rigorous nutrition intervention with medical food powders and dietary supplements and fasting
- Requires clean, organic foods (can be expensive)

Elimination Diet

Elimination diets are the gold standard for assessing food sensitivities. There are certain foods that cause most of the reactions, and these foods are eliminated, all at once, and then reintroduced one at a time after symptoms improve usually in 3 months. The primary goal is to reduce inflammation and allow greater sensitivity to inflammatory foods once reintroduced one at a time. The list of foods that are eliminated should be tailored to the patient if there are any suspicions about foods that are not typically reactive but seem to be for the individual. Food sensitivity testing can be used to help individualize the list of foods removed; however, these tests are not 100 % reliable and discretion is advised. Generally, adding in gut-healing foods and supplements during the elimination can hasten gut healing and reduce intestinal permeability which is at the root of the symptoms patients can feel as a result of the food sensitivity which range from brain fog and arthritic pain to acne and itchy skin. See Fig. A.8 for a sample elimination diet food plan.

Benefits are as follows:

- Very effective in dealing with food allergies. The kind of foods involved and completeness of their avoidance are important factors in reestablishing tolerance [20].

Warnings are as follows:

- Restrictive.

VEGETABLES Non-starchy — **Carbs**

Servings/day____

Brassicales (i.e. Cruciferous)
- Arugula
- Broccoflower
- Broccoli
- Broccoli sprouts
- Brussels sprouts
- Cabbage
- Cauliflower
- Horseradish
- Kohlrabi
- Radishes

Detoxifying Leafy Greens
- Bok choy
- Chard/Swiss chard
- Chervil
- Cilantro
- Endive
- Escarole
- Greens: Beet, collard, dandelion, kale, mustard, turnip, etc.
- Microgreens
- Parsley
- Radicchio

Thiols
- Chives
- Daikon radishes
- Garlic
- Leeks
- Onion
- Scallions
- Shallots

Liver & Kidney Support
- Artichokes
- Asparagus
- Celery
- Sprouts, all

Other Non-Starchy Vegetables
- Bamboo shoots
- Bean sprouts
- Beets (not canned)
- Carrots
- Cucumbers
- Eggplant ●■
- Fennel
- Green beans
- Jicama
- Kimchi ●▲
- Lettuce, all
- Mushrooms ●
- Okra
- Peppers, all ■
- Salsa ●■
- Sauerkraut ●▲
- Sea vegetables
- Shirataki noodles
- Snap peas/snow peas
- Spinach ●
- Squash: Delicata, pumpkin spaghetti, yellow, zucchini, etc.
- Tomato ●■
- Turnip
- Watercress

1 serving = ½ c, 1 c raw greens = 25 calories, 5 g carbs
NO STARCHY VEGETABLES (root vegetables)

Organic, non-GMO fruits, vegetables, herbs and spices preferred

FRUITS — **Carbs**

Servings/day____

Unsweetened, no sugar added
- Blackberries–¾ c
- Blueberries–¾ c
- Cherries ●–12
- Cranberries–¾ c
- Kiwi–1 med
- Pomegranate seeds–½ c
- Raspberries ●–1 c
- Strawberries ●–1¼ c

1 serving = 60 calories, 15 g carbs
NO OTHER FRUITS ALLOWED

HERBS & SPICES

- Basil
- Bay leaf
- Black pepper
- Cayenne pepper ●■
- Chili powder ●■
- Cilantro
- Cinnamon ●
- Cloves ●
- Cacao powder ● (100% raw)
- Coriander seed
- Cumin
- Curry powder ●■
- Dill
- Fenugreek
- Garlic powder
- Ginger
- Himalayan salt
- Nutmeg ●
- Onion powder
- Oregano
- Parsley
- Paprika ●■
- Pumpkin spice
- Red curry paste ●
- Rosemary
- Sage
- Sea salt
- Thyme
- Turmeric
- Vanilla bean (whole)

BEVERAGES

Unsweetened, no sugar added
- Broth (organic): Bone ● meat, ● vegetable
- Coconut water kefir ●▲
- Filtered water
- Seltzer water
- Tea (decaffeinated): ● Green, herbal
- Vegetable juice (fresh, raw, cold pressed)

NO COFFEE, ALCOHOL, CAFFEINE, SODA

CONDIMENTS

- Coconut aminos ●▲
- Lemon/lime juice (fresh) ●
- Miso ●▲
- Mustard: ● Dijon, stone ground
- Tamari ●▲
- Vinegars: ●▲ Apple cider, balsamic, white, etc.

Use sparingly, suggest 1 T or less per serving.
NO SUGARS, NATURAL SWEETENERS, OR ARTIFICIAL SWEETENERS, INCLUDING (BUT IS NOT LIMITED TO) ASPARTAME, SPLENDA, STEVIA, AND SUGAR ALCOHOLS.

KEY
● High Histamine ■ Nightshades ▲ Fermented Foods

In collaboration with
◇ IFM — Cleveland Clinic Center for Functional Medicine
© 2021 The Institute for Functional Medicine

ReNew Food Plan

PROTEINS — **Proteins**

Servings/day____

Lean, free-range, grass-fed, organically grown animal protein; non-GMO, organic plant protein; and wild-caught, low-mercury fish preferred.

Animal Protein:
- Egg ●–1
- Fish: Anchovies, ● cod, flounder/sole, herring, ● halibut, salmon, sardines, ● trout, etc.–1 oz
- Meat: Beef, buffalo, elk, lamb, venison, ostrich, etc.–1 oz
- Poultry (skinless): Chicken, Cornish hen, duck, pheasant, turkey, etc.–1 oz

Plant Protein:
- Black soybeans ●–¼ c
- Edamame–¼ c
- Hemp tofu–1½ oz

1 serving as listed = 35–75 calories, 5–7 g protein, 3–5 g fat, 0–4 g carbs
Average protein serving is 3–4 oz (size of palm of hand).

- Mung bean/ Edamame pasta ●– ½ oz
- Natto ●▲–1 oz
- Spirulina–2 T
- Tofu (firm/extra firm) ●–1½–2 oz
- Tofu (soft/silken) ●– 3 oz
- Tempeh ●▲–1 oz

Protein Powder:
- Check label for # grams/scoop (1 protein serving = 7g protein)
- Bovine collagen, egg, ● hemp, pea

DAIRY ALTERNATIVES — **Proteins/Carbs**

Servings/day____

Unsweetened, organic preferred
- Yogurt: Coconut (plain) ●▲–4-6 oz
- Kefir: Coconut (plain) ●▲–4-6 oz
- Nut/seed milk: Almond, cashew, ● coconut, flaxseed, hazelnut, hemp–8 oz

1 serving = 25–90 calories, 1–9 g protein, 1–4 g carbs (nutritional values vary)
NO DAIRY ALLOWED

NUTS & SEEDS — **Proteins/Fats**

Servings/day____

Unsweetened, unsalted, organic preferred
- Almonds–6
- Brazil nuts–2
- Cashews ●–6
- Chia seeds–1 T
- Coconut (dried)–3 T
- Coconut wraps (raw, vegan)–1 wrap
- Flaxseed (ground)– 2 T
- Hazelnuts–5
- Hemp seeds–1
- Macadamias–2-3
- Nut and seed butters: Almond, cashew, ● macadamia, pecan, sunflower, ● tahini, walnut ●–½ T
- Pecan halves–4
- Pine nuts–1 T
- Pistachios–16
- Pumpkin seeds–1 T
- Sesame seeds–1 T
- Sunflower seeds ●– 1 T
- Walnut halves ●–4

1 serving = 45 calories, 5 g fat

FATS & OILS — **Fats**

Servings/day____

Minimally refined, cold pressed, organic, non-GMO preferred
- Avocado ●–2 T or ⅛ whole
- Coconut butter (raw)–1 t
- Coconut milk, regular (BPA-free canned or boxed)–1½ T
- Ghee/clarified butter (grass-fed)–1 t
- Oils, cooking: Avocado, coconut, ghee/clarified butter, olive (extra virgin), sesame)–1 t
- Oils, salad: Almond, avocado, flaxseed, hempseed, olive oil (extra virgin), sesame, walnut–1 t
- Olives: ● Black, green, kalamata–8
- Pesto (olive oil)–1 t

1 serving = 45 calories, 5 g fat

KEY
● High Histamine ■ Nightshades ▲ Fermented Foods

Notes: Nutritional amounts are based on average values for the variety of foods within each food category.
Dietary prescription is subject to the discretion of the health practitioner.

NO LEGUMES (Except those specifically listed) and NO GRAINS (Bread, pasta, cereal, oats, etc.)

Version 7

In collaboration with
◇ IFM — Cleveland Clinic Center for Functional Medicine
© 2021 The Institute for Functional Medicine

Fig. A.8 Elimination Diet food plan [39]. Used with permission from the Institute for Functional Medicine (IFM), a global leader in functional medicine and a collaborator in the transformation of healthcare. IFM is a 501(c)(3) nonprofit organization that believes functional medicine can help every individual reach their full potential for health and well-being. Under no circumstances may the whole or any part of the materials be translated into another language, nor may you create derivative or other works without IFM's prior written permission (for permission, please contact permissions@ifm.org)

- Not meant for long-term dieting.
- Allergies and intolerances change with age; elimination diet may need to be repeated [20].
- With long-term use, it may cause lower levels of Ca, Zn, and vitamin B2 (milk allergy); of vitamins A, B1, and B2, niacin, and cholesterol (egg); and lower levels of Ca, P, Fe, K, Zn, vitamins B2 and B6, and niacin (wheat and soybean) [20].

Vegan Diet

Plant-exclusive diets, called Vegan, have ample research supporting a reduction in heart disease, type 2 diabetes, obesity, and other health conditions [21]. By following the "power plate" approach (see Fig. A.9), the vegan diet includes fruits, vegetables, grains, and beans and excludes animal products (meat, dairy, and eggs) and added oils (Fig. A.10).

Benefits are as follows:

- Have been shown to both prevent and treat type 2 diabetes:

  - Weight is a major risk factor for the development of T2D; vegans are less likely to develop T2D because of their lower weight [23].

Fig. A.9 The power of your plate [22]

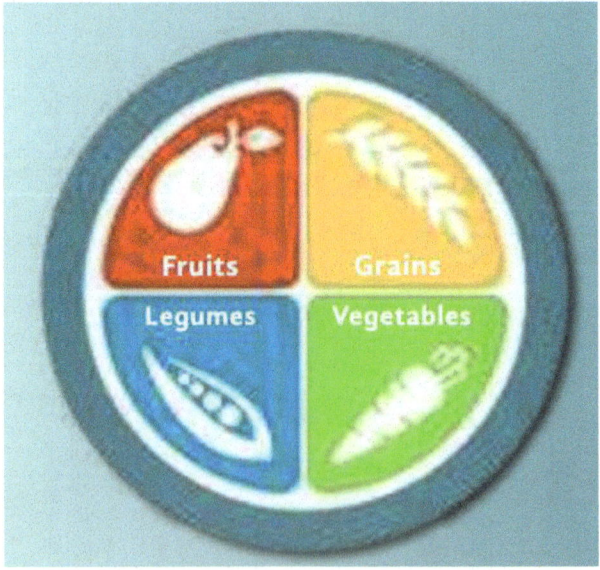

② STOCK UP **Prep Your Pantry**

It's time to stock up on healthful plant-based foods! Here are some staples to look for at the grocery store:

Produce: The bright colors you see in the produce aisle reflect different phytochemicals that benefit health, so be sure to choose a variety of fruits and vegetables. Look for fresh herbs, too, which can add flavors and spices to recipes without extra calories and fat.

Dried Foods: Dried beans and peas, brown rice, whole-wheat pasta, quinoa, barley, oats, cereals, and other whole grains are all great choices.

Canned Foods: Beans, plant-based soups, and vegetables can all be found in the canned foods aisle. Remember to keep your diet low in sodium and read ingredient lists carefully for animal additives like chicken broth or milk.

Refrigerated Foods: Tofu, tempeh, hummus, bean- and lentil-based salads, and plenty of nondairy plant milks and yogurts can be found in this section.

Frozen Foods: Frozen fruits and vegetables are a great way to save time and money! They're just as nutritious as fresh vegetables and last for much longer. Most stores are also now well stocked with low-fat, frozen plant-based meals like pizzas, pasta dishes, burritos, and veggie burgers. Remember to check labels for hidden animal ingredients, like cheese or egg.

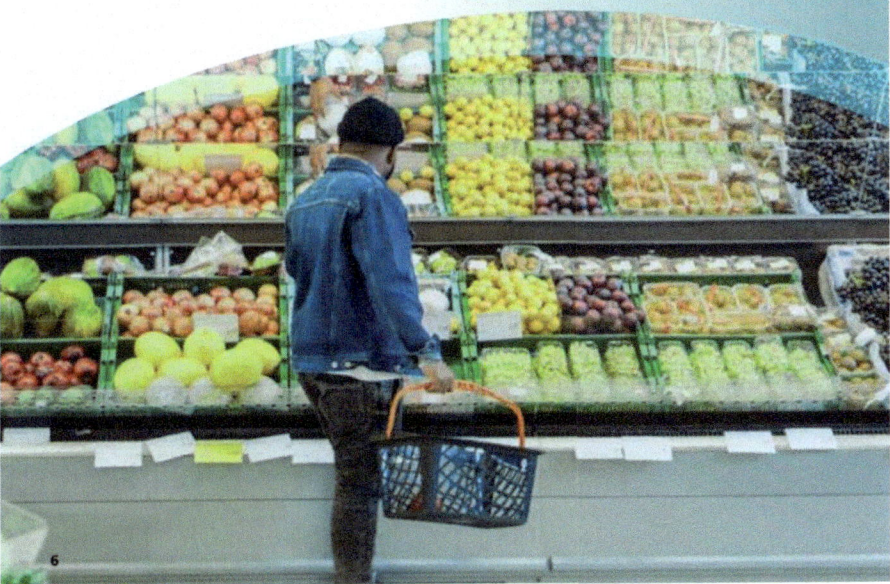

Fig. A.10 Sample vegan food plan [22]

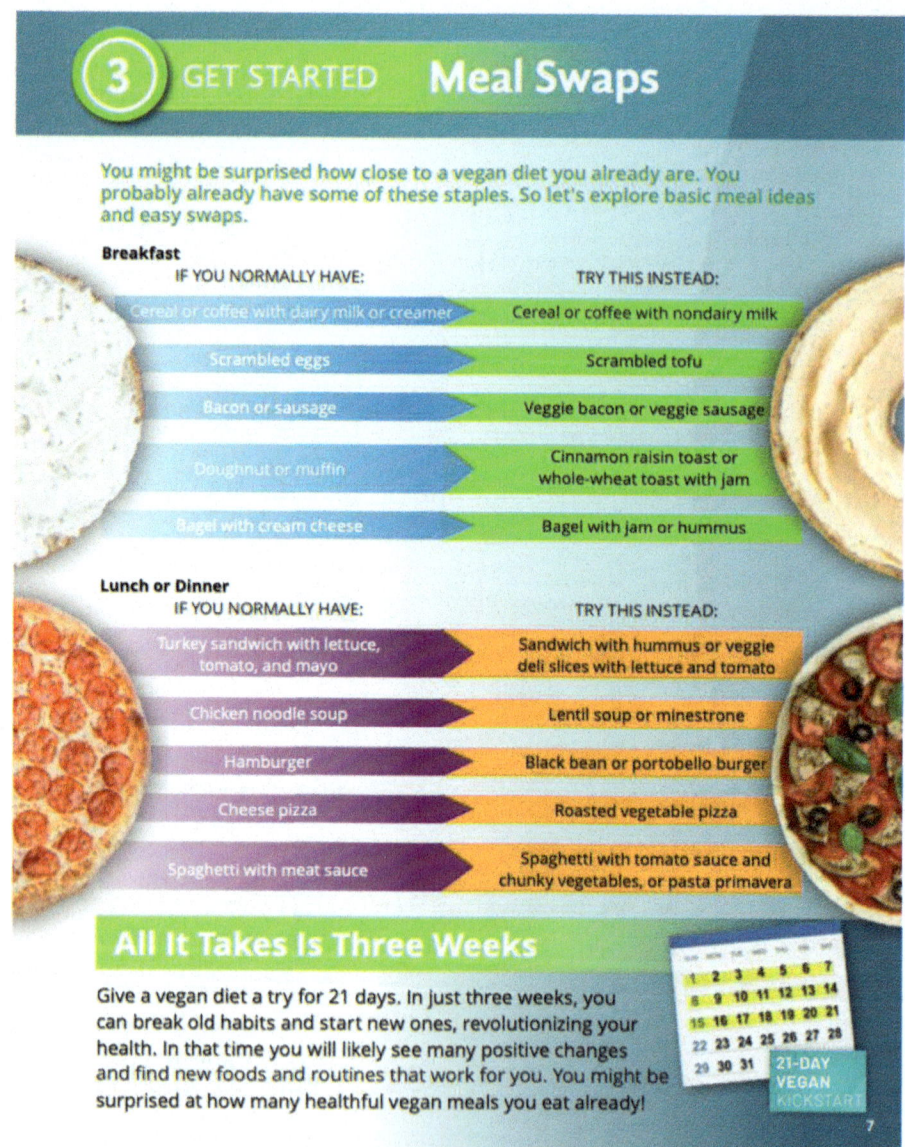

Fig. A.10 (continued)

- Key components of a vegan diet (no red or processed meat, more whole grains and nuts) also have been associated with reduced diabetes risk [24, 25].
- Has been shown to lower total and LDL cholesterol by controlling lipid levels and reducing triglycerides [26].

- Promotes cardiovascular health:

  - Large meta-analysis found that vegetarians had a 29 % lower mortality risk for ischemic heart disease, when compared to omnivores [27].
- Lowers blood pressure:

  - Self-reported hypertension is lowest among vegans [28].
- Highly probable that many vegan diets are less likely to cause cancer than other diets are [29]
- Reduced risk of diverticular disease [30]

  Warnings are as follows:

- Vegans have been shown to have an increased fracture risk, when calcium intake was less than 525 mg per day. When vegans consumed more than 525 mg of calcium per day, their fracture rate was about the same as other groups [31].
- Vegan may have high circulating concentrations of uric acid, which can contribute to development of gout, chronic kidney disease, cardiovascular disease, and cancer [32].
- Diet can be bulky due to increased consumption of dietary fiber.
- Particular macronutrients and micronutrients may be lacking without careful dietary choices: protein, calcium, vitamin B12, vitamin D, essential fatty acids, zinc, iodine, and iron [33–35].

*Intermittent Fasting (IF)

IF is defined by the regular restriction of the eating window and reduction in caloric intake that occurs on a scheduled rhythm. The primary goal of IF is to allow the body to rest from the digestive process and turn its attention to processes that result in a deep cellular cleansing. There are several ways that IF can be done and all of them appear to provide the same results [36].

Of note, IF is not a good fit for everyone. Avoid in patients that have a history of any kind of eating disorder, reactive hypoglycemia, chronic fatigue, or other energy deficits such as from chronic Lyme disease. Please see Fig. A.11 for a sample intermittent fasting food plan.

Top IF approaches are as follows:

1. *Prolon fasting-mimicking diet (FMD)*: research shows FMD to improve body mass index, blood pressure, fasting glucose, IGF-1, triglycerides, total and low-density lipoprotein cholesterol, and C-reactive protein [37]. Patients receive a kit that contains all of the food needed for each day of the 5-day fast. Positive results can occur after one fast; however, three cycles with 1 month in between are what the research is based on. After the 3 months, providers can recommend a continued monthly schedule until health goals are met or reduce the frequency to every other month and then 3–4 times per year. For more information, visit https://prolonfast.com/.

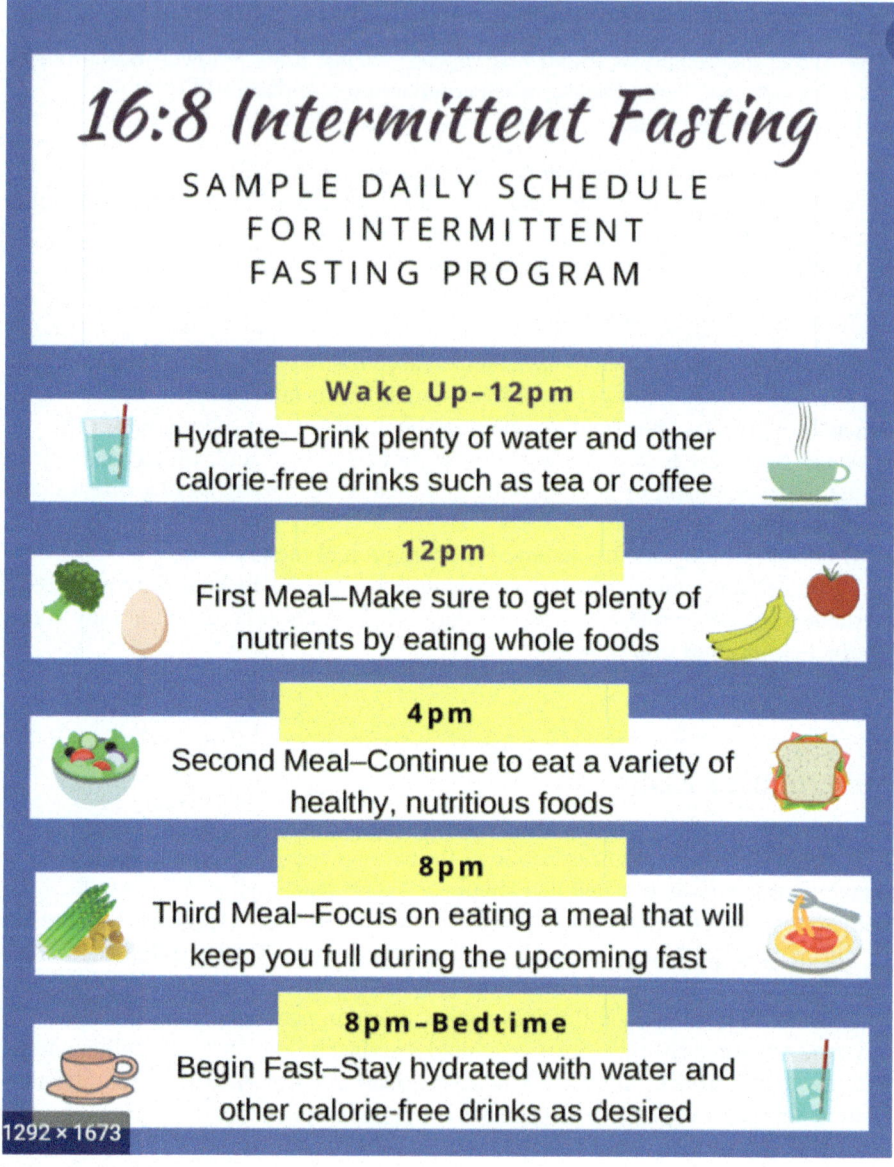

Fig. A.11 Intermittent fasting food plan [42]

2. Fast diet 5:2: the 5:2 diet cycles over the course of 1 week where patients have 5 days of normal eating and 2 days of reduced calorie intake (500 for men and 600 for women). Week after week, this approach produces improvements in body composition, blood lipids, and fasting glucose and insulin.
3. Daily 13–16-h fasting: likely the easiest to follow, nightly fasting from dinner to the first meal of the next day can produce benefits without as much disruption in

the lifestyle. Recent research shows that 13-h nightly fast provides the benefits of the fast and that longer fasts do not have added benefit. Some therapeutic programs related to cognition encourage a 16-h fast which allows additional time for the breakdown of amyloid beta plaque by the insulin-degrading enzyme [38]. The trick with this short eating window is to highly optimize the diet such that all nutrients can be obtained in that 8-h window. Supplements are often needed to ensure adequate intake.

Recommended Therapeutic Food Plans

Used with permission from the Institute for Functional Medicine (IFM), a global leader in functional medicine and a collaborator in the transformation of health-care. IFM is a 501(c)(3) nonprofit organization that believes functional medicine can help every individual reach their full potential for health and well-being. Under no circumstances may the whole or any part of the materials be translated into another language, nor may you create derivative or other works without IFM's prior written permission (for permission, please contact permissions@ifm.org)

References

1. Tuso PJ, Ismail MH, Ha BP, Bartolotto C. Nutritional update for physicians: plant-based diets. Perm J. 2013;17(2):61–6.
2. Estruch R, Ros E, Salas-Salvadó J, Covas M-I, Corella D, Arós F, et al. Primary prevention of cardiovascular disease with a Mediterranean diet. N Engl J Med. 2013;368(14):1279–90.
3. Morris MC, Tangney CC, Wang Y, Sacks FM, Barnes LL, Bennett DA, et al. MIND diet slows cognitive decline with aging. Alzheimers Dement. 2015 Sep;11(9):1015–22.
4. Schwingshackl L, Schwedhelm C, Galbete C, Hoffmann G. Adherence to Mediterranean diet and risk of cancer: an updated systematic review and meta-analysis. Nutrients. 2017;9(10).
5. Bonaccio M, Bes-Rastrollo M, de Gaetano G, Iacoviello L. Challenges to the Mediterranean diet at a time of economic crisis. Nutr Metab Cardiovasc Dis. 2016;26(12):1057–63.
6. Mediterranean Diet Handout [Internet]. Oldways preservation and exchange trust. 2009 [cited 2021 May 28]. Available from: https://memory.ucsf.edu/sites/memory.ucsf.edu/files/MediterraneanDietHandout.pdf.
7. Monash University. FODMAPs and irritable Bowel Syndrome [Internet]. Monash University. 2021 [cited 2021 May 19]. Available from: https://www.monashfodmap.com/about-fodmap-and-ibs/.

8. Nanayakkara WS, Skidmore PM, O'Brien L, Wilkinson TJ, Gearry RB. Efficacy of the low FODMAP diet for treating irritable bowel syndrome: the evidence to date. Clin Exp Gastroenterol. 2016 Jun 17;9:131–42.

9. Hill P, Muir JG, Gibson PR. Controversies and Recent Developments of the Low-FODMAP Diet. Gastroenterol Hepatol (N Y). 2017;13(1):36–45.

10. Bellini M, Tonarelli S, Nagy AG, Pancetti A, Costa F, Ricchiuti A, et al. Low FODMAP diet: evidence, doubts, and hopes. Nutrients. 2020;12(1).

11. Gunsalus KTW, Tornberg-Belanger SN, Matthan NR, Lichtenstein AH, Kumamoto CA. Manipulation of host diet to reduce gastrointestinal colonization by the opportunistic pathogen Candida albicans. mSphere. 2016;1(1).

12. Patil S, Rao RS, Majumdar B, Anil S. Clinical appearance of oral candida infection and therapeutic strategies. Front Microbiol. 2015;6:1391.

13. Pizzo G, Giuliana G, Milici ME, Giangreco R. Effect of dietary carbohydrates on the in vitro epithelial adhesion of Candida albicans, Candida tropicalis, and Candida krusei. New Microbiol. 2000;23(1):63–71.

14. Masood W, Annamaraju P, Uppaluri KR. Ketogenic Diet. StatPearls. Treasure Island (FL): StatPearls Publishing: 2021.

15. Batch JT, Lamsal SP, Adkins M, Sultan S, Ramirez MN. Advantages and disadvantages of the ketogenic diet: a review article. Cureus. 2020;12(8):e9639.

16. The keto diet: pros, cons, and tips [Internet]. The Portland Clinic. 2021 [cited 2021 Apr 20]. Available from: https://www.theportlandclinic.com/the-keto-diet-pros-cons-and-tips/.

17. Broom GM, Shaw IC, Rucklidge JJ. The ketogenic diet as a potential treatment and prevention strategy for Alzheimer's disease. Nutrition. 2019;60:118–21.

18. Whalen KA, McCullough ML, Flanders WD, Hartman TJ, Judd S, Bostick RM. Paleolithic and Mediterranean Diet Pattern Scores Are Inversely Associated with Biomarkers of Inflammation and Oxidative Balance in Adults. J Nutr. 2016;146(6):1217–26.

19. IFM. Detox Food Plan; Comprehensive Guide. 2017.

20. Kim J, Kwon J, Noh G, Lee SS. The effects of elimination diet on nutritional status in subjects with atopic dermatitis. Nutr Res Pract. 2013;7(6):488–94.

21. Medawar E, Huhn S, Villringer A, Veronica Witte A. The effects of plant-based diets on the body and the brain: a systematic review. Transl Psychiatry. 2019;9(1):226.

22. Physicians Committee for Responsible Medicine. Vegan Starter Kit [Internet]. Physicians Committee for Responsible Medicine. 2021 [cited 2021 May 28]. Available from: https://www.pcrm.org/veganstarterkit.

23. Tonstad S, Butler T, Yan R, Fraser GE. Type of vegetarian diet, body weight, and prevalence of type 2 diabetes. Diabetes Care. 2009;32(5):791–6.

24. Pan A, Sun Q, Bernstein AM, Schulze MB, Manson JE, Willett WC, et al. Red meat consumption and risk of type 2 diabetes: 3 cohorts of US adults and an updated meta-analysis. Am J Clin Nutr. 2011;94(4):1088–96.

25. Marsh K. Nuts and diabetes. Diabetes Management: A journal for general practitioners and other health professionals. 2011;36(16).

26. Jenkins DJA, Kendall CWC, Faulkner DA, Nguyen T, Kemp T, Marchie A, et al. Assessment of the longer-term effects of a dietary portfolio of cholesterol-lowering foods in hypercholesterolemia. Am J Clin Nutr. 2006;83(3):582–91.

27. Huang T, Yang B, Zheng J, Li G, Wahlqvist ML, Li D. Cardiovascular disease mortality and cancer incidence in vegetarians: a meta-analysis and systematic review. Ann Nutr Metab. 2012;60(4):233–40.

28. Orlich MJ, Singh PN, Sabaté J, Jaceldo-Siegl K, Fan J, Knutsen S, et al. Vegetarian dietary patterns and mortality in Adventist Health Study 2. JAMA Intern Med. 2013;173(13):1230–8.

29. Key TJ, Appleby PN, Spencer EA, Travis RC, Allen NE, Thorogood M, et al. Cancer incidence in British vegetarians. Br J Cancer. 2009;101(1):192–7.

30. Crowe FL, Appleby PN, Allen NE, Key TJ. Diet and risk of diverticular disease in Oxford cohort of European Prospective Investigation into Cancer and Nutrition (EPIC): prospective study of British vegetarians and non-vegetarians. BMJ. 2011;343:d4131.

31. Appleby P, Roddam A, Allen N, Key T. Comparative fracture risk in vegetarians and nonvegetarians in EPIC-Oxford. Eur J Clin Nutr. 2007;61(12):1400–6.

32. Schmidt JA, Crowe FL, Appleby PN, Key TJ, Travis RC. Serum uric acid concentrations in meat eaters, fish eaters, vegetarians and vegans: a cross-sectional analysis in the EPIC-Oxford cohort. PLoS ONE. 2013;8(2):e56339.

33. Might a vegan diet be healthy, or even healthier? - Animal (de)liberation: should the consumption of animal products be banned? - NCBI Bookshelf [Internet]. [cited 2021 Apr 27]. Available from: https://www.ncbi.nlm.nih.gov/books/NBK396513/.

34. Foster M, Chu A, Petocz P, Samman S. Effect of vegetarian diets on zinc status: a systematic review and meta-analysis of studies in humans. J Sci Food Agric. 2013;93(10):2362–71.

35. Clarys P, Deliens T, Huybrechts I, Deriemaeker P, Vanaelst B, De Keyzer W, et al. Comparison of nutritional quality of the vegan, vegetarian, semi-vegetarian, pesco-vegetarian and omnivorous diet. Nutrients. 2014;6(3):1318–32.

36. Cho Y, Hong N, Kim K-W, Cho SJ, Lee M, Lee Y-H, et al. The effectiveness of intermittent fasting to reduce Body Mass Index and glucose metabolism: a systematic review and meta-analysis. J Clin Med. 2019;8(10).

37. Wei M, Brandhorst S, Shelehchi M, Mirzaei H, Cheng CW, Budniak J, et al. Fasting-mimicking diet and markers/risk factors for aging, diabetes, cancer, and cardiovascular disease. Sci Transl Med. 2017;9(377).

38. Bredesen D. The end of Alzheimer's program: the first protocol to enhance cognition and reverse decline at any age. Illustrated. Avery; 2020.

39. IFM. Food Plans [Internet]. Institute for Functional Medicine. 2021 [cited 2021 May 30]. Available from: https://www.ifm.org/learning-center/?hsa_kw=institute%20for%20functional%20medicine&hsa_net=adwords&hsa_grp=79398164764&hsa_cam=6479100630&hsa_acc=4746158419&hsa_tgt=aud-882708901821:kwd-421125532922&hsa_ver=3&hsa_ad=434238175600&hsa_mt=e&hsa_src=g&gclid=Cj0KCQjw78yFBhCZARIsAO

xgSx12dSsJ75FKuzL_M3nI1sC7isDAKz9V0uS4v8vfPRaPH1nrekUYl3Qa-
AnXuEALw_wcB&gclsrc=aw.ds.

40. Sutter Health. Mediterranean diet made easy [Internet]. Sutter Health. 2021 [cited 2021 May 31]. Available from: https://www.sutterhealth.org/health/nutrition/mediterranean-diet.

41. Monash University. 3 step FODMAP Diet guide [Internet]. Monash University. 2019 [cited 2021 May 31]. Available from: https://www.monashfodmap.com/3_step_fodmap_diet/.

42. Carr E. A beginner's guide to intermittent fasting [Internet]. University of Michigan School of Public Health. 2021 [cited 2021 May 31]. Available from: https://sph.umich.edu/pursuit/2019posts/beginners-guide-to-intermittent-fasting.html.

43. Trescott. Paleo autoimmune protocol print-out guides [Internet]. Autoimmune Wellness. 2019 [cited 2021 May 31]. Available from: https://autoimmunewellness.com/paleo-autoimmune-protocol-print-out-guides/.

Appendix B: Supplement Table

Nutriceuticals, or supplements, play an important role in integrative nutrition due to their ability to help support treatment goals such as overcoming dietary limitations, alter a disease process, support a nutrigenomic impairment, and shift the biochemistry of a patient toward greater health. Due to the therapeutic potential, practitioners that use supplements need to understand the details of how to use them effectively in order for them to support the treatment objectives.

The supplement industry is regulated by the FDA as a food, rather than a drug, under the Dietary Supplement Health and Education Act (DSHEA) of 1994 [1]. "Under DSHEA, a firm is responsible for determining that the dietary supplements it manufactures or distributes are safe and that any representations or claims made about them are substantiated by adequate evidence to show that they are not false or misleading. This means that dietary supplements do not need approval from FDA before they are marketed [2]." In short, the FDA puts the onus on the manufacturer to ensure that the products are safe. Research has shown that this is not a reliable approach to making sure supplements are safe and of high, therapeutic quality. Therefore, it's important that practitioners seek out supplement brands that produce high-quality products that are tested by third parties for quality, purity, and potency [3].

Emerson Ecologics is one of the largest reputable supplement distributors. Emerson qualifies for the gold standard partnership, which means that there is "analytical testing on each batch of Raw Material or Finished Product for: identity, potency (label claim) and microbiological contaminants as well as all other applicable analytical tests on ingredients at risk for certain impurities (e.g., solvents for concentrates, pesticides for non-organics, melamine for animal proteins, aflatoxin for high risk herbs/foods, adulterants" [4].

Table B.1 includes common dietary supplements with their associated uses, dosing, and any relevant provider comments.

J. Wendt et al., *Integrative Geriatric Nutrition*,
https://doi.org/10.1007/978-3-030-81758-9

Table B.1 Common supplements and associated uses

Name	Primary uses	Comments	Dosing
Vitamin C	Oxidative stress Immune support Cancer (high-dose IV)	There are many forms of vitamin C; choose buffered forms to avoid stomach irritation. Ascorbic acid is an adequate form; flavonoids may provide additional benefit	2–5 g/day
Omega-3	Cardiovascular Mood (higher EPA/DHA ratio) Cognition (higher DHA/EPA)	Be sure to look at the actual amount of EPA/DHA rather than just the total omega-3 because ALA requires conversion and has very low bioavailability compared to EPA/DHA	2,000–4,000 mg/day
GLA	Skin issues Gut inflammation	Analysis of fatty acids can test for GLA levels	240 mg/day
Magnesium	Anxiety (glycinate form) Muscle cramps (topical) Sleep (glycinate form) Cognition (threonate form) Constipation (citrate, oxide forms)	Magnesium is indicated where calming is needed	400–600 mg/day
Vitamin D3	Immune support Bone health Cognition	Best if used in combination with vitamin K	25–100 mg/day
Vitamin K2 *See below for K1 vs. K2 explanation*	Immune support Bone health	Used in combination with vitamin D. Primary supplement form is K2, MK4 and MK7	15–40 mg (MK4) 50–500 mcg (MK7)
Zinc	Immune support (picolinate) Gut healing (carnosine)	The optimal ratio between zinc and copper is 2:1	8–11 mg
Potassium	Activates a number of enzymes involved in energy metabolism, antioxidant defense, and repair Supports blood pressure, bone health, and kidney health	People with diabetes, insulin resistance, and impaired kidney function or who are using ACE inhibitors, ARBs, potassium-sparing diuretics, alpha- or beta-blockers, digitalis, heparin, Bactrim, pentamidine, and NSAIDs should not take potassium supplements without consulting with their doctor [5]	4.7 g [6]

Table B.1 (continued)

Name	Primary uses	Comments	Dosing
Multi-strain probiotics	Immune support Gut health	There are spore-based probiotics as well as bacteria and yeast-based probiotics. In some cases such as with bacterial overgrowth, better choice is spore-based multi-strain probiotics	Post-antibiotic dosing should be 100B CFUs, general maintenance dosing between 10 and 50B CFUs
Saccharomyces boulardii	Immune support Gut inflammation	This is a beneficial yeast, helpful with balancing candida in the gut Probiotic activity has helped improve gut barrier function, pathogen competitive exclusion, production of antimicrobial modulation, immune modulation, and trophic effects [7]	$>1 \times 10^9$ [8]
Digestive enzymes	Gut health	Break down proteins, carbohydrates, and lipids. Animal-derived enzymes represent standard of care, but growing research in plant-based and microbe-derived enzymes offers great promise [9]	Varies by enzyme [9]
Calcium	Bone health Vascular contraction and dilation Muscle function Nerve transmission Intracellular signaling Hormonal secretion	<1% of total body calcium is needed to support these critical metabolic functions. The remaining 99 % of the body's calcium supply is stored in bones and teeth to support structure and function [10]	1200 mg [11]
Multivitamin and trace minerals (especially for bone health)	Foundational health	Avoid supplements with cyanocobalamin or folic acid as metabolism varies (dictated by MTHFR gene) [12]	One MTV daily (doses of individual vitamins vary by vitamin)

(continued)

Table B.1 (continued)

Name	Primary uses	Comments	Dosing
Protein powder	Foundational health Hair, skin, and nail support Weight loss or gain Anti-inflammatory	Sources vary widely. Animal sources provide a complete source of protein (all essential amino acids), when vegetable sources generally lack one or more essential amino acids. Animal sources often have more saturated fat compared to vegetable sources. Processing specifics can vary significantly [13]	Start at 20 gm
Curcumin	Anti-inflammatory Antihistamine Antioxidant Joint and muscle pain Cognition Improved B-cell function Decreased insulin resistance Decreased diabetic nephropathy and retinopathy and glycemic control	May cause diarrhea, headache, rash, and yellow stool [14]	1000–1500 (depending on indication)
Fiber	Increases plasma HDL, decreases plasma homocysteine, and increases glutathione [15]. Reduces LDL, regulates body weight, improves glucose metabolism, controls blood pressure, and reduces inflammation [15] Support healthy microbiome Improves GI health and regular bowel movements Reduces inflammation	Resistant starch indicated for low SCFAs on stool tests May make IBS symptoms worse	30–35 g
Iron	Fatigue and anemia Supports microbiome Cofactor for DNA synthesis, important role in tissues with high cellular turnover [16] Is essential component of hemoglobin and myoglobin and supports muscle metabolism and healthy connective tissues. Necessary for physical growth, neurological development, cellular functioning, and synthesis of some hormones	Can interact with certain medications (levodopa, levothyroxine, PPIs) [17]	8 mg [17]

Table B.1 (continued)

Name	Primary uses	Comments	Dosing
Folate	Methyl donor, required for cellular division, as it is involved in synthesis of nucleic acids and metabolism of amino acids [18]	About 85 % of supplemental folic acid, when taken with food, is bioavailable. Without food, nearly 100 % supplemental folic acid is bioavailable. *People with the MTHFR polymorphism may benefit from supplementation with 5-methyl-THF instead* [18]	680–1360 mcg DFE (400 to 800 mcg folic acid)
Vitamin B12	Required for development, myelination, and function of the central nervous system, RBC formation, and DNA synthesis [19]	May interact with certain medications, specifically gastric acid inhibitors (PPIs and H2 blockers) and metformin [19]	50–500 mcg (dose ranges depending on formulation and whether or not B12 is accompanied by other vitamins) [19]
Bacopa monnieri	Cognitive decline Sedative Antiepileptic [20]	*Bacopa* alcohol extract has shown memory-enhancing effects in three double-blind, randomized, placebo-controlled studies. May cause flu-like symptoms or digestive problems [20]	300–1000 mg
Echinacea	Immune health	Available echinacea products differ greatly. The overwhelming majority has not been tested in clinical trials. The use of chemically well-defined preparations is recommended [21]	10.2 g for the first 24 h following cold and 5.1 g following days [21]
Chromium	Might play a role in carbohydrate, lipid, and protein metabolism by potentiating insulin action [22]	Dietary supplements contain many forms of chromium (chromium picolinate, chromium nicotinate, chromium polynicotinate, chromium chloride, chromium histidinate). Absorption is similar across all forms and similar to proportion of chromium absorbed through food [22]	200–500 [22]

(continued)

Table B.1 (continued)

Name	Primary uses	Comments	Dosing
CoQ10	Antioxidant Cardiovascular disease Metabolic support Bone health Multiple sclerosis Fatigue Anti-inflammatory	May experience diarrhea or rash [23]	30–90 mg, taken in divided doses but up to 200 mg per day
Green tea	EGCG: potent antioxidant – polyphenols reduce inflammation [24] Chondroprotective [25] Parkinson's disease Chemoprotective	Both green tea and capsules/powder of EGCG work	400 mg *or* four cups *or* 1 tsp of matcha powder
Milk thistle	Anti-inflammatory and antioxidant	In particular, use with impaired digestion or liver function [26]	70–210 mg TID
5-HTP	Is appetite modifier and influences postmeal satiety [27] Plays major roles in circadian rhythmicity, thermoregulation, emotion, cognition, and nociception [28]	Caution in use with other drugs that increase serotonin level so as to prevent serotonin syndrome [29]	200–900 mg (depending on indication)
Ketones	Type 2 diabetes, can lower blood glucose and lipids [30]	"Keto flu": constipation, headache, halitosis, muscle cramps, diarrhea, and general weakness and rash [31]	3.2–13.2 $mmol.kg^{-1}$ [30]
Melatonin	Immune health Anti-inflammatory Controls eye pigmentation [32] Reduces sleep onset time and increasing sleep duration [33] Neurologic health Chemoprotective at high doses	Physiologic decrease in melatonin in the elderly [32]	0.1–5 mg [34] 3–5 mg sublingual or time-released formula for sleep [33]
Mushrooms	Anti-inflammatory Immune support Modify cytokines, direct anticancer agents, and interact with chemotherapeutic agents [35]	*Agaricus blazei*, *Cordyceps sinensis*, *Grifola frondosa*, *Ganoderma lucidum*, and *Trametes versicolor* [35]	1.5–3 g [36]
Quercetin	Antihistamine Immune support Anti-inflammatory Antioxidant Antinociceptive [37]	No significant side effects	500–1000 mg [38]

Table B.1 (continued)

Name	Primary uses	Comments	Dosing
Glutathione and NAC	Use in cases of liver damage and oxidative stress and inflammation Replenishes intracellular glutathione and cysteine levels and treats wide range of infections by restoring antioxidants [39]	Urine should be tested for sulfites. If positive, glutathione is contraindicated [40] Use extra caution in sun	600–1200 mg [41]
Therapeutic foods			
Garlic	Immune support Anti-inflammatory (supports glutathione) Antihypertensive Supports sulfation, a necessary step in liver detoxification	Rare GI disturbances [42]	180–960 mg (depending on indication) [42, 43]
Apple cider vinegar	GERD Probiotic, assists in protein utilization Stimulates digestion [44] Immune support	Often taken prophylactically	1–2 tsp 3× daily [44]
Adaptogens			
Ashwagandha	GABA mimetic effect, promotes formation of dendrites [45] Hypothyroid Anti-inflammatory Antioxidant Sleep	As an adaptogenic herb, beneficial effects take 2–3 weeks to be noticed	100–250 mg (thyroid) 125–600 (sleep) [46]
Astragalus	Immune support Supports chondrocyte proliferation [47] Topical use improves blood flow and wound healing Nephrotic syndrome	Rare rash, itching, and nasal or GI symptoms [48]	1.3 g [49]
Bacopa	Neural tonic Memory enhancer [50]	Rare side effects include nausea, increased intestinal motility, and GI upset [50]	300–1000 mg
Schizandra	Anticancer Antidiabetic Anti-obesity Protective against skin photoaging, osteoarthritis, sarcopenia, senescence, and mitochondrial dysfunction. It improves physical endurance and cognitive/behavioral functions [51]	No known side effects [51]	Dose not yet defined in humans

(continued)

Name	Primary uses	Comments	Dosing
Rhodiola	Cardiovascular disease [52] Depression [53]	Possible side effects include dizziness, dry mouth, or excessive saliva production [54]	50–680 mg (cardiovascular disease) [55] 340–1360 mg daily (depression)
Herbs			
Oregano	Antimicrobial SIBO [56] Antioxidant Anti-inflammatory Antidiabetic Cancer suppressant [57]	Can be used as a steam for sinus infections, careful to keep eyes closed	Dose not yet determined in humans
Berberine	SIBO [56] Immune support Diabetes support [58]	May cause GI disturbance [58]	500 mg, 2–3x daily
Olive leaf	Antimicrobial, antioxidant, and antiviral [59]	Bioavailability still uncertain	500–1000 mg [60]

Table B.2 below explains the difference between Vitamin K1 and K2.

Table B.2 Vitamin **K1 and K2 [61]**

	Vitamin K1	Vitamin K2, menaquinone-4 (MK4)	Vitamin K2, menaquinone-7 (MK7)
Function	Participates in blood clotting, cofactor for carboxylation	Osteocalcin (synthesized in the bone) serves as matrix GLa protein, involved in calcium transport, and helps improve bone density	As for MK4 but long-chain form with longer half-life
Source	Green leafy vegetables and some plant oils	Butter, eggs, yolks, lard, and animal-based foods. Synthesized by bacteria in the intestinal tract	Fermented foods and some cheese
Dose	100–500 mcg *Must be avoided if warfarin is co-administered*	15–45 mg *Caution is advised with warfarin; check INR within 2 weeks after initiating*	50–500 mcg *Caution is advised with warfarin; check INR within 2 weeks after initiating*

Secondary Supplements

Name	Primary uses	Comments	Dosing
Bee pollen	Immune support [62] Antifungal, antimicrobial, antiviral, anti-inflammatory, hepatoprotective, anticancer immunostimulating, and local analgesic [63]	Take before eating [63]	20–40 g [63]
Grapefruit essential oil	Depression Antimicrobial Anticancer Antioxidant [64] Anti-obesity [65]	Best antimicrobial effect on *Bacillus subtilis*, *Escherichia coli*, *Staphylococcus aureus*, and *Salmonellaty phimurium* [64]	Median effective dose 130.09 mg/mL [64]
Lavender	Anxiety Sleep Anti-inflammatory Antioxidant [66]	Oral capsules and aromatherapy are effective	80–160 mg [67]
CBD	Pain Anxiety Sleep Digestion	At the time of this writing, availability of CBD and *Cannabis* varies from state to state Best guidance is to start small and slowly increase to determine therapeutic dose	CBD 15–50 mg BID, if using low-dose THC then keep CBD/THC ratio at 10:1 or more. Often adding low-dose THC can boost CBD effectness

References

1. FDA. Dietary supplements [Internet]. US FDA. 2020 [cited 2021 Apr 14]. Available from: https://pubmed.ncbi.nlm.nih.gov/33412717/.
2. FDA. Questions and answers on dietary supplements [Internet]. US FDA. 2019 [cited 2021 Apr 15]. Available from: https://www.fda.gov/food/information-consumers-using-dietary-supplements/questions-and-answers-dietary-supplements.
3. Wheatley VM, Spink J. Defining the public health threat of dietary supplement fraud. Comp Rev Food Sci Food Safety. 2013;12(6):599–613.

4. Emerson Ecologics. EQP standards [Internet]. Emerson Ecologics. 2020 [cited 2021 May 27]. Available from: https://www.emersonecologics.com/blog/post/eqp-standards.

5. Masterjohn C. The Vitamins and Minerals 101 Cliff Notes. 2021.

6. Staruschenko A. Beneficial effects of high potassium. Hypertension. 2018;71(6):1015–22.

7. Pais P, Almeida V, Yılmaz M, Teixeira MC. Saccharomyces boulardii: what makes it tick as successful probiotic? J Fungi (Basel). 2020;6(2).

8. McFarland LV. Systematic review and meta-analysis of Saccharomyces boulardii in adult patients. World J Gastroenterol. 2010;16(18):2202–22.

9. Ianiro G, Pecere S, Giorgio V, Gasbarrini A, Cammarota G. Digestive enzyme supplementation in gastrointestinal diseases. Curr Drug Metab. 2016;17(2):187–93.

10. Institute of Medicine (US) Committee to Review Dietary Reference Intakes for Vitamin D and Calcium. Dietary reference intakes for calcium and vitamin D. In: Ross AC, Taylor CL, Yaktine AL, Del Valle HB, editors. Washington, DC: National Academies Press (US); 2011.

11. NIH. Calcium [Internet]. NIH Office of Dietary Supplements. 2021 [cited 2021 Apr 1]. Available from: https://ods.od.nih.gov/factsheets/Calcium-HealthProfessional/.

12. MTHFR Gene, Folic Acid, and Preventing Neural Tube Defects I CDC [Internet]. [cited 2021 May 25]. Available from: https://www.cdc.gov/ncbddd/folicacid/mthfr-gene-and-folic-acid.html.

13. Hoffman JR, Falvo MJ. Protein - which is best? J Sports Sci Med. 2004;3(3):118–30.

14. Hewlings SJ, Kalman DS. Curcumin: a review of its effects on human health. Foods. 2017;6(10).

15. Mietus-Snyder ML, Shigenaga MK, Suh JH, Shenvi SV, Lal A, McHugh T, et al. A nutrient-dense, high-fiber, fruit-based supplement bar increases HDL cholesterol, particularly large HDL, lowers homocysteine, and raises glutathione in a 2-wk trial. FASEB J. 2012;26(8):3515–27.

16. Thompson JM, Mirza MA, Park MK, Qureshi AA, Cho E. The role of micronutrients in alopecia areata: a review. Am J Clin Dermatol. 2017;18(5):663–79.

17. NIH. Iron [Internet]. NIH Office of Dietary Supplements. 2020 [cited 2021 Mar 5]. Available from: https://ods.od.nih.gov/factsheets/Iron-HealthProfessional/.

18. NIH. Folate [Internet]. National Institutes of Health Office of Dietary Supplements. 2020 [cited 2020 Dec 30]. Available from: https://ods.od.nih.gov/factsheets/Folate-HealthProfessional/.

19. Vitamin B12 [Internet]. NIH National Institutes of Health Office of Dietary Supplements. 2020 [cited 2021 Jan 2]. Available from: https://ods.od.nih.gov/factsheets/VitaminB12-HealthProfessional/.

20. Calabrese C, Gregory WL, Leo M, Kraemer D, Bone K, Oken B. Effects of a standardized Bacopa monnieri extract on cognitive performance, anxiety, and depression in the elderly: a randomized, double-blind, placebo-controlled trial. J Altern Complement Med. 2008;14(6):707–13.

21. Karsch-Völk M, Barrett B, Kiefer D, Bauer R, Ardjomand-Woelkart K, Linde K. Echinacea for preventing and treating the common cold. Cochrane Database Syst Rev. 2014;(2):CD000530.

22. NIH. Chromium [Internet]. NIH Office of Dietary Supplements. 2020 [cited 2021 Jan 31]. Available from: https://ods.od.nih.gov/factsheets/chromium-Consumer/.

23. Saini R. Coenzyme Q10: the essential nutrient. J Pharm Bioallied Sci. 2011;3(3):466–7.

24. Chacko SM, Thambi PT, Kuttan R, Nishigaki I. Beneficial effects of green tea: a literature review. Chin Med. 2010;5:13.

25. Leong DJ, Choudhury M, Hanstein R, Hirsh DM, Kim SJ, Majeska RJ, et al. Green tea polyphenol treatment is chondroprotective, anti-inflammatory and palliative in a mouse post-traumatic osteoarthritis model. Arthritis Res Ther. 2014 Dec 17;16(6):508.

26. Silybum marianum (milk thistle). Altern Med Rev. 1999;4(4):272–4.

27. Halford JCG, Harrold JA, Lawton CL, Blundell JE. Serotonin (5-HT) drugs: effects on appetite expression and use for the treatment of obesity. Curr Drug Targets. 2005;6(2):201–13.

28. Rancillac A. Serotonin and sleep-promoting neurons. Oncotarget. 2016;7(48):78222–3.

29. Cangiano C, Ceci F, Cascino A, Del Ben M, Laviano A, Muscaritoli M, et al. Eating behavior and adherence to dietary prescriptions in obese adult subjects treated with 5-hydroxytryptophan. Am J Clin Nutr. 1992;56(5):863–7.

30. Stubbs BJ, Cox PJ, Evans RD, Santer P, Miller JJ, Faull OK, et al. On the metabolism of exogenous ketones in humans. Front Physiol. 2017;8:848.

31. Harvey CJDC, Schofield GM, Williden M. The use of nutritional supplements to induce ketosis and reduce symptoms associated with keto-induction: a narrative review. PeerJ. 2018;6:e4488.

32. Yi C, Pan X, Yan H, Guo M, Pierpaoli W. Effects of melatonin in age-related macular degeneration. Ann N Y Acad Sci. 2005;1057:384–92.

33. Srinivasan V, Pandi-Perumal SR, Trahkt I, Spence DW, Poeggeler B, Hardeland R, et al. Melatonin and melatonergic drugs on sleep: possible mechanisms of action. Int J Neurosci. 2009;119(6):821–46.

34. Bahrampour Juybari K, Pourhanifeh MH, Hosseinzadeh A, Hemati K, Mehrzadi S. Melatonin potentials against viral infections including COVID-19: current evidence and new findings. Virus Res. 2020;287:198108.

35. Guggenheim AG, Wright KM, Zwickey HL. Immune modulation from five major mushrooms: application to integrative oncology. Integr Med (Encinitas). 2014;13(1):32–44.

36. Weil A. Integrative Geriatric Medicine. Kogan M, editor. Oxford University Press; 2018.

37. Valério DA, Georgetti SR, Magro DA, Casagrande R, Cunha TM, Vicentini FTMC, et al. Quercetin reduces inflammatory pain: inhibition of oxidative stress and cytokine production. J Nat Prod. 2009;72(11):1975–9.

38. Li Y, Yao J, Han C, Yang J, Chaudhry MT, Wang S, et al. Quercetin, inflammation and immunity. Nutrients. 2016;8(3):167.
39. Neag MA, Mocan A, Echeverría J, Pop RM, Bocsan CI, Crişan G, et al. Berberine: botanical occurrence, traditional uses, extraction methods, and relevance in cardiovascular, metabolic, hepatic, and renal disorders. Front Pharmacol. 2018;9:557.
40. Prousky J. The treatment of pulmonary diseases and respiratory-related conditions with inhaled (nebulized or aerosolized) glutathione. Evid Based Complement Alternat Med. 2008;5(1):27–35.
41. Minich DM, Brown BI. A review of dietary (phyto)nutrients for glutathione support. Nutrients. 2019;11(9).
42. Ried K, Frank OR, Stocks NP. Aged garlic extract reduces blood pressure in hypertensives: a dose-response trial. Eur J Clin Nutr. 2013;67(1):64–70.
43. Ried K, Travica N, Sali A. The effect of kyolic aged garlic extract on gut microbiota, inflammation, and cardiovascular markers in hypertensives: the gargic trial. Front Nutr. 2018;5:122.
44. Gunnars K. 6 Health Benefits of Apple Cider Vinegar, Backed by Science [Internet]. Healthline. 2020 [cited 2021 Mar 4]. Available from: https://www.healthline.com/nutrition/6-proven-health-benefits-of-apple-cider-vinegar.
45. Singh N, Bhalla M, de Jager P, Gilca M. An overview on ashwagandha: a Rasayana (rejuvenator) of Ayurveda. Afr J Tradit Complement Altern Med. 2011;8(5 Suppl):208–13.
46. Pratte MA, Nanavati KB, Young V, Morley CP. An alternative treatment for anxiety: a systematic review of human trial results reported for the Ayurvedic herb ashwagandha (Withania somnifera). J Altern Complement Med. 2014;20(12):901–8.
47. Song J, Lee SH, Lee D, Kim H. Astragalus extract mixture HT042 improves bone growth, mass, and microarchitecture in prepubertal female rats: a micro-computed tomographic study. Evid Based Complement Alternat Med. 2017;2017:5219418.
48. Astragalus | NCCIH [Internet]. [cited 2021 May 27]. Available from: https://www.nccih.nih.gov/health/astragalus
49. Kogan M, Weil A. Common rheumatic diseases in the elderly. In: Integrative geriatric medicine. Oxford Online; 2018. p. 463.
50. Aguiar S, Borowski T. Neuropharmacological review of the nootropic herb Bacopa monnieri. Rejuvenation Res. 2013;16(4):313–26.
51. Nowak A, Zakłos-Szyda M, Błasiak J, Nowak A, Zhang Z, Zhang B. Potential of Schisandra chinensis (Turcz.) Baill. in human health and nutrition: a review of current knowledge and therapeutic perspectives. Nutrients. 2019;11(2).
52. Maslova LV, Kondrat'ev BI, Maslov LN, Lishmanov IB. [The cardioprotective and antiadrenergic activity of an extract of Rhodiola rosea in stress]. Eksp Klin Farmakol. 1994;57(6):61–3.

53. Mao JJ, Li QS, Soeller I, Xie SX, Amsterdam JD. Rhodiola rosea therapy for major depressive disorder: a study protocol for a randomized, double-blind, placebo- controlled trial. J Clin Trials. 2014;4:170.
54. NIH. Rhodiola [Internet]. NIH National Center for Complementary and Integrative Health. 2020 [cited 2021 Jan 16]. Available from: https://www.nccih.nih.gov/health/rhodiola.
55. What is Rhodiola Rosea? [Internet]. Examine. 2021 [cited 2021 Jan 16]. Available from: https://examine.com/supplements/rhodiola-rosea/.
56. Chedid V, Dhalla S, Clarke JO, Roland BC, Dunbar KB, Koh J, et al. Herbal therapy is equivalent to rifaximin for the treatment of small intestinal bacterial overgrowth. Glob Adv Health Med. 2014;3(3):16–24.
57. Leyva-López N, Gutiérrez-Grijalva EP, Vazquez-Olivo G, Heredia JB. Essential oils of oregano: biological activity beyond their antimicrobial properties. Molecules. 2017;22(6).
58. Yin J, Xing H, Ye J. Efficacy of berberine in patients with type 2 diabetes mellitus. Metab Clin Exp. 2008;57(5):712–7.
59. Lockyer S, Yaqoob P, Spencer JPE, Rowland I. Olive leaf phenolics and cardiovascular risk reduction: physiological effects and mechanisms of action. NUA. 2012;1(2):125–40.
60. Kandola A. Health benefits of olive leaf extract [Internet]. Medical News Today. 2019 [cited 2021 Mar 9]. Available from: https://www.medicalnewstoday.com/articles/324878.
61. Mangano KM, Sahni S, Kerstetter JE. Dietary protein is beneficial to bone health under conditions of adequate calcium intake: an update on clinical research. Curr Opin Clin Nutr Metab Care. 2014;17(1):69–74.
62. Tukua D. 6 amazing health benefits of local, raw honey [Internet]. Farmers Almanac. 2020 [cited 2021 Mar 9]. Available from: https://www.farmersalmanac.com/local-raw-honey-22439.
63. Komosinska-Vassev K, Olczyk P, Kaźmierczak J, Mencner L, Olczyk K. Bee pollen: chemical composition and therapeutic application. Evid Based Complement Alternat Med. 2015;2015:297425.
64. Deng W, Liu K, Cao S, Sun J, Zhong B, Chun J. Chemical composition, antimicrobial, antioxidant, and antiproliferative properties of grapefruit essential oil prepared by molecular distillation. Molecules. 2020;25(1).
65. Dosoky NS, Setzer WN. Biological Activities and Safety of Citrus spp. Essential Oils. Int J Mol Sci. 2018;19(7).
66. Koulivand PH, Khaleghi Ghadiri M, Gorji A. Lavender and the nervous system. Evid Based Complement Alternat Med. 2013;2013:681304.
67. Malcolm BJ, Tallian K. Essential oil of lavender in anxiety disorders: ready for prime time? Ment Health Clin. 2017;7(4):147–55.

Appendix C: Drug-Nutrient Interactions

Many commonly used medications can cause alterations in nutrient balance. Table C.1 summarizes the effect of these medications along with associated risk factors.

Table C.1 Drug-nutrient interactions and known risk factors [1]

Drug category	Name	Nutrients	Effect on nutrient status	Risk factors
Acid-suppressing drugs	Proton pump inhibitors	Vitamin B12 Vitamin C Iron Calcium Magnesium Zinc β-Carotene	Decrease	Advanced age, *Helicobacter pylori* infection, genetics, vegetarians, iron deficiency, women, dose/duration of drug use
NSAIDs	Aspirin	Vitamin C Iron	Decrease	Advanced cold virus, advanced age, *H. pylori* infection, dose/duration of drug use
Anti-hypertensives	Diuretics (loop, thiazide, potassium-sparing), ACE inhibitors, calcium channel blockers	Calcium Magnesium Thiamin Zinc Potassium Folate Zinc Potassium Iron Folate Potassium	Decrease (loop)/ increase (thiazide) Decrease (loop and thiazide) Decrease (loop) Decrease (thiazide) Decrease (thiazide) Decrease Decrease Increase N/A Decrease Increase	Formation of loop diuretic, advanced age, women, heart failure, low magnesium intake, alcohol use, women, low thiamin intake, cirrhosis, diabetes mellitus, dose/ duration of drug use

(continued)

© The Editor(s) (if applicable) and The Author(s), under exclusive license to Springer Nature Switzerland AG 2021
J. Wendt et al., *Integrative Geriatric Nutrition*,
https://doi.org/10.1007/978-3-030-81758-9

Table C.1 (continued)

Drug category	Name	Nutrients	Effect on nutrient status	Risk factors
Hypercholesteremia	Statins	Coenzyme Q10 Vitamin D Vitamin E/B-Carotene	Decrease Increase/Decrease Increase/Decrease	Advanced age, statin-associated myopathy, heart disease, Vitamin D deficiency, dose/duration of drug use
Hypoglycemia	Biguanides (Metformin) Thiazolidinediones	Vitamin B12 Calcium/vitamin D	Decrease Decrease	Advanced age, vegetarians, women, low calcium/vitamin D intake, dose/duration of drug use
Corticosteroids	Glucocorticoids (oral)	Calcium/vitamin D Sodium/Potassium Chromium	Decrease Increase (Na)/decrease (K) Decrease	Low calcium/vitamin D intake, at risk for bone fracture/loss
Bronchodilators	Corticosteroids (inhaled)	Calcium/vitamin D	Decrease	Presence of COPD, smoking, at risk for bone fracture/loss, low calcium/vitamin D intake
Antidepressants	SSRIs	Folate Calcium/vitamin D	Increase Decrease	Low folate intake, genetics (MTHFR variants), alcoholism, at risk for bone fracture/loss, low calcium/vitamin D intake

Reference

1. Mohn ES, Kern HJ, Saltzman E, Mitmesser SH, McKay DL. Evidence of drug-nutrient interactions with chronic use of commonly prescribed medications: an update. Pharmaceutics. 2018;10(1).

Appendix D: Functional Testing

Below please find key lab testing for toxicities, food sensitivities, digestive issues, toxicities, and nutrient deficiencies. For complete information (and additional functional lab testing), please see *Integrative Geriatric Medicine* [1].

Nutritional testing can be helpful in a myriad of patient concerns including the following:

- Behavioral or mood imbalances (depression, anxiety, ADD/ADHD, OCD)
- Chronic fatigue or fibromyalgia
- Cognitive decline, Alzheimer's disease
- Headaches/migraines
- Weight loss/gain resistance
- Heartburn
- Insomnia/sleep disorders
- Irritable bowel syndrome (IBS) and irritable bowel disease (IBD)
- Gastrointestinal tract disorders (constipation, diarrhea, gas, bloating)
- Autoimmune disease
- Hormonal imbalances
- Cardiovascular disease
- Arthritis
- Chemical sensitivities
- Eczema, psoriasis, and atopic dermatitis

Food Sensitivities

There is no one best way to diagnose food sensitivities. IgE tests, RAST/blood tests, and skin prick tests are most common. These look for type 1 acute hypersensitivity reactions. IgG (blood) and IgA (blood, stool, or saliva) tests along with lymphocyte

J. Wendt et al., *Integrative Geriatric Nutrition*,
https://doi.org/10.1007/978-3-030-81758-9

reactivity assays or other non-antibody-mediated cytotoxicity tests look for type 1 acute hypersensitivity reactions. Of note, IgG tests are covered by many insurance companies but tend to have a high false-positive rate. Type 3 and 4 hypersensitivity tests are the most difficult to test for, as the reactions themselves are more complicated. Of note, since the COVID-19 pandemic, patients can conduct many of these tests at home through a finger prick. As such, we have seen an increase in direct to consumer allergy testing.

There is a long list of conditions that may benefit from food sensitivity testing. These include, but are not limited to, GI disorders, neurological symptoms, respiratory disease, metabolic/endocrine disorders, etc. For a complete list, please refer to Integrative Geriatric Medicine (Chapter 25) [2].

The gold standard in food sensitivity testing is the elimination and reintroduction diet. Potential trigger foods should be avoided for a minimum of 3–6 weeks before reintroduction to determine reactivity. It should be acknowledged that elimination diets can be difficult in the geriatric population due to reduced access to nutrients and requires expertise to implement.

Nutritional Status

Fundamental to functional lab testing is understanding the nutrients and metabolites in blood cells, plasma, urine, and hair. Functional lab tests help guide providers in recommendations on nutrient supplementation, microbiome status, neurotransmitter metabolism, energy production and mitochondrial function, vitamin and mineral metabolism, detoxification, and oxidative stress. A wide range of conditions may benefit from functional lab testing. For a complete list, please refer to *Integrative Geriatric Medicine* (Chapter 25) [2].

Toxicities

Part of the integrative approach to nutrition includes understanding the environment we live in. Unfortunately, this environment can be responsible for hosting toxic chemicals and elements that show up in the food we eat, air we breathe, and space we occupy. Toxins can come from the outside world or be produced from within by pathogenic bacteria. They can wreak havoc on many organ systems, interrupt metabolism, and interfere with homeostasis. Many chronic conditions (e.g., autoimmune, neurodegenerative, cancer, and diabetes) have been associated with toxin exposure (Sears and Genuis 2012). Functional labs help quantify exposure to such toxins, such as mercury, lead, arsenic, and persistent organic pollutants (POPs). Functional labs can also help us determine the effectiveness of our natural detoxification system, the liver. For more information on labs beneficial in understanding toxic exposures, please refer to *Integrative Geriatric Medicine* (Chapter 25) [1]. For recommendations on how to minimize these toxic exposures, please see the Environmental Working Group (http://www.ewg.org/).

Digestive

Stool Testing

Typical digestive analysis in a traditional outpatient setting is the ova and parasite test. While it is helpful, this test misses a wide range of digestive issues, including testing for digestive function, microbiome balance, digestive tract inflammation, or bacteria and yeast growth. These are evaluated by looking at digestive enzyme breakdown products, inflammatory markers, short-chain fatty acids, DNA-identified or cultured bacteria, cultured yeast, ova and parasite microscopy, pH, occult blood, PCR-DNA analysis, intestinal permeability, hydrogen/methane breath tests, and more. A wide range of conditions may benefit from the use of functional digestive lab testing. For a complete list, please refer to *Integrative Geriatric Medicine* (Chapter 25) [2].

Breath Testing

Assessment of small intestinal bacterial overgrowth (SIBO) via breath testing can often elucidate the root cause of many patients suffering from IBS. The gold standard test is a 3-h methane/hydrogen breath test which can be ordered by a gastroenterologist or through specialty functional lab companies such as Genova Diagnostics and Aerodiagnostics.

Below, please find suggested functional laboratory testing based on macronutrient or micronutrient of interest (Fig. D.1).

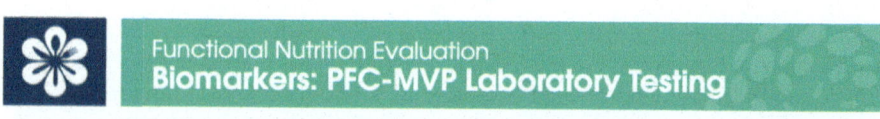

Functional Nutrition Evaluation
Biomarkers: PFC-MVP Laboratory Testing

	1st Tier Clinically Useful, More Cost Effective	2nd Tier Clinically Useful, Less Cost Effective	3rd Tier Unique Associated Patterns, May Be Less Cost Effective
P = Protein			
	▪ Total Protein ▪ Albumin ▪ Globulin	▪ Prealbumin – Transthyretin ▪ Plasma Amino Acids ▪ Carnitine	▪ Urinary Amino Acids ▪ Transferrin ▪ Fibronectin ▪ Somatomedin C ▪ 3-Methylhistadine ▪ Serum Proteins Electrophoresis
F = Fats			

	▪ Lipid Profile and Ratios
	  Total Cholesterol (TC)
	  Low Density Lipoprotein (LDL)
	  High Density Lipoprotein (HDL)
	  Triglycerides (TG)
	▪ Lipid Particle Number, Size and Subfractions
	▪ TG/HDL Ratio
	▪ Apolipoprotein B (ApoB)
	▪ Apolipoprotein A1 (ApoA1)
	▪ ApoB/A1 Ratio
		▪ Red Blood Cell Essential Fatty Acid Panel (RBC EFA)
		▪ Omega 3 Index
		▪ Plasma Essential Fatty Acid (EFA) Panel
		▪ Oxidized LDL	

C = Carbohydrates			
	▪ Fasting Blood Glucose ▪ Fasting Insulin Homeostatic Model Assessment of Insulin Resistance (HOMA-IR) Score ▪ Hemoglobin A1c (HgA1c) ▪ Triglycerides ▪ Gamma-Glutamyl Transferase (GGT) ▪ Uric Acid	▪ Adiponectin ▪ Fructosamine	▪ ½ hour Glucose Tolerance Test (gtt) for glucose and insulin ▪ 1 and 2 hour gtt for glucose and insulin levels
M = Minerals			
Foundational	▪ Complete Blood Count with differential (CBC w/diff) ▪ Comprehensive Metabolic Panel (CMP)		
Calcium	▪ Serum Calcium (Ca^{2+}) ▪ Ionized Calcium		▪ Parathyroid Hormone (PTH) ▪ 1,25-Dihydroxy Vitamin D_3 (1,25 OH$_2$ D_3) ▪ 25-Hydroxy Vitamin D_3 (25 OH D_3) ▪ Urinary Calcium

Version 9   © 2017 The Institute for Functional Medicine

Fig. D.1 Functional nutrition evaluation Biomarkers: BFC-MVP Laboratory Testing [3]. Used with permission from the Institute for Functional Medicine (IFM), a global leader in functional medicine and a collaborator in the transformation of healthcare. IFM is a 501(c)(3) nonprofit organization that believes functional medicine can help every individual reach their full potential for health and well-being. Under no circumstances may the whole or any part of the materials be translated into another language, nor may you create derivative or other works without IFM's prior written permission (for permission, please contact permissions@ifm.org)

Functional Nutrition PFC-MVP Biomarkers

Vitamin E		• Serum Vitamin E
		  ○ Alpha Tocopherol
		  ○ Gamma Tocopherol	

Vitamin K	• Prothrombin Time (PT) • Partial Thromboplastin Time (PTT)	• Serum Phylloquinone (Vitamin K1) • Under-Carboxylated Osteocalcin	
Water Soluble			

Vitamin B1
(Thiamine)
	• Plasma Thiamine	• Red Blood Cell (RBC) Transketolase Index	• Urine Alpha Ketoacids
			  ○ Isovalerate
			  ○ Isocaproate
			  ○ Methylvalerate
			• Plasma Isoleucine

Vitamin B2
(Riboflavin)
	• Plasma Riboflavin		• Urine Alpha Ketoacids
			  ○ Methyl succinate
			  ○ Ethylmalonate

Vitamin B3 (Niacin)			• Urine Lactate • Urine Pyruvate • N-Methylnicotinamide
Vitamin B6 (Pyridoxine)	• Homocysteine • Plasma Pyridoxal-5 Phosphate (P5P)	• Urine Xanthurenate • Urine Kynurenate	• Tryptophan Load Test • Methionine Load Test • Cystathionine-Beta-Synthase (CBS) SNPs*
Vitamin B7 (Biotin)		• Urine Alpha and Beta Hydroxyisovalerate	
Vitamin B9 (Folate)	• Serum Folate • Homocysteine • Mean Corpuscular Volume (MCV)	• Red Blood Cell (RBC) Folate • Urine Formiminoglutamic acid (FIGLU)	• Unmetabolized Folic Acid • Methylenetetrahydrofolate reductase (MTHFR) (677, 1298,...) SNPs* • Catechol-O-Methyltransferase (COMT) SNPs*
Vitamin B12 (Cobalamin)	• Serum B12 • Homocysteine • Methylmalonic Acid (MMA) • Mean Corpuscular Volume (MCV) • Mean Corpuscular Hemoglobin (MCH)		• Methionine Synthase (MTR) SNPs* • Methionine Synthase Reductase (MTRR) SNPs*
Vitamin C (Ascorbic Acid)			• Serum Vitamin C • White Blood Cell (WBC) Vitamin C
P = Phytonutrients			
		• Lipid Peroxides • Oxidized LDL • 8-Hydroxydeoxyguanosine (8-OHdG) • Total Antioxidant Capacity	• Red Blood Cell (RBC) Glutathione • Serum Coenzyme Q10 (CoQ10)

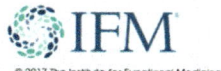

*SNPs = Single nucleotide polymorphisms

© 2017 The Institute for Functional Medicine

Fig. D.1 (continued)

Functional Nutrition PFC-MVP Biomarkers			
Calcium (cont.)			• Bone Resorption Markers (N-Telopeptide, 24 Hour Urine Calcium, 24 Hour Urine Protein, Pyridinium Crosslinks, Deoxypyridinoline,....)
Copper	• Serum Copper • Ceruloplasmin	• Red Blood Cell (RBC) Copper	
Iodine		• Spot First Morning Urine Iodine • 24 Hour Urine Iodine	

Iron	• Serum Iron
	• Transferrin
	• Total Iron Binding Capacity (TIBC)
	• Ferritin
	• Complete Blood Count (CBC)
	  - Hemoglobin (Hgb)
	  - Hematocrit (Hct)
	  - Mean Corpuscular Volume (MCV)
	  - Mean Corpuscular Hemoglobin (MCH)
	• Hemachromatosis (HFE) Gene Panel		

Magnesium	• Serum Magnesium (Mg^{2+}) • Red Blood Cell (RBC) Magnesium	• Buccal Cell Magnesium • Ionized Magnesium by Nuclear Magnetic Resonanace (NMR) • Urinary Magnesium – 24 hour	• Magnesium Load
Phosphorus	• Serum Phosphorus		
Selenium	• Serum Selenium	• Red Blood Cell (RBC) Selenium	• Glutathione Peroxidase
Zinc	• Plasma Zinc (Zn^{2+})	• Red Blood Cell (RBC) Zinc • Urinary Zinc – 24 hour	• Serum Metallothionein

V = Vitamins			
Foundational	• Complete Blood Count with differential (CBC w/diff)		
Fat Soluble			
Vitamin A		• Serum Beta Carotene • Serum Retinol	• Retinol Binding Protein
Vitamin D	• Serum 25-Hydroxy Vitamin D_3 (25 OH$_2$ D_3)	• Serum 1,25-Dihydroxy Vitamin D_3 (1,25 OH$_2$ D_3)	• Parathyroid Hormone (PTH) • Ionized Calcium • Vitamin D Receptor (VDR) Gene Panel – Fok1, Taq1, Bsm1 SNPs*

*SNPs = Single nucleotide polymorphisms

Fig. D.1 (continued)

References

1. Weil A. Integrative geriatric medicine. Kogan M, editor. Oxford University Press; 2018.
2. Weil A, Kogan M. Functional laboratory studies. In: Oxford, editor. Integrative geriatric medicine. 2018. p. 503–15.
3. IFM. Functional Nutrition Evaluation [Internet]. Institute for Functional Medicine. 2021 [cited 2021 May 30]. Available from: https://www.ifm.org/learning-center/?hsa_kw=institute%20functional%20medicine&hsa_net=adwords&hsa_grp=79398164764&hsa_cam=6479100630&hsa_acc=4746158419&hsa_tgt=aud-882708901821:kwd-358094946884&hsa_ver=3&hsa_ad=434238175600&hsa_mt=p&hsa_src=g&gclid=Cj0KCQjw78yFBhCZARIsAOxgSx3WSaE8380DsnYtq3QQCo2Djttg_RSfhoEN8oa9VYxNkw3dZzHwymYaAqwaEALw_wcB&gclsrc=aw.ds.

Appendix E: Micronutrient Deficiencies

Micronutrients play a critical role in cellular health as they are key cofactors required to run our biochemical reactions. Deficiencies in micronutrients impact the ability of the cell to function optimally, and over time, insufficient micronutrients create cells that are dysfunctional which then create tissues that do not work well, and with enough time, we can see the degradation of organs, and subsequently the disease process is born. Integrative nutrition always begins with an assessment of cellular health, and micronutrients take center stage!

There are some key abbreviations that are helpful to understand when it comes to micronutrients because their distinction is meaningful [1]:

- Recommended dietary allowance (RDA) : The FDA defines RDA as "the average amount of a nutrient a healthy person should get each day. RDAs vary by age, gender and whether a woman is pregnant or breastfeeding. RDAs are developed by the Food and Nutrition Board at the Institute of Medicine of the National Academies."
- Adequate intake (AI): The FDA sets AI when evidence is insufficient to develop an RDA and is set at a level assumed to ensure nutritional adequacy.
- Tolerable upper intake level (UL) is defined by the FDA as the "maximum daily intake unlikely to cause adverse health effects."

The Institute of Medicine uses these three measurements to create a dietary reference intake (DRI) which the National Institutes of Health's Office of Dietary Supplements maintains on their website at https://ods.od.nih.gov/HealthInformation/Dietary_Reference_Intakes.aspx. These are based on population studies for general health and are not appropriate when using nutrient therapeutically to alter a disease process or accommodate for genetic variations that create inefficiencies in how cofactors are used.

Personalized medicine is no doubt the future of medicine. The ability to personalize nutrition is within the scope of integrative nutrition, and we have shared various tools by which that is accomplished such as nutrigenomic testing, functional nutrition testing, physical examination, toxicity testing, and standard laboratory assessment. Using a patient's actual biomarkers to determine how much of a micronutrient is needed is personalized nutrition. We now have the tools to do this if we know it's possible. Thus throughout the book, our recommended supplement dosing to impact therapeutic responses will be different in many cases from the RDA or DRI.

Deciphering nutritional labels can be challenging for anyone. There are a few pieces of the label that are most important to understand. The first is the information on serving size. Oftentimes, containers or packages contain more than one serving, and one serving can be smaller than we think. Second, the calories show the energy consumed in each serving. The third and largest portion of the label, nutrients, explains the micronutrients and macronutrients included in each serving. Saturated fat, sodium, and added sugars are some of the nutrients we should be consuming less of. Dietary fiber, vitamin D, calcium, iron, and potassium are some of the nutrients we should be getting more of. Fourth and final is the % daily value, the percentage of the daily value that each nutrient in a serving of food contributes to a total daily diet. This can help you understand if a serving of food is high or low in a particular nutrient [2].

Table E.1 highlights key vitamins and minerals, their function in the body, food sources, and the RDA. Please also see Appendix F for signs, symptoms, and lab findings when these micronutrients are deficient.

Table E.1 Key micronutrients, function, source, and dosing

Vitamin/mineral	Functions	Top food sources	RDA[a]	Comments
Vitamin A: retinoids and carotene [3]	Immune function, vision, reproduction, cellular communication, skin integrity, and sleep health [4]	Beef liver, dairy fat, egg yolks, sweet potato, spinach, pumpkin pie, and carrots. Animal food sources contain retinol, while red, orange, yellow, and green vegetables contain carotenoids (provitamin A) which can be turned into retinol [4]	900 mcg RAE M 700 mcg RAE F (300–500 IU) [4]	Many things can hurt our ability to derive vitamin A from plant foods (too much fiber, deficiencies in vitamin E, protein, iron, zinc) or toxic compounds. Animal foods are a more reliable source of vitamin A [4]
[a]Vitamin D: calciferol [5]	Promotes calcium absorption in the gut, maintains serum calcium and phosphate concentrations to enable normal bone mineralization, reduces inflammation, and modulates cell growth, neuromuscular and immune function, and glucose metabolism	Cod liver oil, trout, salmon, mushrooms, milk, tuna, sardines, swordfish, and egg [6]	800 IU	Sunshine is the best source of vitamin D, best midday [4]. Interplay between serum Ca homeostasis, parathyroid hormone, and 1,25(OH)2D [6]
Vitamin E: alpha-tocopherol [7]	Antioxidant, involved in immune function, cell signaling regulation of gene expression, and other metabolic processes	Wheat germ oil, sunflower seeds, almonds, sunflower oil, safflower oil, and hazelnuts	15 mg	Most do not need a vitamin E supplement, but if you switch from high-PUFA oils to low-PUFA oils, supplementation may be beneficial [4]. Avoid synthetic vitamin E (all-rac or DL-alpha-tocopherol) [4]

(continued)

Table E.1 (continued)

Vitamin/mineral	Functions	Top food sources	RDA[a]	Comments
Vitamin K: phylloquinone and menadione [8]	Vitamin K1: participates in blood clotting, cofactor for carboxylation Vitamin K2: osteocalcin (synthesized in the bone) serves as matrix GLa protein, involved in calcium transport, and helps improve bone density	Vitamin K1: green leafy vegetables and some plant oils Vitamin K2: butter, eggs, yolks, lard, and animal-based foods. Synthesized by bacteria in the intestinal tract	Vitamin K1: 100–500 mcg Vitamin K2 (MK4): 15–45 mg Vitamin K2 (MK7) [8]	If supplementing with more than 500 mcg/d (excluding natural K found in food), balance each additional 500 mcg with 3000 IU vitamin A, 900 IU vitamin D, and 5 IU vitamin E [4]
[a]Vitamin B1: thiamin [9]	Has critical role in energy metabolism, is antioxidant, and supports methylation [4]. Growth of cells [6]	Rice, breakfast cereals, egg noodles, pork chop, trout, black beans, nutritional yeast, legumes, mussels, tuna, acorn squash, and sunflower seeds [4, 6]	1.2 mg M 1.1 mg F	Will retain and activate more vitamin B1 if taken with meals [4]. Measured indirectly via transketolase [6]
Vitamin B2: riboflavin [10]	Plays major role in energy production, cellular function, growth and development, and metabolism of fats, drugs, and steroids, is antioxidant, and supports methylation [4]	Beef liver, breakfast cereals, oats, yogurt, milk, beef, and clams	1.3 mg M 1.1 mg F	Free riboflavin is best for most (rather than riboflavin 5'-phosphate), taken with meals and spread out evenly throughout the day [4]
Vitamin B3: niacin [11]	Required in most metabolic redox processes, genome integrity and expression, and cellular communication. Supports the mind, gut, and skin. Provides antioxidant and anti-inflammatory support and neurotransmitter support [4]	Beef liver, chicken, marinara, turkey breast, salmon, tuna, pork, and nutritional yeast [4]	16 mg NE M 14 mg NE F	If used to lower cholesterol, avoid snacking on carbs 3–6 h post-dose and pair with glycine and trimethylglycine If used for antiaging, use nicotinamide riboside, nicotinamide mononucleotide, or nicotinamide and pair with TMG If used in multivitamin or B complex form, look for forms of nicotinamide or nicotinic acid or nicotinate [4]

Vitamin B5: pantothenic acid [12]	Key player in fatty acid synthesis. Supports acne, high cholesterol, anemia, and poor wound healing [4]	Beef liver, breakfast cereals, shiitake mushrooms, sunflower seeds, and nutritional yeast	5 mg	Large amounts can interfere with absorption of biotin and lipoic acid. Best to take B5 away from foods rich in these two nutrients [4]
[a]Vitamin B6: pyridoxine [13]	Involved in numerous enzyme reactions, including protein, carbohydrate, and lipid metabolism, cognitive development, gluconeogenesis, glycogenolysis, and immune function and neurotransmitter synthesis [6]	Chickpeas, beef liver, tuna, salmon, chicken, potatoes, turkey, banana, and breakfast cereals [6]	1.7 mg M 1.5 mg F	Pyridoxal 5'phosphate (P5P) is the best supplement [4]. Can be conditionally deficient when B9 and B12 are deficient. Functional marker is homocysteine (as well as B12) [6]
Vitamin B7 (biotin)	Required for energy metabolism, fatty acid synthesis, and hair and skin health [4]	Egg yolks, beef liver, chicken liver, peanuts, sunflower seeds, almonds, and walnuts [4]	30 mcg [14]	Can interfere with absorption of B5 and lipoic acid, best to take biotin away from these two nutrients [4]
[a]Vitamin B9: folate [15]	Methyl donor, required for cellular division, as it is involved in synthesis of nucleic acids and metabolism of amino acids	Beef liver, spinach, black-eyed peas, breakfast cereals, rice asparagus, brussels sprouts, romaine lettuce, avocado, broccoli, and mustard greens [6]	400 mcg DFE	Variations in folate-related genes can make it difficult to use synthetic folic acid (e.g., MTHFR gene) [4]

(continued)

Table E.1 (continued)

Vitamin/mineral	Functions	Top food sources	RDA[a]	Comments
[a]Vitamin B12: cobalamin [16]	Required for development, myelination, and function of the central nervous system, RBC formation, and DNA synthesis	Beef liver, clams, tuna, nutritional yeast, salmon, beef, milk, and trout	2.4 mcg	Hydroxocobalamin is preferred; methylcobalamin can support methylation system [4]. Blood markers of functional deficiency are elevated methylmalonic acid and homocysteine (as well as B6) [6] Less common form adenosylcobalamin is also available. Therapeutic doses can be in 1–5 mg/day in oral, sublingual, or subcutaneous or intramuscular injections
Vitamin C: ascorbic acid [17]	Is required for the biosynthesis of collagen, L-carnitine, and certain neurotransmitters, involved in protein metabolism, is antioxidant, has important role in immune function, and improves absorption of nonheme iron	Red pepper, orange juice, orange, grapefruit, kiwifruit, green pepper, and broccoli	90 mg M and 75 mg F	People with a history of kidney stones, of hemochromatosis, and of G6PD deficiency should take caution with vitamin C supplements [4]
Boron [18]	May have beneficial effects on reproduction and development, calcium metabolism, bone formation, brain function, insulin and energy substrate metabolism, immunity, and function of steroid hormones	Prune juice, avocado, raisins, peaches, and grape juice	Insufficient data to derive an RDA. The WHO estimates 1–3 mg/day is "acceptable"	No known medication interaction, side effects, or specifics about formulations

	Function	Sources	Amount	Notes
Choline [19]	Required for cell membrane structure, needed to produce acetylcholine, an important neurotransmitter for memory, mood, muscle control, and other brain and nervous system functions. Also plays important roles in modulating gene expression, cell membrane signaling lipid transport and metabolism, and early brain development	Beef liver, egg, beef, soybeans, and chicken	550 mg M 425 mg F	Alpha-GPC is best supplement for neurological health, anxiety, and muscle strength. Trimethylglycine is the best supplement for methylation. Betaine HCl is used for digestion. Phosphatidylcholine is best for liver health and fat digestion [4]
Calcium [20]	Required for vascular contractions and vasodilation, muscle function, nerve transmission, intracellular signaling, and hormonal secretion	Yogurt, orange juice, mozzarella, sardines, cheese, and milk	1200 mg	Calcium absorption from different foods is widely variable; best sources are dairy, bones, napa cabbage, Chinese mustard greens, and bok choy [4]
Chloride	Maintains osmotic and acid-base balance, muscular and nervous activity, and movement of water and solutes between fluid compartments [21]	Sodium chloride [21]	2300 mg [22]	Usually consumed with sodium in the form of sodium chloride
Chromium [23]	Might play a role in carbohydrate, lipid, and protein metabolism by potentiating insulin action	Grape juice, ham, English muffin, and brewer's yeast	30 mcg M 20 mcg F	May interact with insulin, metformin, other antidiabetes medications, and levothyroxine [23]

(continued)

Table E.1 (continued)

Vitamin/mineral	Functions	Top food sources	RDA[a]	Comments
Copper [24]	Involved in energy production, iron metabolism, neuropeptide activation, connective tissue synthesis, neurotransmitter synthesis, angiogenesis, neurohormone homeostasis, regulation of gene expression, brain development, pigmentation, and immune system functioning, antioxidant	Beef liver, oysters, baking chocolate, potatoes, mushrooms, and cashews	900 mcg	Zinc supplements can cause copper deficiency. Avoid zinc supplements over 50 mg/d unless you have a compelling reason otherwise. If supplementing with zinc, ensure the zinc-to-copper ratio is around 10–20:1 [4]
Fluoride [25]	Inhibits or reverses the initiation and progression of dental caries and stimulates new bone formation	Black tea, coffee, water with added fluoride, shrimp, and raisins	4 mg M and 3 mg F	Fluoridated drinking water prevents dental caries in both children and adults [25]
Iodine [26]	Essential component of thyroid hormones, required for proper skeletal and central nervous system development in fetuses and infants	Seaweed, bread, cod, yogurt, oysters, and milk	150 mcg	Goitrogenic foods (cruciferous vegetables), sulforaphane, fluoride, chlorine, and bromine can all interfere with iodine function [4]
[a]Iron [27]	Is essential component of hemoglobin and myoglobin and supports muscle metabolism and healthy connective tissues. Necessary for physical growth, neurological development, cellular functioning, and synthesis of some hormones and energy cycle [6]	Breakfast cereals, oysters, white beans, dark chocolate, beef liver, lentils, spinach, tofu, and kidney beans [6]	8 mg	Keeping inflammation low and getting plenty of copper and riboflavin are necessary to proper iron usage [4]. Iron from food comes in heme (animal) and nonheme (plant) forms. Heme iron is more bioavailable [6] Avoid prescribing for long periods of time if not deficient. Excess iron adds to free radical load

[a]Magnesium [28]	Cofactor in more than 300 enzyme reactions, including protein synthesis, muscle and nerve function, blood glucose control, blood pressure regulation, energy production, oxidative phosphorylation, and glycolysis [6]	Pumpkin seeds, chia seeds, almonds, spinach, cashews, peanuts, cereal, soymilk, black beans, wheat, edamame, avocado, potato, and brown rice	420 mg M 320 mg F	Alcoholism, diabetes, antacids, digestive problems, and increased urination can increase magnesium needs. Supplemental doses higher than 350 mg/d may cause GI side effects (softened stools, diarrhea) [4]. It is difficult to measure Mg status as most is in bones and blood; best test is Mg RBC, which still misses some patients with functional deficiency. Key signs of deficiency are muscle twitches and cramps, nervous tension, and difficulty sleeping [6]
Manganese [29]	Involved in amino acid metabolism; cholesterol, glucose, and carbohydrate metabolism; reactive oxygen species scavenging; bone formation; reproduction; and immune response, blood clotting, and hemostasis	Mussels, hazelnuts, pecans, brown rice, oysters, clams, and chickpeas	2.3 mg M 1.8 mg F	Manganese supplements should not be given to those with chronic liver disease or iron deficiency [4]
Molybdenum [30]	Supports metabolism of sulfur-containing amino acids, purines, and pyrimidines	Black-eyed peas, beef liver, lima beans, yogurt, milk, and potato	45 mcg	Diets rich in animal protein and poor in legumes are at risk for molybdenum deficiency (carnivore, paleo, keto, low carb, high protein) [4]

(continued)

Table E.1 (continued)

Vitamin/mineral	Functions	Top food sources	RDA[a]	Comments
Phosphorus [31]	Components of bones, teeth, DNA, and RNA. Key component of cell membrane structure and body's energy source. Key role in regulation of gene transcription, activation of enzymes, maintenance of normal pH in extracellular fluid, and intracellular energy storage	Yogurt, milk, salmon, scallops, cheese, chicken, and lentils	700 mg	Largely a risk of mostly fat diets, refeeding, anorexia, or other long-term decreases in food intake. Be sure to check vitamin D and calcium levels when assessing phosphorus levels [4]
Potassium [32]	Required for normal cell function due to its role in maintaining intracellular fluid volume and transmembrane electrochemical gradients	Apricots, lentils, prunes, squash, raisins, and potato	3,400 mg M 2,600 mg F	Those eating keto or low-carb high-fat diets need to eat large volumes of high-potassium, low-carb vegetables, while carnivores need to keep fat low and consume all meat juices [4]
[a]Selenium [33]	Plays critical role in reproduction, thyroid hormone metabolism, DNA synthesis, and protection from oxidative damage and infection	Brazil nuts, tuna, halibut, sardines, ham, shrimp, macaroni, beef steak, turkey, and beef liver	55 mcg	Vitamin B6, folate, B12, choline, protein, iodine, vitamins E and C, zinc, copper, manganese, and iron are all important to utilizing selenium effectively. Hashimoto's, Graves', and HIV are conditions where supplementation may be helpful [4]. No more than two Brazil nuts should be consumed per day to avoid risk of selenosis [6]
Sodium	Controls fluid balance and maintains blood volume and blood pressure [34]	Smoked, cured, salted, or canned meat/fish/poultry, frozen breaded meats and dinners, canned entrees, salted nuts, and canned beans	1,500 mg [22]	Keeping potassium in the 4700–11,000 mg/d range will allow most people to consume appropriate amounts of salt [4]

Sulfur	Builds and repairs DNA, antioxidant, synthesizes protein, regulates gene expression, and maintains integrity of connective tissues [35]	Organ meats, shrimp, scallops, legumes, nuts and seeds, whole eggs, and cheddar [35]	1000 mg (methionine) [36]	Methionine and cysteine are both sulfur-containing amino acids, but methionine cannot be synthesized by the body; it must be supplemented by the diet [36]
[a]Zinc [37]	Critical role in immune function, protein synthesis, wound healing, DNA synthesis, and cell division. Supports normal growth and development during pregnancy, childhood, and adolescence, required for proper taste and smell	Oysters, beef, crab, lobster, pork chop, and baked beans	11 mg M 8 mg F	Vegetarians and vegans must pay special attention to zinc intake. Sugar and fat can both displace zinc in diet. Moderating sweets using honey and molasses and focusing on high-fat top-tier zinc foods (oysters, liver, red meat) will help [4]. Three ounces of oysters contains nearly 500 % of the RDA for zinc. Functional deficiency symptoms include poor wound healing, decreased taste or smell, skin disorders, and depressed immune function [6]
[a]Hydrochloric acid (HCl)	Denatures proteins, increases absorption of minerals, and kills pathogens [6]	Apple cider vinegar [6]	1–2 tsp 3× daily [38]	GERD is usually a function of low stomach acid and an insufficient lower esophageal sphincter feedback loop [6]

[a]Indicates key nutritional deficiencies in older adults

References

1. NIH. Nutrient recommendations: dietary reference intakes [Internet]. NIH Office of Dietary Supplements. 2021 [cited 2021 May 29]. Available from: https://ods.od.nih.gov/HealthInformation/Dietary_Reference_Intakes.aspx.
2. FDA. How to understand and use the nutrition facts label [Internet]. FDA. 2020 [cited 2021 May 31]. Available from: https://www.fda.gov/food/new-nutrition-facts-label/how-understand-and-use-nutrition-facts-label.
3. NIH. Vitamin A [Internet]. Vitamin A. 2020 [cited 2021 Jan 30]. Available from: https://ods.od.nih.gov/factsheets/VitaminA-HealthProfessional/.
4. Masterjohn C. The vitamins and minerals 101 Cliff Notes. 2021.
5. NIH. Vitamin D [Internet]. NIH National Institutes of Health Office of Dietary Suppolements. 2020 [cited 2020 Dec 31]. Available from: https://ods.od.nih.gov/factsheets/VitaminD-HealthProfessional/
6. Weil A. Integrative geriatric medicine. Kogan M, editor. Oxford University Press; 2018.
7. NIH. Vitamin E [Internet]. NIH Office of Dietary Supplements. 2020 [cited 2021 Jan 30]. Available from: https://ods.od.nih.gov/factsheets/VitaminE-HealthProfessional/.
8. Mangano KM, Sahni S, Kerstetter JE. Dietary protein is beneficial to bone health under conditions of adequate calcium intake: an update on clinical research. Curr Opin Clin Nutr Metab Care. 2014;17(1):69–74.
9. NIH. Thiamin [Internet]. National Instiues of Health Office of Dietary Supplements. 2020 [cited 2021 Jan 16]. Available from: https://ods.od.nih.gov/factsheets/Thiamin-HealthProfessional/#:~:text=Food%20sources%20of%20thiamin%20include,major%20source%20of%20the%20vitamin.
10. NIH. Riboflavin [Internet]. NIH Office of Dietary Supplements. 2021 [cited 2021 Mar 18]. Available from: https://ods.od.nih.gov/factsheets/Riboflavin-HealthProfessional/.
11. NIH. Niacin [Internet]. NIH Office of Dietary Supplements. 2021 [cited 2021 Mar 5]. Available from: https://ods.od.nih.gov/factsheets/Niacin-HealthProfessional/.
12. NIH. Pantothenic Acid [Internet]. NIH Office of Dietary Supplements. 2021 [cited 2021 May 6]. Available from: https://ods.od.nih.gov/factsheets/PantothenicAcid-HealthProfessional/.
13. NIH. Vitamin B6 [Internet]. National Institutes of Health Office of Dietary Supplements. 2020 [cited 2020 Dec 30]. Available from: https://ods.od.nih.gov/factsheets/VitaminB6-HealthProfessional/#:~:text=The%20richest%20sources%20of%20vitamin,1%2C3%2C5%5D.
14. NIH. Biotin [Internet]. NIH Office of Dietary Supplements. 2020 [cited 2021 Feb 12]. Available from: https://ods.od.nih.gov/factsheets/Biotin-HealthProfessional/.
15. NIH. Folate [Internet]. National Institutes of Health Office of Dietary Supplements. 2020 [cited 2020 Dec 30]. Available from: https://ods.od.nih.gov/factsheets/Folate-HealthProfessional/.

16. Vitamin B12 [Internet]. NIH National Institutes of Health Office of Dietary Supplements. 2020 [cited 2021 Jan 2]. Available from: https://ods.od.nih.gov/factsheets/VitaminB12-HealthProfessional/.

17. NIH. Vitamin C [Internet]. National Institutes of Health Office of Dietary Supplements. 2020 [cited 2020 Dec 30]. Available from: https://ods.od.nih.gov/factsheets/VitaminC-HealthProfessional/.

18. NIH. Boron [Internet]. NIH Office of Dietary Supplements. 2021 [cited 2021 Apr 1]. Available from: https://ods.od.nih.gov/factsheets/Boron-HealthProfessional/#:~:text=The%20main%20sources%20of%20boron,cheese%20%5B6%2C20%5D.

19. NIH. Choline [Internet]. NIH Office of Dietary Supplements. [cited 2021 May 6]. Available from: https://ods.od.nih.gov/factsheets/Choline-HealthProfessional/.

20. NIH. Calcium [Internet]. NIH Office of Dietary Supplements. 2021 [cited 2021 Apr 1]. Available from: https://ods.od.nih.gov/factsheets/Calcium-HealthProfessional/.

21. EFSA Panel on Nutrition, Novel Foods and Food Allergens (NDA), Turck D, Castenmiller J, de Henauw S, Hirsch-Ernst K-I, Kearney J, et al. Dietary reference values for chloride. EFSA J. 2019;17(9):e05779.

22. Strohm D, Bechthold A, Ellinger S, Leschik-Bonnet E, Stehle P, Heseker H, et al. Revised reference values for the intake of sodium and chloride. Ann Nutr Metab. 2018;72(1):12–7.

23. NIH. Chromium [Internet]. NIH Office of Dietary Supplements. 2020 [cited 2021 Jan 31]. Available from: https://ods.od.nih.gov/factsheets/chromium-Consumer/.

24. NIH. Copper [Internet]. NIH Office of Dietary Supplements. 2020 [cited 2021 Mar 9]. Available from: https://ods.od.nih.gov/factsheets/Copper-HealthProfessional/.

25. NIH. Fluoride [Internet]. NIH Office of Dietary Supplements. 2021 [cited 2021 May 6]. Available from: https://ods.od.nih.gov/factsheets/Fluoride-HealthProfessional/.

26. NIH. Iodine [Internet]. NIH Office of Dietary Supplements. 2021 [cited 2021 May 6]. Available from: https://ods.od.nih.gov/factsheets/Iodine-HealthProfessional/.

27. NIH. Iron [Internet]. NIH Office of Dietary Supplements. 2020 [cited 2021 Mar 5]. Available from: https://ods.od.nih.gov/factsheets/Iron-HealthProfessional/.

28. NIH. Magnesium [Internet]. National Institutes of Health Office of Dietary Supplements. 2020 [cited 2020 Dec 30]. Available from: https://ods.od.nih.gov/factsheets/Magnesium-HealthProfessional/#:~:text=Magnesium%20is%20widely%20distributed%20in,cereals%20and%20other%20fortified%20foods.

29. NIH. Manganese [Internet]. NIH Office of Dietary Supplements. 2021 [cited 2021 May 6]. Available from: https://ods.od.nih.gov/factsheets/Manganese-HealthProfessional/.

30. NIH. Molybdenum [Internet]. NIH Office of Dietary Supplements. 2021 [cited 2021 May 6]. Available from: https://ods.od.nih.gov/factsheets/Molybdenum-HealthProfessional/.
31. NIH. Phosphorus [Internet]. NIH Office of Dietary Supplements. 2021 [cited 2021 May 6]. Available from: https://ods.od.nih.gov/factsheets/Phosphorus-HealthProfessional/.
32. NIH. Potassium [Internet]. NIH Office of Dietary Supplements. 2021 [cited 2021 May 5]. Available from: https://ods.od.nih.gov/factsheets/Potassium-HealthProfessional/.
33. NIH. Selenium [Internet]. NIH Office of Dietary Supplements. 2020 [cited 2021 Jan 30]. Available from: https://ods.od.nih.gov/factsheets/Selenium-HealthProfessional/.
34. Guidelines for a Low Sodium Diet [Internet]. UCSF Health. [cited 2021 May 5]. Available from: https://www.ucsfhealth.org/education/guidelines-for-a-low-sodium-diet.
35. All You Need to Know About Sulfur-Rich Foods [Internet]. Healthline. 2021 [cited 2021 May 5]. Available from: https://www.healthline.com/nutrition/foods-with-sulfur.
36. Nimni ME, Han B, Cordoba F. Are we getting enough sulfur in our diet? Nutr Metab (Lond). 2007;4:24.
37. NIH. Zinc [Internet]. NIH Office of Dietary Supplements. 2020 [cited 2021 Feb 5]. Available from: https://ods.od.nih.gov/factsheets/Zinc-HealthProfessional/.
38. Gunnars K. 6 Health Benefits of Apple Cider Vinegar, Backed by Science [Internet]. Healthline. 2020 [cited 2021 Mar 4]. Available from: https://www.healthline.com/nutrition/6-proven-health-benefits-of-apple-cider-vinegar.

Appendix F: Integrative Nutrition Assessment Guide

There are often subtle cues to imbalances in the body that provide critical insights into the nutritional status of the patient which either will not show up in standard laboratory tests or when they do show up, the imbalance has created a level of dysfunction that requires medical intervention. When the provider is aware of how to assess nutritional imbalance before it gets to a critical state, the patient can get the support needed to re-establish optimal function (Table F.1).

Table F.1 Nutritional assessment tools for the geriatric population [1]

Region/subject	Indication	Assessment	Clinical notes	Therapeutic foods
Physical assessment	*Tongue* Red and inflamed Coated Bald, slick, and red	Niacin deficiency Digestive enzymes, probiotics, and fiber B vitamins, cobalamin, and iron		Brewer's yeast, rice and wheat bran, liver, peanuts, sesame and sunflower seeds, oysters, white beans, dark chocolate, and lentils
	Mouth Cheilosis	Riboflavin and iron		Oysters, white beans, dark chocolate, beef liver, lentils, spinach, tofu, brewer's yeast, almonds, wheat germ, and rice
	Ears Hard earwax Vertical lobe crease Sound sensitivity Tinnitus	Omega-3 Magnesium, B complex, omega-3, and CoQ10 Mg and Zinc Niacinamide, pyridoxine	Allergies Cardiovascular risk Temporomandibular joint disorders	Fatty fish, leafy greens, oysters, nuts, pumpkin seeds, ginger, kelp, molasses, buckwheat, and wheat
	Eyes Burning, itching, and bloodshot Dry, soft cornea, and xerosis Eyelid pallor Iris: copper ring Vision dysfunction	Riboflavin Vitamin A and zinc Iron Zinc Omega-3, and thiamine	Excess copper, Wilson's disease Hypoadrenalism	Prioritize foods with high zinc content and limit foods with high copper Liver, chili peppers, dandelion root, carrots, dried apricots, and leafy greens
	Hair Lackluster Thinning/loss	Biotin Essential fatty acids Protein Zinc	Screen for hypothyroid and excess vitamin A	Brewer's yeast, liver, soy, rice, peanuts, nuts, fatty fish, and oysters
	Nails White spots Pale nail beds	Zinc Iron deficiency		Oysters, pumpkin seeds, ginger, pecans, split peas, Brazil nuts, wheat, rye, and oats
	Skin Acne, eczema, dermatitis, and psoriasis Peeling hands/feet Rosacea	Zinc; vitamins A, D, and B; and niacin Omega-3, vitamins A and D, and zinc Riboflavin + B complex	Consider food sensitivities, especially dairy	Oysters, mushrooms, fatty fish, red palm oil, nuts and seeds, and leafy greens
	Sinusitis	Vitamins C, A, and B5, zinc, quercetin, and B-carotene	Allergies, especially dairy	Acerola, chili peppers, guavas, sweet peppers, leafy greens, onions, apples, and pomegranate

Subjective testing	Decreased taste and/or smell	Use zinc tally test to assess zinc sufficiency	RA related to zinc deficiency Medications influence zinc status Toxins block zinc
	Metallic taste		Excess zinc, toxic metals
Objective testing	Mini Nutritional Assessment – Short Form (MNA-SF)		In a 2012 prospective cohort study, MNA-SF scores of 11 or below correlated with nutritional malnutrition that was confirmed with biochemical workup of albumin, cholesterol, and vitamins A and D
	SNAQ (Simplified Nutritional Assessment Questionnaire)	Anorexics at risk of weight loss over the next 6 months	
	All patients	Genetic testing (www.23andme.com)	Use full genetic code in various interpretive online applications to assess SNPs that respond well to directed nutritional interventions such as COMT, MTHFR, CBS, MAO, and DAO
	Urinary 8-OHdG	Increase food-based antioxidants	Oxidative stress marker that is adversely involved in aging process
	Uric acid elevation	Essential fatty acid deficiency	Associated with antioxidant deficiency and high-sugar diet or diabetes
	Bioimpedance analysis		Inexpensive and noninvasive technology to estimate body composition (fat, water, bone)
	Complete blood count	Transferrin (half-life of 8 days) Prealbumin (half-life of 17–21 days) Albumin (half-life of 17–21 days) Hypocholesterolemia Iron-Iron-binding capacity Total lymph count	

Modified with permission from Dana Lake

Reference

1. Weil A. Integrative geriatric medicine. Kogan M, editor. Oxford University Press; 2018.

Appendix G: Health Coaching Handouts to Support the Change Process

Likely the hardest part of integrative medicine is the lifestyle change process that is imperative to the success of the approach. A 2013 meta-analysis studying the changes to lifestyle over 9 years found that only 13 % of participants maintained a change in exercise patterns [1]. The most radical aspect of integrative medicine rests in the principle that lifestyle change happens each moment that you choose your health over the status quo. Each time a patient chooses to go for a walk or eat a salad, they are saying yes to their health and longevity. However, there isn't one change or one effort alone that will reward them. It's the day-in and day-out process of choosing to live in a health-focused way that will ultimately reward them with the best of health and longevity. This goes against human nature! Therefore, a critical role that must be filled is that steady reminder of why they are making these efforts.

It's imperative that providers understand precisely how hard lifestyle changes can be for all patients but even more so the aging adult that has been accustomed to the problematic habits for 6–7 decades! Once we providers embrace this as a critical step, the ability to adequately support the change process can be integrated into the care model.

There are many approaches to supporting lifestyle change. Many offices employ a health coach specifically trained to support change for their patients which allows the provider to create the plan and the health coach to play the role of implementation support. We are providing some helpful tools here to give you an idea of what type of structure is helpful, and we encourage each provider to make something similar to help support the lifestyle changes that are at the root of integrative medicine.

Below, please see Figs. G.1, G.2, and G.3 for diet journals, goal setting worksheets, and functional coaching plans to be used as tools to support an integrative lifestyle.

Used with permission from the Institute for Functional Medicine (IFM), a global leader in functional medicine and a collaborator in the transformation of health-care. IFM is a 501(c)(3) nonprofit organization that believes functional medicine can help every individual reach their full potential for health and well-being. Under no circumstances may the whole or any part of the materials be translated into another language, nor may you create derivative or other works without IFM's prior written permission (for permission, please contact permissions@ifm.org)

© The Editor(s) (if applicable) and The Author(s), under exclusive license to
Springer Nature Switzerland AG 2021
J. Wendt et al., *Integrative Geriatric Nutrition*,
https://doi.org/10.1007/978-3-030-81758-9

Diet, Nutrition, and Lifestyle Journal – 1 Day

Patient Name_____ Date_____

Food Plan Type:_____

Day 1

Day Event	Food & Drink Intake (include type, amount, brand)	Macronutrients (PFC) and Phytonutrients
Rising Time		
Breakfast Time		_____P_____F_____C □R □O □Y □G □B/P/BL □W/T/BR
Mid-AM Snack Time		_____P_____F_____C □R □O □Y □G □B/P/BL □W/T/BR
Lunch Time		_____P_____F_____C □R □O □Y □G □B/P/BL □W/T/BR
Mid-PM Snack Time		_____P_____F_____C □R □O □Y □G □B/P/BL □W/T/BR
Dinner Time		_____P_____F_____C □R □O □Y □G □B/P/BL □W/T/BR
PM Snack Time		_____P_____F_____C □R □O □Y □G □B/P/BL □W/T/BR
Bed Time		

P: Proteins; **F**: Fats; **C**: Carbohydrates; **R**: Red; **O**: Orange; **Y**: Yellow; **G**: Green; **B/P/BL**: Blue/Purple/Black; **W/T/BR**: White/Tan/Brown

Sleep & Relaxation	Exercise & Movement	Stress	Relationships
Sleep Quantity: _____ (hours) Quality: □Poor □Fair □Good **Relaxation** □Yes □No Type/Amount:	Type, Duration, & Intensity □Aerobic: □Strength: □Flexibility:	Stress Reduction Practices: Stressors:	Supporting: Non-supporting:

Mental	Emotional	Spiritual

Fig. G.1 Diet, nutrition, and lifestyle journal [2]. Used with permission from the Institute for Functional Medicine (IFM), a global leader in functional medicine and a collaborator in the transformation of healthcare. IFM is a 501(c)(3) nonprofit organization that believes functional medicine can help every individual reach their full potential for health and well-being. Under no circumstances may the whole or any part of the materials be translated into another language, nor may you create derivative or other works without IFM's prior written permission (for permission, please contact permissions@ifm.org)

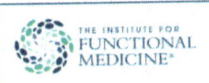

Goal Setting for Behavior Change

"A goal properly set is halfway reached."   —*Zig Ziglar*

Changing habits to consciously improve your health is no small undertaking, and making the decision to change is just the first step. Actively thinking about and planning for change will help prepare you for the process and motivate you to stay on track.

When you're ready to make a change, it is often helpful to set tangible goals. These goals can be short-term (daily, weekly, monthly) or long-term (6–12 months). When goal setting for behavior change, it's also helpful to set goals that are SMART—specific, measurable, attainable, realistic, and timely. The table below lists some examples of SMART goals.

SMART Goal Component	Example
Specific State the desired outcome as explicitly as possible, and target a specific area for improvement. This is the "who, what, where, when, which, and why" of your goal.	I will walk at least five days per week in the evenings to lower my cholesterol.
Measurable Identify the ways in which you will track your progress, and be as specific as possible. This is the "how" of your goal.	I will meditate for 30 minutes a day five times a week in order to lower my stress levels and blood pressure.
Attainable Start with small, achievable goals that are easily outlined into specific steps that will enable you to complete the goal. Then, as you meet those smaller goals, work up to intermediate goals and goals that are more difficult to achieve.	I will make an effort to move my body for at least 15 minutes three days a week, increasing my time each week by five minutes until I reach 30 minutes per day. I will add an extra day every two to four weeks until I reach 30-60 minutes for five days a week.
Realistic Create a goal that you are both willing and able to accomplish.	I will begin my bedtime ritual one hour before bedtime, which will help me fall asleep faster each night.
Timely Set a deadline or time for achieving your goal to help keep you motivated.	Over the next month, I will start eating breakfast every day. For the first week, I will make breakfast (or prepare it ahead the night before) twice per week. In the second week, I will make breakfast three times per week. In the third week, I will make breakfast five times per week. In the fourth week, I will make breakfast every day.

To begin setting your own SMART goals, flip the page and fill in the information in the template provided.

Fig. G.2 Goal setting for behavior change [2]. Used with permission from the Institute for Functional Medicine (IFM), a global leader in functional medicine and a collaborator in the transformation of healthcare. IFM is a 501(c)(3) nonprofit organization that believes functional medicine can help every individual reach their full potential for health and well-being. Under no circumstances may the whole or any part of the materials be translated into another language, nor may you create derivative or other works without IFM's prior written permission (for permission, please contact permissions@ifm.org)

SMART HEALTH GOALS

Date_____

Name_____

SMART Health Goals are:

Specific ▪ Measurable ▪ Attainable ▪ Realistic ▪ Timely

SMART Health Goal	Does the goal require adding or eliminating a behavior?	What is the first action step to accomplish the goal?	What is the start date, timeframe, or deadline for taking action?

References

1. American Council on Exercise. The science supporting the stages of change model. Coaching Behavior Change. 2nd ed. San Diego, CA: American Council on Exercise; 2019. 46–57.
2. Bailey R. Goal Setting and Action Planning for Health Behavior Change. Am J Lifestyle Med. 2017;13(6):615–618. doi:10.1177/1559827617729634

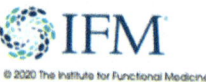

Fig. G.2 (continued)

THE INSTITUTE FOR FUNCTIONAL MEDICINE®

Functional Coaching Plan

Name: ______________________ Session Date: __________

What Do You Want Your Health For? ______________________

Co-created Health Goal(s)

1. ______________________

2. ______________________

3. ______________________

Progress Made Since Last Session: ______________________

Updated Lifestyle Factors	
Sleep & Restoration	
Exercise & Movement	
Nutrition	
Stress	
Relationships	

Comments: ______________________

Next Action Steps	What is the start date or deadline for taking action?
1.	
2.	
3.	
4.	
5.	

Next Session Date/Time: ______________________

Disclaimer: This tool is intended to be used within the scope of your practice.

Version 2

Fig. G.3 Functional coaching plan [2]. Used with permission from the Institute for Functional Medicine (IFM), a global leader in functional medicine and a collaborator in the transformation of healthcare. IFM is a 501(c)(3) nonprofit organization that believes functional medicine can help every individual reach their full potential for health and well-being. Under no circumstances may the whole or any part of the materials be translated into another language, nor may you create derivative or other works without IFM's prior written permission (for permission, please contact permissions@ifm.org)

References

1. Koetaka H, Ohno Y, Morimoto K. The change in lifestyle data during 9 years: the reliability and continuity of baseline health practices. Environ Health Prev Med. 2013;18(4):335–40.
2. IFM. Handouts [Internet]. Institute for Functional Medicine. 2021 [cited 2021 May 30]. Available from: https://www.ifm.org/.

Index

The manufacturer's authorised representative in the EU is Springer
Nature Customer Service Centre GmbH, Europaplatz 3, 69115 Heidelberg,
Germany. If you have any concerns regarding our products, please
contact ProductSafety@springernature.com

Printed and bound by CPI Group (UK) Ltd, Croydon, CR0 4YY
24/04/2026
02096309-0002